MEASUREMENT
IN EXERCISE
ELECTROCARDIOGRAPHY

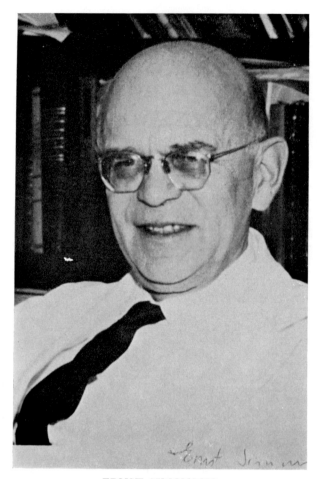

ERNST SIMONSON

MEASUREMENT IN EXERCISE ELECTROCARDIOGRAPHY

The Ernst Simonson Conference

Edited by

HENRY BLACKBURN, M.D.

With a Foreword by

Ancel Keys, Ph.D.
Professor and Director
Laboratory of Physiological Hygiene
University of Minnesota
Minneapolis, Minnesota

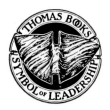

CHARLES C THOMAS · PUBLISHER
Springfield · Illinois · U.S.A.

Published and Distributed Throughout the World by
CHARLES C THOMAS · PUBLISHER
BANNERSTONE HOUSE
301-327 East Lawrence Avenue, Springfield, Illinois, U.S.A.
NATCHEZ PLANTATION HOUSE
735 North Atlantic Boulevard, Fort Lauderdale, Florida, U.S.A.

With THOMAS BOOKS *careful attention is given to all details of
manufacturing and design. It is the Publisher's desire to present books
that are satisfactory as to their physical qualities and artistic possibilities
and appropriate for their particular use.* THOMAS BOOKS *will be true
to those laws of quality that assure a good name and good will.*

Printed in the United States of America
H-2

Contributors

Arnold Adicoff, M. D.

Assistant Professor of Medicine
Department of Medicine
University of Minnesota
Minneapolis, Minnesota

E. Russell Alexander, M. D.

Departments of Medicine and
    Preventive Medicine
University of Washington
Seattle, Washington

Irma Åstrand, M. D.

Associate Professor
Institute of Work Physiology
Stockholm, Sweden

Reuben Berman, M. D.

Director, Coronary Drug Project
Mount Sinai Hospital
Minneapolis, Minnesota

Henry Blackburn, M. D.

Professor
Laboratory of Physiological Hygiene
University of Minnesota
Minneapolis, Minnesota

C. Gunnar Blomqvist, M. D.

Assistant Professor
Department of Internal Medicine
University of Texas
Southwestern Medical School
Dallas, Texas

Chandler McC. Brooks, Ph. D.

Professor and Chairman
Department of Physiology
State University of New York
Downstate Medical Center
Brooklyn, New York

Robert A. Bruce, M. D.

Professor of Medicine
Chief, Division of Cardiology
University of Washington
School of Medicine
Seattle, Washington

Howard B. Burchell, M. D.

Professor of Medicine
University of Minnesota
Minneapolis, Minnesota

J. A. Burdeshaw

Department of Medicine
University of Alabama
    Medical Center
Birmingham, Alabama

Cesar A. Caceres, M. D.

Chief, Medical Systems Development
    Laboratory
Heart Disease and Stroke
    Control Program
National Center for Chronic
    Disease Control
Washington, D.C.

B. N. Chiang, M. D.

National Defense Medical Center
Veterans General Hospital
Taipei, Taiwan

D. V. Conroy

Department of Medicine
University of Alabama
    Medical Center
Birmingham, Alabama

L. H. Dworetzky, M. M. E.

Re-entry Systems
General Electric Company
Philadelphia, Pennsylvania

Alvin H. Freiman, M. D.

*Associate Professor of
    Clinical Medicine
Memorial Hospital
New York, New York*

J. von der Groeben, M. D.

*Department of Anesthesia
Stanford University School
    of Medicine
Palo Alto, California*

Burt B. Hamrell, M. D.

*Medical Officer
Heart Disease and Stroke
    Control Program
National Center for Chronic
    Disease Control
United States Public Health Service
Laboratory of Physiological Hygiene
University of Minnesota
Minneapolis, Minnesota*

Herman Hellerstein, M. D.

*Associate Professor of Medicine
Department of Medicine
Lakeside Hospital
Cleveland, Ohio*

V. Hofer

*Departments of Medicine and
    Preventive Medicine
University of Washington
Seattle, Washington*

T. R. Hornsten, M. D.

*Medical Officer
Heart Disease and Stroke
    Control Program
National Center for Chronic
    Disease Control
United States Public Health Service
University of Washington
Seattle, Washington*

Larry Jackson, M. D.

*Medical Officer
Medical Systems Development
    Laboratory*

*Heart Disease and Stroke
    Control Program
National Center for Chronic
    Disease Control
Washington, D.C.*

L. N. Larkin

*Department of Medicine
University of Alabama Medical Center
Birmingham, Alabama*

Eugene Lepeschkin, M. D.

*Professor of Medicine
Cardiovascular Research Unit
Department of Medicine
University of Vermont
Burlington, Vermont*

Y. B. Li, M. D.

*Veterans General Hospital
National Defense Medical Center
Taipei, Taiwan*

Robert E. Mason, M. D.

*Associate Professor of Medicine
Johns Hopkins University
School of Medicine
Baltimore, Maryland*

Herbert M. Maistelman, M. S.

*Director
Health and Physical Education
    Department
Jewish Community Center
Cleveland, Ohio*

Paul McHenry, M. D.

*Captain, USAF, MC
Internal Medicine Branch
Aerospace Medical Sciences Division
Brooks Air Force Base, Texas*

Jerome Meyers, B. S.

*Human Ecology Section
Cornell Medical Center
New York, New York*

M. D. Perry

*Department of Medicine
University of Alabama Medical
    Center
Birmingham, Alabama*

Norma J. Pitts

Applied Physiology Laboratory
Heart Disease and Stroke
Control Program
National Center for Chronic
Disease Control
United States Public Health Service
Georgetown University Medical
Center
Washington, D.C.

John D. Radke, M. D.

Assigned Trainee
United States Public Health Service
Department of Medicine
Western Reserve University
Cleveland, Ohio

Pentti Rautaharju, M. D., Ph. D.

Professor of Biophysics
Department of Physiology
and Biophysics
Dalhousie University
Halifax, Novia Scotia, Canada

T. Joseph Reeves, M. D.

Professor of Medicine and Associate
Professor of Physiology
Department of Medicine
University of Alabama
Medical Center
Birmingham, Alabama

Ray Ricklin, B. S.

Assistant Director Health and
Physical Education Department
Jewish Community Center
Cleveland, Ohio

Paul G. Rochmis, M. D.

Medical Officer
Heart Disease and Stroke Control
Program
National Center for Chronic
Disease Control
United States Public Health Service
Arlington, Virginia

James A. Ronan, M. D.

Medical Officer
Heart Disease and Stroke
Control Program
National Center for Chronic
Disease Control
United States Public Health Service
Applied Physiology Laboratory
Georgetown University Medical
Center
Washington, D.C.

Stephen H. Salzman, M. D.

Research Associate
Department of Medicine
University Hospitals of Cleveland
Cleveland, Ohio

Otto H. Schmitt, Ph. D.

Professor, Department of
Zoology and Physics
University of Minnesota
Minneapolis, Minnesota

L. Thomas Sheffield, M. D.

Assistant Professor of Medicine
University of Alabama
Medical Center
Department of Medicine
Division of Cardiology
Birmingham, Alabama

Ernst Simonson, M. D.

Director of Medical Electronics
Mount Sinai Hospital
Minneapolis, Minnesota

Ralph E. Smith, M. D.

Consultant in Medicine
Mayo Clinic
Rochester, Minnesota

Raphael F. Smith, M. D.

Lieutenant Commander,
Medical Corps,
U.S. Navy
Assistant Head, Cardiology Branch
Naval Aerospace Medical Institute
Pensacola, Florida

Henry L. Taylor, Ph. D.

Professor
Laboratory of Physiological Hygiene
University of Minnesota
Minneapolis, Minnesota

R. Taylor

Departments of Medicine and
*   Preventive Medicine*
University of Washington
Seattle, Washington

Nong Ting, M. D.

Veterans General Hospital
National Defense Medical Center
Taipei, Taiwan

J. Gerald Toole, M. D.

Chief of Cardiology
Santa Clara Valley
Medical Center
San Jose, California

Naip Tuna, M. D.

Associate Professor of Medicine
406 Variety Club Heart Hospital
University of Minnesota
Minneapolis, Minnesota

Yang Wang, M. D.

Associate Professor of Medicine
University of Minnesota
Minneapolis, Minnesota

Charles S. Weaver, Ph. D.

Research Engineer in
Electrical Engineering
Stanford Engineering Laboratories
Stanford, University
Palo Alto, California

Edwin Westura, M. D.

Chief,
Applied Physiology Laboratory
Georgetown University
*   Medical Center*
Washington, D.C.

C. Ray White

Heart Disease and Stroke
*   Control Program*
National Center for Chronic
*   Disease Control*
United States Public Health Service
Applied Physiology Laboratory
Georgetown University Medical
*   Center*
Washington, D.C.

David Winter, Ph. D.

Department of Physiology and
*   Biophysics*
Dalhousie University
Halifax, Nova Scotia, Canada

Hermann Wolf, M. Sc.

Department of Physiology and
*   Biophysics*
Dalhousie University
Halifax, Nova Scotia, Canada

This conference and its transcript are dedicated to
ERNST SIMONSON,
*physiologist and physician, who has best understood
the need for measurement in electrocardiography, who
has provided the best compendium of quantitative conventional electrocardiography, and who has pioneered
and stimulated development of the new quantitative
electrocardiography.*

Foreword

A SYMPOSIUM dedicated to Ernst Simonson could be arranged around many topics—he has contributed importantly to many fields of medicine—but Henry Blackburn, who conceived of and organized this symposium, made a particularly felicitous choice. Any mention of quantitative analysis of electrocardiograms at once calls to mind the name of Ernst Simonson. Moreover, some of his earliest research concerned exercise physiology and from time to time over the years he returned to work effectively in that same vineyard.

Electrocardiography is one of the more recondite and highly specialized fields; because of its technical complexity only a limited number of devotees contribute to the advance of this subject. Exercise physiology, too, is a restricted specialty demanding training, facilities, and techniques available to only a relatively small number of experts. So a symposium on the application of electrocardiography to exercise physiology might seem to involve super-specialization, particularly when the further specification is added that the aim is *measurement* of the response to the stress of physical activity. Yet in the evaluation of cardiac function and status the importance of the measurement of electrophysiological responses to exercise must be obvious even to the nonspecialist.

We sympathize with physicians who lament the fragmentation of medicine and deplore the intrusion of elaborate instruments between them and their patients. But the aim of the development of sophisticated electrocardiographic and computer techniques applied to exercise tests is to supply a better basis for the art of the physician, not to supplant it; to provide more sensitive and reliable observations from which to draw better conclusions and exercise better judgment. Long ago physicians learned to use their fingers and ears to judge something about the rate, rhythm and force of the heart beat in its response to exercise and to value the crude information obtained in that way. They appreciated the extension of their unaided senses with stethoscopes and sphygmomanometers when those instruments became available, though it may be appropriate to recall that both of those innovations encountered some resistance at first. Electrocardiographic recordings, but not their measurement, are standard in every good medical examination. Exercise tests, too, are now generally accepted as useful even if they are not as widely applied as we should like. We can insist that the subject matter of this symposium should not alienate clinicians and should in fact, be of concern for every cardiologist.

No one can doubt that quantitative electrocardiographic responses to standardized exercise tests should provide extremely valuable data for the evaluation of the diagnostic and functional status of patients and for comparisons between them and with controls. Until recently, the ECG signals recorded during exercise have been so distorted and full of "noise" that little more than impressionistic evaluation was possible in only a fraction of the recordings. Only recovery records could be used. The myocardial events at various recovery intervals are even more obscure and standard conditions less defined than during work. Recordings suitable for truly quantitative analysis are the goal, of course. The necessary technical instrumentation seemed to be "just around the corner" some years ago but formidable difficulties had to be overcome; first to obtain clean and faithful recordings, second to devise suitable computer programs for their analysis. Progress towards these ends, well portrayed in the proceedings of this symposium, has now gone so far that technical refinements rather than fundamental theory seem to be the current outstanding needs.

It appears likely that accurate recordings can or soon will be reliably made without constant ministrations of electronics engineers; and that suitable computer programs are available for quantitative analysis or need only refinement along lines that pose no serious difficulty. But neither electronic nor physiological theory can substitute for the experience to be gained from extensive application of new methods and equipment to a wide variety of subjects and patients. It took half a century of trial, experiment, observation and measurement to arrive at the present state of understanding of the clinical significance of ordinary planar electrocardiograms; the clinical evaluation of vectorcardiograms is not yet that far advanced, and as practiced, is largely qualitative.

The meaning, in terms of the current state of cardiac health, of various findings of the exercise response in electrocardiograms is far from clear; their significance and independent contribution to prognosis is largely conjectural. Progress in these regards can come in part from theoretical advances and technical improvements in the recording and measurement of the electrocardiogram; but long follow-up of large numbers of subjects, with appropriate statistical analysis, is the requisite. In this connection more attention must be given to the conditions involved in the exercise tests. The multiplicity of methods currently advocated for exercise tests is testimony to the unsatisfactory state of the subject. Almost all exercise tests currently used are directed towards the problem of evaluating the degree of cardiorespiratory "fitness" for brief but fairly intense physical work. The *extent* to which such tests provide estimates of long-time endurance or can be used to diagnose underlying disease or prognosticate future cardiovascular health is unknown. This is the business of measurement in exercise electrocardiography.

These papers speak for themselves. They will repay detailed study by all who are actively engaged in research and development of the areas covered. For others, their perusal will indicate the complexity of the problems and the shape of things to come.

ANCEL KEYS

"Minnelea," Pioppi (Salerno), Italy

Preface

WELCOME TO THE Twin Cities. We are here at the Minneapolis Veterans Hospital for two reasons. First, there is a long tradition of academic excellence at this institution combined with a uniquely relaxed feeling of being away from the bustle and from "games people play." We want this conference to be similarly relaxed and open. Second, this is one of the institutions where for many years Ernst Simonson has done research and influenced thinking and where he has trained young internists to use the electrocardiogram wisely.

The title of this conference was initially "Quantitative Exercise Electrocardiography." But to suggest that any of us had arrived at a quantitative cardiography was presumptuous. We wished, however, to emphasize the desirability, indeed necessity to move toward a quantitative approach. The conference title "Measurement in Exercise Electrocardiography," in no way indicates a lack of recognition of many earlier efforts which have brought this field to its present wide concern. The original observations were surely the most exciting. Observance of ST changes in spontaneous and exercise-induced angina pectoris and the adaptation of this observation to electrocardiographic diagnosis are credited to Feil and Seigel, Scherf and Goldhammer, Wood and Wolferth, Master and Dack. Development of functional testing using the electrocardiogram is credited to Sjostrand and to Yu. The important concept that exercise responses predict future disease risk in apparently healthy men is credited to Robb, Marks and Mattingly.

In the end, in every field, establishment of the full role and usefulness of a medical test rests on measurement and quantitative comparison. We anticipate that this conference will represent a milestone in which it is clearly recognized that improved understanding and utilization of the electrocardiographic response to exercise rests on modern methods of faithful recording, precise measurement, fine analysis and efficient handling of numerical data. But there are too

This symposium was held in Minneapolis, Minnesota, September 28-29, 1967.

[xv]

many variables not yet controlled to claim that we can quantify the exercise electrocardiogram.

Each group of investigators represented here has made a contribution to one or more areas of interest, in standardization of the work load and test procedure, in instrumentation, in lead derivation, in noise reduction, in measurement of the signal, in programming the analysis or in validation of the method. None of us has yet found a universally applicable system of quantitative exercise electrocardiography. It may be that no given system is applicable to all experimental conditions or research goals, to diagnosis, function testing, characterization of populations, evaluation of clinical trials, or prediction of future risk. But common principles and standardization within disciplines are needed.

Caution is required even as concept and method approach an ideal: adequate leads simultaneously recorded, excellent skin-electrode preparation, good signal to noise ratio, faithful records, equivalent cardiovascular stress, precise measurement, optimal signal representation, and elegant data treatment. The need for caution derives from the fact that dramatic effects on the discriminatory and predictive power of the exercise ECG result from relatively slight modifications of the lead system, changing the criteria for onset and offset of waves, using fixed-interval sampling points versus points determined by cycle length, using simple amplitude criteria versus curve-fitting terms for ST evaluation and various reclassifications of the clinical groups being compared.

Sharp as the edge of precision may become, dull may the power remain. Here we come close to the classic philosophical battle between science and the humanities. As Pascal says in his *Penseés,* "Truth is so subtle a point that our instruments are too blunt to touch it exactly. When they do reach it, they crush the point and bear down around, *more on the false than on the true."*

The uncertainty principle remains with us. Before we can claim a quantitative cardiography the uncertainty must be assessed by repetition of the observations and of the analysis, by varying the conditions and again repeating the analysis, by arriving at conclusions only when the incongruities and inconsistencies, about which we would never be aware without the repetitions, are whittled down to a minimum.

Many factors underly the current obscurity in the significance of the electrocardiographic response to muscular work. They are the subject of our conference. Not the least of these is our ignorance of the fundamental electrophysiology, of the effect on the cell of oxygen lack, metabolite accumulation or change in substrate activity, and of the principal determinants of myocardial ischemia. This we will take up in the introductory session. Also obvious are the sources of variability in the electrocardiographic response to exercise and the "confounding variables," the personal characteristics of age, sex, body build, blood pressure, state of physical training and posture as well as environmental conditions, all of which have been shown to influence or be associated with different exercise electrocardiographic responses. Of immediate concern are the inadequately considered questions of engineering specifications for stress testing systems and this will be a preoccupation throughout the conference.

Our only commission here is to initiate a vigorous dialogue among those who have made serious efforts to measure the electrocardiographic response to exercise.

HENRY BLACKBURN

Acknowledgments

THE PRINCIPAL SPONSORS of the Ernst Simonson Conference and of these Proceedings, the Minnesota Heart Association and the Heart Disease and Stroke Control Program of the U. S. Public Health Service, shared equally the expenses and the planning for this conference. Helen Bies and the professional staff of the Minnesota Heart Association deserve credit for most of the legwork and they, with the Veterans Hospital Staff, made the physical arrangements possible.

The Ernst Simonson Conference and Banquet were planned by Henry Blackburn, Reuben Berman, Otto H. Schmitt, Arnold Adicoff, Naip Tuna and James Dahl. The Ernst Simonson Banquet was held at the Minneapolis Club through the courtesy of Dr. Karl Anderson. A leather-bound collection of greetings from friends and colleagues of Ernst Simonson around the world was prepared by Lual Sather. The conference manuscripts were prepared for the publisher by Roberta Klock and Marjorie Konopliv.

This symposium was also sponsored by the University of Minnesota, the Veterans Hospital and the Mount Sinai Hospital, Minneapolis, Minnesota.

Contents

PART ONE
ELECTRICAL AND PHYSIOLOGICAL BACKGROUND FOR MEASUREMENT OF THE ELECTROCARDIOGRAPHIC RESPONSE TO EXERCISE

Chapter

PART TWO
METHODS AND EARLY RESULTS OF AUTOMATED COMPUTER PROGRAMS FOR EXERCISE ELECTROGRAPHY

PART THREE

BIOENGINEERING PROBLEMS AND SPECIFICATIONS OF AUTOMATED SYSTEMS OF EXERCISE ELECTROCARDIOGRAPHY

MEASUREMENT
IN EXERCISE
ELECTROCARDIOGRAPHY

PART ONE

ELECTRICAL AND PHYSIOLOGICAL BACKGROUND FOR MEASUREMENT OF THE ELECTROCARDIOGRAPHIC RESPONSE TO EXERCISE

1

Electrophysiological Processes in the Heart
Recordable Consequences of their Abnormality and Failure of their Integration

CHANDLER McC. BROOKS

INTRODUCTORY REMARKS

D R. BLACKBURN, DR. ADICOFF, PROFESSOR SIMONSON—I am honored by your invitation to participate in this conference on Measurement in Exercise Electrocardiography. As the first speaker, I presume I should attempt to identify the problems, state some rather obvious facts about the aims of electrocardiography so that others will not need to do so, and place the present conference in proper perspective by a brief review of the history of this discipline.

The heart is comprised of a population of cells which, though possessing quite diverse characteristics, normally cooperate in a cyclical series of actions. This cycle of events culminates in a cardiac output which is adjusted to meet body needs during rest and exercise by control mechanisms acting on the intrinsic excitatory process, its conduction and the mechanical response elicited thereby. Since the time of William Harvey (1578-1657) and Stephen Hales (1677-1761)— and I should like to point out that these men dealt extensively with measurement—physiologists have been striving to identify the processes basic to these phenomena and to determine the causes of their frequently observed abnormality.

Note: The original work reported was done with the support of grants from the New York Heart Association and from the NIH (PN 7770, 5 R01 HE 10070).

It is well recognized, but probably seldom said, that the cardiologist must deal both with the ultimate minutiae of functional processes, factors maintaining function of the heart as a whole, and consider the integration of heart activity with that of the body. To be more specific, electrocardiography has at least three related purposes: to estimate the normality of total integrated heart action, to identify the nature and precise locus of any abnormalities present, and to judge the normality of heart responses to anticipated or increased body need for a greater minute volume flow of blood. Exercise presents to the heart a need for a greater output. The technical developments we have witnessed during the past decades have been results of attempts either to obtain a better estimation of function as a whole, or to obtain a clearer view of local processes.

Before considering modern developments in this field, I should like to refer briefly to its history. It can be said that there have been three rather distinct phases in the development of electrocardiography. I daresay that those who made the earliest pertinent discoveries did not consider them to be the primitive beginnings of a discipline. A great deal was known about the heart before it became possible to study the electrical phenomena related to its action. It is also true that with primitive equipment much which was developed later had been suggested. I believe, however, that those studies of electrocardiography carried on before the beginning of this century were relatively primitive and approximate in their conclusions.

Electrocardiography could not develop until men realized that electric current flow was generated during tissue activity. Credit can be given to Luigi Galvani (1737-1798) for having derived that idea on September 20, 1786. Alessandro Volta (1745-1827) deserves some credit for having clarified the situation and corrected some of Galvani's mistakes. To be sure, John Hunter had, in 1773, studied electric emissions from the torpedo and the Romans had used the shocks obtained from these selachians or rays (Torpedinidae) for therapeutic purposes but this qualifies less well as a beginning of electrophysiology (1). In 1841 Carlo Matteucci (2) showed that a beating heart produces enough current flow or voltage to excite a nerve laid across its surface. Albert von Kolliker and H. Muller performed this same experiment in 1855 and went on to show, by newly invented instrumentation, that there were two electrical surges, one occurring just before systole and a second weaker deflection at the beginning of diastole. These produce the "R" and "T" waves we know so well.

As early as 1825 Leopoldo Nobili had developed a galvanometer which he used to record the current from activated frog nerve and muscle. Emil Du Bois-Reymond (1818-1896) contributed even more to knowledge by measuring both "resting" and "action potentials" in 1843. He first used the term *action potential* and recorded the voltage and duration of this electric phenomenon with instruments which he had devised and called "rheotomes." This type of instrument, after some improvements by Julius Bernstein, became the first accurate and practical instrument used in electrocardiography. It was used by Marchand in 1877 to record a cardiac electrogram from a frog heart. At this same time Burdon-Sanderson of England was recording the electrical events occurring in the turtle heart. Theodore Wilhelm Engelmann (3) was pursuing similar interests. In 1872 Gabriel Lippmann invented the "capillary electrometer" and Marey, by 1876, had developed a means of photographing its deflections. Finally, Augustus Desire Waller (1856-1922) in 1887, obtained from humans recordings which he called electrograms and cardiograms using this instrument. As a matter of fact, many of the major features of the "electrocardiogram" were known before the late eighteen-hundreds (4).

I think it is appropriate to recognize here that Hugo Kronecker (1839-1914) had begun the study of muscular fatigue and recovery by 1871.

Long before the start of this present century the anatomists also had made many of the contributions essential to interpretation of records obtained of the electrical activity of the heart by external leads. Purkinje had described the fibers now known to comprise the conducting system by 1839. In 1893 His described the atrioventricular connections and the bundle bearing his name. But all this has been better described by others (5,6). This progress I have discussed represents to me the primitive beginnings, the preparation for, rather than the advent of modern electrocardiology.

Ernst Simonson was born toward the end of this first or initial developmental phase of electrocardiology. He probably was not fully aware of its end or the advent of the second period, the beginning of modern electrocardiography, which occurred during the first years of this century but by 1922 he was contributing significantly to this new development (7). Incidentally, this was the year of Waller's death.

It is generally agreed that electrocardiography is a science of this century; at any rate, its modern phase, its modern vocabulary began with the Century. It all started with the invention of the string galvanometer by Willem Einthoven (1866-1927) in 1901. In 1903 Einthoven first made recordings from man, which he called electrocardiograms, using this instrument. In 1908 he published his classical interpretation of the "electrokardiogram"; in 1913 he enunciated his law of the equilateral triangle and its derivation from leads I, II and III. The first textbook of electrocardiography was published in Dusseldorf, Germany, by Augustus Hoffman in 1914. The work of Waller and others had prepared the way for early acceptance of this new discipline of electrocardiography. There were also men of great ability such as Sir Thomas Lewis who were prepared to make maximum use of this new methodology (8).

Alfred Cohn brought the first electrocardiograph machine to reach the United States from Germany to the Mount Sinai Hospital of New York in 1909. Another American, a Minneapolitan, George E. Fahr worked in Leiden with Einthoven from 1911 to 1913 and contributed methods of calculating the electrical axis of the heart. I believe it was Horatio B. Williams and Walter B. James, working with Cohn, who in 1910 published the first American article on work with the electrocardiograph. Other Americans should be mentioned, especially Frank N. Wilson, as having contributed greatly to the instrumentation and theory of this field.

We should, in referring to men, mention Hubert Mann (9) and the advent of vectorcardiography. This is a branch of the subject to which Dr. Simonson has contributed greatly (10). The development of the vacuum tube in the 1920's again revolutionized the recording of electrical correlates of the heart's activity. I should also mention use of suction electrodes in the late 20's and 30's and the recording of the monophasic action potentials from the surface of the heart because records obtained thus gave information confirmed by methods which introduced what I have called the third phase of electrocardiography.

The third phase of electrophysiological study of the heart was made possible by the invention in 1949, by Ling and Gerard, of a micro-electrode method of recording from individual muscle cells. The 3M KCl filled glass pipette which they used as an electrode could penetrate the plasma membrane without seriously damaging the cell. Resting and action potentials could be recorded from individual cells of various types and in 1949 Coraboeuf and Weidmann (11) and slightly later Woodbury, Hecht, and Christopherson (12), and others (13) began intracellular recording from heart cells.

During the last eighteen years many studies have been made of the electrical reactions of cardiac cells *in situ* and in isolation (14). It can be said that this new technique facilitated a long step forward in fulfillment of one purpose of electrocardiography, that of obtaining a record of the minutest details of heart function. It permitted study of cells. It also contributed to the analysis of the factors unifying or integrating activity of the heart's population of cells. The nature and effectiveness of integrative factors and their resistance to stress has been better estimated.

I wish now to discuss some recent contributions made by this technique and some of the new ideas which have been advanced as a result of this last great development in studies of the electrical activity of the heart. The aspects I will concentrate on are those dealing with the integration of activity within the heart's population of cells and the question of how heart function is controlled intrinsically as well as extrinsically.

But before I leave this brief review of history, I wish to correct one impression, if I have created the misconception. I do not believe one phase ends as a new one begins. The beginning of intracellular recording contributed something new, but use of indirect recording and the study of the heart by this means has matured also. Computers, analyzers and filters, to exclude noise and emphasize transients, did not become important to electrocardiologists as early as they did to electroencephalographers because of the more favorable ratio to noise level maintained in electrocardiography. Computer analysis has been used, however, by cardiologists for a number of years. They have been employed, for example, in the study of propagation of impulses through the myocardium (15). A careful perusal of the literature probably would show that cardiologists have attempted to use all types of computers shortly after they have become available, but use has not been extensive. The development of more massive clinical responsibilities and heavier patient-physician loads, the desire to detect latent cardiac disease, the need for continual surveillance of men under stress now necessitate a greater reliance on computers and a new evaluation of procedures to be followed in their use. This is a natural development of procedures begun by Waller, Einthoven, Thomas Lewis and the early electrocardiographers rather than something completely new. The "new" generally has been anticipated and the old does not cease to be important. The division of history into eras or the development of a science into phases is somewhat hazardous and is worthy of only limited attention here.

I will, therefore, turn to the progress which has been made in recent years in studies of the basic processes of action and integration of behavior.

PACEMAKER ACTION AND ITS CONTROL

The heart beats rhythmically because of its pacemaker, and as pacemaker action accelerates, heart rate rises. External control is exerted on the heart through its pacemakers. We also know that integrated action of the heart can be maintained by subsidiary pacemakers normally dominated by the primary pacemaker cells of the sinoatrial node.

The new studies of cells and membranes have revealed much concerning the characteristics of pacemakers. I will not repeat the discussion of ion fluxes or changes in permeability to potassium ion thought to explain the generation of pacemaker potential (14,16). I will attempt, however, to deal with some obvious questions such as the following:

What factors tend to maintain the rhythmic action of the pacemaker and relate its rate to cardiac response?

1. There is evidence to suggest that the action potential itself has an effect which helps determine rhythm. Let us turn back to Mateucci and those who showed that the heart's action potential could excite adjacent nerves. Autonomic nerves containing mediators at their terminals are imbedded in heart tissue, concentrating in the nodal regions. Is it not logical to assume that these nerves might be excited by the heart's action potential thus discharging acetylcholine and catechola-

mines on to the pacemaker cells with each heartbeat? Certainly, if one implants an artificial pacemaker in the sinus area and drives the heart with even a minimal level of current pulse, ACh and catecholamines can be shown to be liberated (17,18). It is well known that the effects of ACh, though more powerful than catecholamines, are more transient. I suggest that the rhythm of the pacemaker is maintained *in part* or made secure by this autogenic feedback; the ACh liberation preventing too early a pacemaker cell depolarization and the catecholamines eventually encouraging it. This is an intrinsic phenomenon underlying tonic activity of extrinsic nerves and the augmentation of directives (neural and humoral) coming during exercise to change the rate of heart action (19).

2. I would like to mention another example of ancient knowledge supplemented by new information which has permitted a new hypothesis to be suggested. Bainbridge in 1915 suggested that acceleration of the heart in exercise might be due to increased venous return and greater filling. That conclusion has been rejected in part or in totality many times, but it has been shown by many persons here in Minnesota and elsewhere (20,21) that stretching of pacemaker tissues accelerates their rates of firing and microelectrode studies have shown this to be associated with a partial depolarization and possibly a resulting increase in Na^+ permeability.

There undoubtedly is an eventual acceleration of venous return during exercise and any rate of venous return stretches atrial tissues to some degree. Why not then assume that the distention caused by a venous return causes a localized stretch which ultimately might, in the absence of other primary and more potent factors, favor pacemaker acceleration? It is bad physiology to think only of one cause, one factor, one or two variables in any physiological process. I think it is good physiology to assume that something known to occur might have functional significance. I am willing to suggest that venous return which stretches the atrial chambers and great veins might act to prevent too long a delay in sinus pacemaker action—thus helping to assure a rhythmicity. A stretch of less than 10 per cent (prolongation of length) will accelerate firing of pacemaker cells in an isolated node.

3. A final pacemaker problem I wish to discuss is the matter of

the dominance of the primary pacemaker over potential pacemakers which we know reside within the AV node and the specialized conducting system. When they become dominant we have nodal or idioventricular rhythms. When they escape from dominance, arrhythmias tend to result. Is the SA node merely faster than other pacemakers or does it actually also hold them under suppression? The latter is true, I believe. I will not repeat all the evidence, some of which is familiar to you.

It suffices to say that if the SA node is suddenly blocked, subsidiary pacemakers do not act immediately but develop control slowly. Also, pacemakers are depressed by overdriving. On cessation of overdrive, a period of asystole is followed by a gradual development and acceleration of pacemaker action. The sinoatrial node is more resistant to depression by overdrive than are the AV node and idioventricular pacemakers. The idioventricular pacemaker is also somewhat difficult to depress and all nodes are more difficult to depress by retrograde (driving from below) than orthograde drive. This suppression by drive from a faster pacemaker is imposed by liberation of acetylcholine, potassium ion and the produced hyperpolarizing effects (14,17,18). Much more could be said about interaction and control of pacemakers, but it is clear that subsidiary pacemakers are normally *suppressed* by action of a dominant pacemaker. I believe I have made my point that microelectrode studies of cell performance have added a new perspective to electrocardiography during the last half-century.

CARDIAC INJURY AND MAINTENANCE OF HEART ACTION

The electrocardiogram reveals cardiac lesions and their locus. Even before the advent of cardiac cell recording, it was shown by Wiggers (1937) that ischemic tissue initially repolarizes faster than do normal tissues in the surround. This has been amply confirmed and one would expect this earlier repolarization, caused by ischemia, to establish a source-sink relationship and current flow, an outward flow, which seemingly could cause an immediate new depolarization of the tissue. It is known also that these tissues are initially hyperexcitable after a coronary occlusion (22). Extrasystoles frequently are generated and fibrillation frequently does result, but not inevitably.

The question of why injuries, ischemias, do not always cause arrhythmias and fibrillation is as interesting as why they often do. Why do antifibrillatory drugs give protection? Newer techniques have given some suggestions or partial answers. In dealing with this question new information obtained a long time ago must be considered. Keith Lucas (1907), A. V. Hill (1936) and others observed that accommodation to applied current flow of long duration can occur in nerve and muscle tissues. Of recent years it has been shown that this is true of heart muscle also (23). Similarly, tissues possess minimal gradient requirements for excitation. Unless applied currents have a certain rate of rise to threshold intensity, they will not excite. The power of accommodation and minimal gradient requirements can be greatly affected by conditions maintaining, such as tissue temperature, drugs applied and ionic concentration changes (24, 25). It is known that some agents and circumstances which reduce minimal gradient requirements and power of accommodation do contribute a vulnerability to fibrillation. It is known that some agents which have an antifibrillatory action raise threshold potential requirement for excitation, prolong postexcitation refractoriness and augment minimal gradient requirements for excitation. Thus although, as a result of localized permanent or transient myocardial ischemias, sufficient charge differences may exist to generate adequate voltages and current flow to excite, the rate of rise is slow, accommodation may occur and minimal gradient requirements may not be met. Even isolated tissues can accommodate to long duration flow. These processes can be considered to be mechanisms protecting the heart from happenings which would otherwise disorganize activity in the myocardium and inactivate the pumping action of the heart.

Shifts in the ST segment and changes in the T wave with myocardial ischemia and injury indicate cardiac abnormality but also potentially greater trouble. Analysis of this proceeds somewhat as follows: There is a vulnerable period during the heart cycle in the region of or at the time of the T complex. It is commonly agreed that arrhythmias indicate irregularity and lack of uniformity in the tissues response. Since the T wave indicates recovery or repolarization, one can infer that there is a tendency toward greater variation in cells during recovery from, than in the activation reaction. This is correct.

Ischemia, constant current flow, ionic abnormalities, action of cate-cholamines, etc. affect the phase of maintained depolarization (the plateau of the heart cells action potential) and the rate of the terminal repolarization process most selectively. Furthermore, various types of heart cells are affected to different degrees by rate changes, ischemia, acetylcholine, catecholamines, and by plasma ion concentrations. It is not surprising, therefore, to find that in studies of heart muscle strips, those containing diverse types of fibers (atrial and sinus tissues, ventricular muscle and conducting fibers) are vulnerable to fibrillation, and multiple beats or fibrillation result from single stimuli applied in the recovery phase (T wave segment of electrocardiogram). Strips of uniform fibers (papillary muscle, etc.) cannot be induced to give multiple responses out of phase by stimuli applied at any time until some fibers sustain injury. Any treatment asymmetrically given renders the bundles vulnerable to disorganization.

When the entire ventricle is under study, it has a vulnerable period especially when the cyclical activities of the diverse cells comprising it are made more diverse by exercise, catecholamine or other factors which accelerate processes in some cells more than in others. Differences tend to become greater under stress when ion fluxes, exchange pump actions, are driven to maximum rates. In extreme depression they also become more diverse. Nevertheless, arrhythmias are harder to create in a healthy heart than in one in which injury or ischemia have created diversities outside the normal span. Following ischemia or injury, some fibers become relatively fast in recovery and others relatively slower, thus reentry is possible or a varied latency occurs in beat origin which is augmented by a growing diversity in conduction rate as one beat precedes another.

The normal ECG can be said to indicate a uniformity as well as occurrences of phases of myocardial state. Any ST depression, change in ST junction or T wave amplitude might be due to a loss of population uniformity. Of course when one comes right down to attempting electrocardiogram analysis in terms of what is happening in the heart, one has to admit no activity is precisely identified by any element in the complex. There is no deflection indicating onset of activity in the sinoatrial node or the onset and completion of recovery of that tissue. There is no precise identification of possible variations of spread of activity over the atrium and through the atrioventricular node or recovery therefrom. The P wave indicates activity presumably spreading in one direction and the T wave, when seen, indicates a degree of uniformity in atrial repolarization. Spread of activity through the His-Purkinje system is not recorded, although the U wave may indicate a special sequence in recovery (repolarization). Activation of the ventricle gives the QRS complex; its duration, amplitude and composition reveals a direction, uniformity and time duration of activation. The ST segment is a potential indicating balance, an isopotential, which is affected by imbalance in the sequence of repolarization, asymmetry in the coincidence of activation and repolarization. This segment corresponds roughly to the plateau phase of the myocardial cell action potential. If the plateau phase is shortened in some cells, then the balance shifts up or down. Since the left ventricle is dominant, dissimilarities within its muscle walls are more likely to change the balance.

The T wave shape, duration, amplitude is likewise reflective of a balance as well as changes in cells, in their terminal phases of repolarization. One difficulty in trying to transfer from the ECG record to what is happening in the heart is due to the fact that changes in individual cell action potentials, changes in conduction path or relative rates and changes in sequence and uniformity of cell population action all affect the record and similar changes might be due to somewhat different occurrences.

The non-clinically-oriented physiologist believes that the reason that electrocardiography has been so useful is due to the fact that all changes indicate some injury or abnormality and just precisely where it is, or what it is in detail, is relatively less important than knowing injury or failure is there. Also, the uniformity of anatomy, circulatory structure and locus of low safety permit use of electrocardiography with success. It does seem, however, that indirect leading gives such an approximate record (the ECG) of change that elaborate and costly analysis of configurations is not very desirable. Record of the occurrence of change would be more instructive and a better signal than the nature of any ultimate picture. The full analysis of an ultimate picture in terms of what has occurred in the heart requires a much more elaborate monitoring of the minutiae of change in all parts of the myocardium than is possible at present.

The ECG is certainly a record of electrical and not mechanical events in the heart. However, the contractile process does affect blood flow, and this effect is probably greater on channels coursing through the myocardium. Failure of contraction in one region and compensatory strength and rate changes elsewhere might affect blood flow creating marginal ischemias in specific regions, especially where flow may initially be subnormal. This would modify durations of action potentials there. Such shortening could in turn change the electrocardiographic picture.

The essence of the ischemic ST segment change seems to be augmentation of the ST shift by exercise. The abnormality in the ischemic ECG seems to those of us who work with cellular potential to be due to the faster repolarization and eventually the lower voltage in the ischemic area relative to normal tissue. This possibly is occasioned by the oxygen lack but is more probably due to the abnormal handling of metabolites, in particular potassium fluxes. It is inescapable that the dissimilarity between normal and ischemic tissue is augmented by exercise, improvement in flow being proportionately greater in the normal tissue. The accumulation of metabolites and external potassium becomes proportionately greater in exercise and the action potential is more drastically changed in the abnormal tissue, throwing the balances more out of line than during rest.

EXCITATION-CONTRACTION COUPLING

Normally the mechanical response is so well integrated with the electrical that records of the latter suffice as indicators of normality and abnormality. However, in pulsus alternans this integration is impaired and it is now possible to analyze its processes and its resistance to stress. There are adaptive mechanisms which tend to maintain this normal association. These can be studied also. Finally, it has been found that there are mysterious disparities between configurations of electrical and mechanical responses.

In exercise, heart rates accelerate markedly especially if the vagus-breaking mechanism is impaired. Above certain rates of drive, at rates of 200 per minute in some cases, which are not much in excess of those occurring normally, a pulsus alternans develops. Figure 1-1 is an example of this type of integrative failure. One of the interesting but not understood related phenomena is the compensatory adjust-

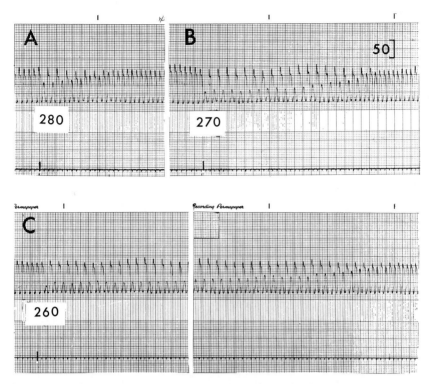

FIGURE 1-1. Compensatory abolition of pulsus alternans. *A*. Cycle length (280 msec—rate 214 beats/min) at which alternation begins. Note slower recovery at faster rates of drive in *B* (270 msec cycle—224 beats/min) and *C* (260 msec cycle—231 beats/min). Blood pressure maintained above 90 mm Hg. Pulse calibration = 50 mm Hg. Electrically driven dog heart.

ments which occur. At threshold rates, those which produce alternation, the alternation gradually disappears as though the mechanical cycle of contraction and relaxation can gradually be accelerated. Also, this process, whatever it is, has a temporal duration because when the heart is accelerated much above the threshold rate for alternation and then decelerated to the alternation threshold rate, the alternation does not begin again for several seconds (26). These same phenomena occur in isolated tissues, and the compensatory mechanisms, therefore, cannot be due entirely to extrinsic factors although there is evidence that they do play a part (27). Sympathetic nerve fibers to the ventricle have a much stronger action on the inotropic responses than

on ventricular pacemakers (28). Norepinephrine, the transmitter liberated from sympathetic nerve terminals, and the catecholamines
improve coupling and raise the critical rate of dissociation. A calcium ion flux is known to be involved in triggering contraction following the electrical response. A reduction in calcium ion in perfusing
fluids or blood weakens coupling while an increase in calcium ion
concentration raises the "threshold rate" of coupling failure. Ouabain
has a similar action, and it is of interest that blocking of catecholamine
and of calcium flux does not fully abolish the compensation (29).
Thus, recent studies have shown that those reactions associated with
the coupling of electrical and mechanical events are complex, contain
factors of safety and require more study. It is of interest that integration is so well protected even at this seemingly weakest link.

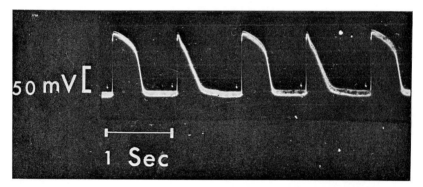

FIGURE 1-2. Alternation of intracellularly recorded action potential. Voltage
and time as indicated. Cat papillary muscle held at room temperature. (From
H-H. Lu—see reference 27.)

I should like to show (Fig. 1-2) another phenomenon. This is an
example of electrical response alternation. In this alternation of reactions the stronger, longer-lasting mechanical response is produced by
the action potential of seemingly briefest duration. This more effective
action potential differs little in peak voltage, rise in time or ultimate
duration from the less effective electrical response; but its initial phase
of repolarization is briefer, and it is very difficult to explain how this
could be responsible for the discrepancy in effect. Presumably, the
failure of the contractile materials to bind the Ca^{++} creates a higher
$[Ca]_o$ and prolongs alternate potentials (27).

Thus, the microanalysis proceeds. We now know that the basic processes whereby the electrical responses trigger the mechanical actions are much more complex than originally assumed.

Finally, I wish to suggest another cycle in our interests and our philosophies.

AUTONOMIC NERVE ACTIONS IN EXERCISE

In the early days of this century when Dr. Simonson and I were young, the concept that breadth of knowledge was required of physiologists dominated the discipline. For some time now, however, the theory of specialization has dominated, and there have been those who think that a person with broad interests is a dilettante. But the wheel turns and the old becomes new again. The heart is in the environment of the body and he who would study the heart must study the nervous system and receptors too.

I would like to give as my final point an illustration of this from the field of cardiac control study.

It has been recognized for many years that central control mechanisms activate the sympathico-adrenal system as a whole during exercise and under stressful circumstances. These nerves and their transmitters can bring about compensatory action of the heart by effects upon its pacemakers and contractile processes. I will not elaborate upon this well-known subject, but here too there have been new developments. An unexpected corollary of nerve action in the heart has been discovered; we now know that autonomic fibers innervate the carotid sinus and carotid bodies. Their discharge sensitizes these two receptor systems as indicated by increased rates of firing in afferents of the ninth cranial nerve (30). The physiological implication of this is that as reflex action increases, to give an increase in cardiac output in exercise for example, protection against excessive blood pressure is strengthened. At the same time, chemoreceptors become more sensitive to blood O_2 and CO_2 or pH levels, adjusting respiratory action to cooperate more delicately in meeting body needs for oxygen and CO_2 elimination.

It is probably unnecessary for me to point out to you, if you have seen any list of Dr. Simonson's papers, that he has conducted studies in more than one field. He would not neglect to consider the totality of any reaction. In this he belongs to the old but also to the coming generation.

Advances occur in new fields and in old at a bewildering rate. New techniques have created new concepts and revealed new problems. Older techniques, used to test new ideas, have uncovered unexpected integrative and adaptive reactions, many of which must become effective during exercise. Certainly, the last quarter of this century holds as much promise as did the first. Electrocardiography has progressed, but there is no end in view. Possibly, our greater knowledge instead of bringing solutions has merely brought a greater appreciation of the complexities of the life processes. This is progress and it does not dismay those who have, like Dr. Simonson, accepted the life of perpetual quest for knowledge.

REFERENCES

1. GARRISON, F.H.: *History of Medicine.* Philadelphia, Saunders, 1913, pp. 327-328.
2. MATTEUCCI, C.: Note sur les phénomènes électriques des animaux. *CR Acad Sci (Paris), 13*:540, 1841.
3. ENGELMANN, TH. W.: Ober de electromotorische verschijnselen van het hart. Proc. verb. Kon. Akad. Wetensch. te Amsterdam, 1873.
4. WALLER, AUGUST D.: A demonstration on man of electromotive changes accompanying the heart's beat. *J Physiol, 8*:229, 1887.
5. WILLIUS, F.A., and KEYS, T.E.: *Classics of Cardiology.* New York, Dover, 1941.
6. FULTON, J.F.: *Selected Readings in the History of Physiology.* Springfield, Thomas, 1930.
7. SIMONSON, E.: Beobachtungen über die Herzbewegung. *Pflueger Arch Ges Physiol, 165*:1922.
8. LEWIS, T.: *Mechanism and Graphic Registration of the Heart Beat.* London, Shaw and Sons, 1925.
9. MANN, H.: A method of analyzing the electrocardiogram. *Arch Intern Med, 25*:283, 1920.
10. SIMONSON, E.; TUNA, N.; OKAMOTO, N., and TOSHIMA, H.: Diagnostic accuracy of the vectorcardiogram and electrocardiogram. *Amer J Cardiol, 17*:829, 1966.
11. CORABOEUF, E., and WEIDMANN, S.: Potential de repos et potentiels d'action du muscle cardique, mesurés a l'aide l'électroes internes. *CR Soc Biol (Paris), 143*:1329, 1949.
12. WOODBURY, L.A.; HECHT, H.H., and CHRISTOPHERSON, A.R.: Membrane resting and action potentials of single cardiac muscle fibers of the frog ventricle. *Amer J Physiol, 164*:307, 1951.

13. Brooks, C.McC.; Hoffman, B.F.; Suckling, E.E., and Orias, O.: *Excitability of the Heart.* New York, Grune, 1955.

14. Sano, T.; Mizuhira, V., and Matsuda, K.: *Electrophysiology and Ultrastructure of the Heart.* Tokyo, Bunkodo, 1967.

15. Scher, A.M.: Excitation of the heart. *Handbook of Physiology.* Amer. Physiol. Soc., Washington, D.C., 1962, Sect. 2 (Circulation), p. 287.

16. Hoffman, B.F., and Cranefield, P.F.: *Electrophysiology of the Heart.* New York, McGraw, 1960.

17. Lange, G.: Action of driving stimuli from intrinsic and extrinsic sources on *in situ* cardiac pacemaker tissues. *Circ Res, 17*:449, 1966.

18. Lu, H-H.; Lange, G., and Brooks, C.McC.: Factors controlling pacemaker actions in cells of the sinoatrial node. *Circ Res, 17*:460, 1966.

19. Brooks, C.McC.; Gilbert, J.F.; Badeer, H.S.; Ryo, U.Y.; Krellenstein, D., and Pliam, M.: Basic physiological processes related to fibrillation. Presented 17th General Assembly of the Japanese Medical Congress, 1967 (in press).

20. Brooks, C.McC.; Lu, H-H; Lange, G.; Mangi, R.; Shaw, R.B., and Geoly, K.: Effects of localized stretch of the sinoatrial node region of the dog heart. *Amer J Physiol, 211*:1197, 1966.

21. Lange, G.; Lu, H-H.; Chang, A., and Brooks, C.McC.: Effect of stretch on the isolated cat sinoatrial node. *Amer J Physiol, 211*:1192, 1966.

22. Brooks, C.McC.; Gilbert, J.L.; Greenspan, M.E.; Lange, G., and Mazzella, H.M.: Excitability and electrical response of ischemic heart muscle. *Amer J Physiol, 198*:1143, 1960.

23. Brooks, C.McC.; Gilbert, J.L.; Kavaler, F.; Suckling, E.E.; Ang, M.K., and Lange, G.: The phenomenon of accommodation in the ventricular myocardium. *Arch Kreislaufforsch, 33*:102, 1960.

24. Ushiyama, J., and Brooks, C.McC.: Hypothermia and minimal gradient requirements for excitation of cardiac muscle. *Amer J Physiol, 200*:718, 1961.

25. Ushiyama, J., and Brooks, C.McC.: Electrotonic and chemical effects on minimal gradient requirements for cardiac muscle. *Amer J Physiol, 202*:245, 1962.

26. Brooks, C.McC.; Gilbert, J.L.; Janse, M.J.; Lu, H-H., and Pinkston, J.O.: Production and abolition of alternation in mechanical action of the ventricle. *Amer J Physiol, 209*:945, 1965.

27. Lu, H-H.; Lange, G., and Brooks, C.McC.: Comparative studies of electrical and mechanical alternation in heart cells. *J Electrocardiol,* 1968 (in press).

28. Vassalle, M.; Levine, M.J., and Stuckey, J.H.: Sympathetic control of ventricular automaticity; effects of direct and reflex sympathetic excitation. In preparation for publication, 1968.

29. Badeer, H.S.; Ryo, U.Y.; Gassner, W.F.; Kass, E.J.; Cavaluzzi, J.; Gilbert, J.L., and Brooks, C.McC.: Factors affecting pulsus alternans

in the rapidly driven heart and papillary muscle. *Amer J Physiol,* 1968 (in press).

30. KOIZUMI, K., and SATO, A.: The influence of sympathetic innervation of the carotid sinus on baroreceptor activity in the Virginia opossum (*Didelphis virginiana*). *Amer J Physiol,* 1968.

DISCUSSION

Dr. Bruce: I was indeed intrigued with this recitation. May I ask how much change in temperature is necessary to bring about these adverse effects? Many have witnessed sudden death as a result of cooling. One man, for example, with an ischemic ST response exercised frequently with no adverse effects. He was even active at handball. On one occasion he went to the gym on a cold day and was just beginning to warm up when he dropped dead. Of course we started resuscitation, but to no avail, presumably because of ventricular fibrillation and the magnitude of the atherosclerotic disease. The room temperature at this time was definitely lower than usual.

Dr. Brooks: It is a difficult question. I would doubt that my reasoning would be of much help in that case because I was talking of heart temperature. External temperature may create more autonomic activity, adrenergic material release, which might have contributed in the case described. A rise in temperature does not change accommodation significantly. When temperature drops the heart must change in temperature a few degrees before one need concern himself about a decreased accommodation. I will say that it takes less current to excite an infarcted area than is required for normal tissue. It might be that in this situation described, an increased excitability maintained in one area at a time when there was an epinephrine discharge of unusual magnitude. This, plus a lack of uniformity in the myocardium, could have created a graver condition than would occur in normal tissue. One could draw all sorts of diagrams and not happen upon anything that would entirely explain the problem. A number of factors would have been involved in the situation you described.

Dr. Wolf: Would exposure to cold change the rate of accommodation?

Dr. Brooks: Not by direct action. Ischemia could have been enough to change the rate of accommodation. What always impresses me is the higher excitability in the area which receives less blood. It can be assumed that when blood is cut off, the metabolic maintenance of the membrane state is weakened and one gets a greater responsiveness. One visualizes creation of a circus movement. If there is an ischemic area, there is during the cycle a disparity of cellular states; the normal action potential may be something like 300 msec, while in the ischemic area, the duration might fall to 100 msec. That leaves 200 msec for current to flow out of normal tissue into the ischemic and this might start an ectopic beat. Since this ischemic area is more excitable than the other areas, it takes less current to excite change. Also, the approaching current may jump into the ischemic area so that excitation there precedes excitation in other normal tissue since there is a lower excitability there. Conduction may be faster in one area than in another. Then there may be reentry. All this could occur because the unity of this tissue's state and its integration is broken. Thus, weakening of its blood supply reduces the stability of the cell membranes. The basic danger is that segments of the myocardium get out of phase and go into fibrillation.

Another failure in integrative mechanisms may occur thus: Suppose a rapid arrhythmia—a very rapid beat occurs and suddenly this ceases—a suppressed pacemaker results. When this occurs a fibrillation may result. Also a very rapid drive may result in a pacemaker suppression. If it doesn't recover fast enough, there may be an escape of other pacemakers and this may disorganize the myocardium. When one is defibrillating a heart, one wants a pacemaker in the operating room to get it started again—it does not always start readily. The pacemaker has its own intrinsic excitatory mechanism and this is reduced by a fast drive.

Question: To what degree does the heart temperature have to drop before it will react as you said? Frequently, infants have a temperature drop to 96° or 95° F. It is clear that infants have much more ventricular fibrillation.

Dr. Brooks: I would say that five degrees was quite signifiant as a minimum requirement. There is a critical temperature band of two to ten degrees—beginning at five or six degrees. Below this band the heart is inactivated by cold, but my experience is only with the dog and separated tissue, I would say a critical fall is 5° C.

Question: Are there any mechanics to lengthen the flow of acteylcholine?

Dr. Brooks: Yes, by administering anti-cholinesterase.

Question: Does one wish to reduce the acetlycholine or to stop the sympathetic transmitter production?

Dr. Brooks: If one has an acetylcholine-produced depression of the pacemaker, atropine will reduce it and anticholinesterase increase it. If adrenergic material is given, it counteracts depression. Although I am a little uncertain of the theory that the beat of the heart liberates acetylcholine, it can be proved that overdrive by a pacemaker produces liberation of acetylcholine and also an excessive potassium discharge from the coronary sinus. There is evidence that in the beating heart actions occur which act back on the pacemaker to affect its rate of action.

Question: As to the initiation of arrhythmia, potassium is present in the coronary sinus and also in the lymph and coronary cells. When potassium is given rapidly, it can bring the myocardium closer to the critical stage, and in the long range, depolarization becomes so great that the excitability decreases. Can rapid potassium administration do so?

Dr. Brooks: Yes, some potassium tends to destroy stability and favor arrhythmia, but larger applications will depolarize and stop cardiac action.

Mr. Wolf: How much of the normal fluctuation of the heart can be attributed to the potassium: Can one quantitate the relative amount of effect on K release that stretch of the SA node would have?

Dr. Brooks: We have been thinking of doing this but I do not know quite how this could be done. Perhaps one might attach some kind of a strain gauge to the sinus to see how much it is stretched in filling. One might relate degree of stretch to potassium flux but this would be more easily done in isolated tissue.

Question: How does acetylcholine compare with adrenergic material in effect on accommodation?

Dr. Brooks: I do not know how these compounds could compete in their effect on accommodation. We talk about two things in accommodation. If we are talking about minimal gradient requirements, let us say the threshold for a rectangular pulse is five milliamps, and current strength is brought up slowly to the same threshold it may not excite. If one then gives epinephrine, this gradient requirement moves in one direction; if one gives acetylcholine, it goes in the other direction. How epinephrine competes with choline—this has not been tried. Epinephrine might even be protective; in certain circumstances epinephrine can be protective against arrhythmias. It increases excitability and then reduces it: if one can get past the bad area, one has a protection by epinephrine against excitation. Competition may have something to do with it, but I cannot really answer the question.

Question: Can you explain the relationships of the fast drive of the pacemaker to postdrive effects?

Dr. Brooks: There is a great compensation in the pacemaker. If one drives very fast, one does get a greater depression than if one drives slightly above the normal rate. However, there is a limit. If one overdrives for five minutes, one gets a certain degree of depression; if one overdrives for fifteen minutes, one gets a much longer-lasting depression. If one overdrives for thirty minutes, one gets the maximum depression. If one overdrives beyond thirty minutes, depression is less; some sort of adaptation occurs. Either one reduces the acetylcholine liberation or a desensitization occurs. Do not quote me, but it is my opinion that one does not play with a pacemaker; if it is used, it should be permitted to drive a long time rather than five minutes; one should not flick it off and on.

Question: How fast does one have to drive the heart in order to observe the failure of the mechanical response to follow the electrical response?

Dr. Brooks: It depends. It generally starts at 200 beats a minute. Some show alternans temporarily; it disappears after a while at rates up to 150 beats a minute. It depends on the condition and temperature of the animal. At a lower temperature, coupling fails very easily. If the heart is cooled a few degrees below normal, one gets uncoupling at rates of only slightly above 100.

Dr. Blackburn: We have seen alternate beats with ST depression. Do you know if that is associated with mechanical alternans?

Dr. Brooks: I should think mechanical alternation should be greater than electrical.

2

Anatomic and Physiologic Factors Affecting Cardiac Performance and Myocardial Perfusion

Yang Wang

THE CAPACITY FOR sustained exertion is dependent primarily on an adequate rate of delivery of oxygen to the exercising tissues by the cardiopulmonary system. Delivery is modified by the adequacy of muscle strength, the integrity of the central nervous system, the motivation of the individual, and by other factors concerning which data have been accumulated and which will be discussed later. It is clear that the most important factor limiting sustained physical exercise is the maximal rate of oxygen delivery to the exercising tissues. There is as yet no convincing evidence that the rapid transit time through the pulmonary capillary bed at high levels of exercise might be insufficient to allow adequate reoxygenation of the venous return. Normally the lungs are probably not a limiting factor. Furthermore, the diffusion capacity of the lungs rises significantly with exercise. Though pulmonary diseases may be a serious limiting factor to complete oxygenation of blood this discussion will be limited to cardiovascular factors.

The ability to achieve and sustain a cardiac output appropriate to the level of work is clearly the major determinant in the capacity to perform sustained work at that level. The cardiac output at any level of exercise is largely determined by the oxygen needs of the exercising tissues and the magnitude of the skin blood flow serving as thermoregulatory mechanism. A substantial sparing of cardiac effort is effected by redistribution of regional blood flow such that the exercising tissues are the primary beneficiaries of the increase in cardiac output, while others are temporarily deprived.

[26]

The cardiac output is the volume of blood ejected by the left ventricle per minute; or the product of stroke volume and heart rate in beats per minute. Under steady state conditions the stroke volume shows remarkably little change over a wide range of physical effort. At rest the upright stroke volume is less than the supine and less than the upright exercising stroke volume. There is also evidence that at a physical effort resulting in a maximal oxygen intake the stroke volume may increase 15 per cent over that at submaximal levels. With these exceptions, the pulse rate is thus a reasonably linear guide to changes in cardiac output providing steady state conditions obtain throughout the course of observation. Since the cardiac output is linearly related to the minute oxygen consumption, at least at submaximal levels of exercise, changes in pulse rate provide a useful estimate of changes in oxygen uptake.

Under standardized conditions the pulse rate, cardiac output and oxygen consumption at a given level of exercise show relatively small variation in the same individual. However, factors of training, changes in ambient temperature and humidity, emotional and motivational factors, the type of work and pharmacologic agents such as catecholamines may cause significant deviations. Training tends to decrease the pulse rate and increase the stroke volume but has little effect on cardiac output at a given work level in the same individual. Emotional factors may be related to the action of catecholamines. Different types of work often call into play different groups of large muscle masses. Nevertheless, in the same individual such variables appear not to change the maximal oxygen intake, which for a given individual remains remarkably constant over a wide range of conditions, varing from day to day little more than 50 to 75 ml of oxygen per minute.

Maximal oxygen intake should be determined by stepwise graded exercise, measuring oxygen consumption at each level until it plateaus despite increases in external work. At this level the pulse rate is usually 180 to 200 beats per minute, whether the individual be sedentary or athletic, while the cardiac output will increase three to four times from the resting value in sedentary subjects and five to seven times in athletes. The maximal oxygen intake is a useful concept, a reasonable biological constant, and is minimally affected by perturbating factors, including motivation. Because it is a time-consuming procedure, and many subjects cannot attain this level of exercise because of physical or motivational reasons, extrapolative methods often have been used to predict maximal oxygen intake from performance at submaximal levels of exercise. It is well to remember that such methods rest on the assumption that many factors of variability are not operative at these submaximal levels, an assumption which is not always justified.

The ability to increase cardiac output relative to peripheral needs is the most crucial factor in cardiac performance. Central to this ability is the regulation of coronary blood flow which is modified by the presence of organic heart disease.

In man there are usually two coronary arteries: the right is dominant in 48 per cent of the cases, the left is dominant in 18 per cent, and in 34 per cent the distribution is balanced. In the left ventricle branches of the coronary arterial tree penetrate perpendicularly from the epicardium to subendocardium. During early systole there is a sudden marked increase in intramyocardial tension and a slight reversal of flow in the larger coronary arteries, followed by forward coronary blood flow largely paralleling the aortic systolic pressure. However, most of the left ventricular coronary flow occurs during diastole, especially early diastole, when compression of the coronary vascular bed is at a minimum. Thus rapid heart rate, ventricular hypertrophy and elevated diastolic pressures will compromise coronary flow to the left ventricle. Coronary flow to the right ventricle is of a similar pattern but occurs fairly uniformly through both systole and diastole because of lower right ventricular pressures. Collateral vessels are potentially present but do not become functional until stenotic gradients develop in the coronary arteries, or probably from the stimulus of metabolites resulting from local tissue ischemia.

The coronary circulation is unique in the completeness with which oxygen is extracted during a single circulation, even in the resting state. Thus, increased oxygen delivery to the myocardium is for all practical purposes possible only through an increase in coronary blood flow mediated by a fall in the coronary vascular resistance. Experimental evidence points to an efficient autoregulatory mechanism related to local tissue hypoxia, but the exact interrelationship of mechanical, neural and humoral factors in such autoregulation needs more elucidation. Changes in coronary perfusion pressure over the physiologic range apparently have only a transient effect. The vagi have little or no direct effect providing the heart rate is kept constant even though acetylcholine is a coronary vasodilator. There is no evidence that endogenous acetylcholine plays a role in autoregulation of coronary circulation. Sympathetic stimulation has a mixed effect, the net result of which is an increased coronary blood flow. Catecholamines directly injected into the coronary arteries cause arteriolar vasoconstriction initially and thus a decrease in coronary flow. This is more than overcome by their effect in increasing the mechanical and metabolic activities of the myocardium and coronary vasodilation secondary to this. The paradox of the exercising heart is in all likelihood similarly explained—exercise-induced tachycardia which alone would tend to impede coronary blood flow is counterbalanced by increased metabolic activity of the myocardium, with resulting vasodilation and a net increase in coronary flow. The role of ions and polypeptides in vasodilation have been studied with little success. However, there is some evidence that adenine nucleotides or their breakdown products may be direct vasodilating agents, their accumulation resulting from local myocardial hypoxia secondary to either increased metabolic activity or arterial oxygen unsaturation, or both.

Under resting conditions, myocardial oxygen consumption is about 8 to 10 ml/min/100 gm of left ventricle. Two important variables influence changes in oxygen requirements of the myocardium: the tension developed by the contraction or the time integral of systolic force, and the velocity of shortening of the myocardial fibers. It should be noted that the time integral of systolic force implies that the heart tolerates volume work more effectively than pressure work. For identical products of cardiac output and aortic mean pressure (and hence identical external work), myocardial oxygen consumption is much greater for increased pressure work. The internal work of the heart has so far been considered negligible—that is, the work involved in shortening muscle fiber length and changing the ventricular configuration during systole. However certain conditions, most notably ischemia and scarring, may cause cardiac dyssynergy so that part of the internal cardiac work is squandered in such efforts as stretching of a ventricular aneurysm; the velocity of contraction is altered. Such

dyssynergy thus clearly decreases cardiac efficiency by increasing myocardial oxygen requirements without a corresponding increase, or even
a decrease, in external work. Increased myocardial oxygen consumption is effected through an increase in coronary blood flow up to five-
fold, which under normal conditions meets the demands imposed by
maximal effort. In subjects with normal hearts, there is little or no
change in the oxygen content of coronary sinus blood even during
fairly severe exercise. Under conditions where the coronary circulation is compromised, increased oxygen demands are met in a very
limited degree by greater oxygen extraction, since extraction is already high in the coronary circulation. Where demands exceed this
mechanism, glycolysis results in lactate production detectable in coronary sinus blood. This mechanism is limited because the myocardium
is incapable of significant anerobic metabolism. Pain occurs presumably when oxygen demands exceed the available supply. Myocardial
hypoxia may be generalized, as in aortic stenosis or diffuse severe
coronary atherosclerosis, or localized as in localized coronary disease.
This pain, angina pectoris, becomes a significant limiting factor in
achieving higher sustained work levels, although higher levels at dis-
continuous work may be feasible. The clinical picture of myocardial
ischemia may be complicated by the presence of emotional factors,
paroxysmal tachydysrhythmias, myocardial dyssynergy and ventricular
failure, any of which increase myocardial oxygen consumption or
affect coronary blood flow with or without concomitant increase in
physical work.

3

Panel Discussion on Determinants of Myocardial Oxygen Consumption

T. JOSEPH REEVES, *Chairman*, HOWARD BURCHELL
and C. GUNNAR BLOMQVIST

Dr. Reeves: The question of the myocardial oxygen consumption really relates very closely to exercise electrocardiography, specifically in the design of the stress test that is to be used, and most specifically if one is concerned with quantitation of that stress in relationship to the challenge that might be offered by it to the coronary circulation.

I think that it might help actually to write a simple equation to give us a little focus at the beginning. $O_2 = M + E + P$. The O_2 consumption of the myocardium could be considered to be the sum of several metabolic processes related to several specific activities of the heart. One is just the O_2 cost of maintaining an inactive myocardial cell, that is, the plain cost of keeping it alive, and we might list that as "M," or maintenance cost. I think that one also has to consider the oxygen cost of electrical activation, and we might list that as "E," and finally, one must consider the cost of mechanical activity, which is something the heart does—if it is doing its job well it is continuously active; it pumps, it relaxes and it pumps.

Now, the maintenance cost has been studied and measured in arrested tissue and arrested hearts. It is a relatively small percentage of the total oxygen cost of the heart. It is changed, however, by such things as varying concentrations of myocardial catecholamines.

The oxygen cost of electrical activation has also been studied. This also is a relatively small percentage of the total and it is changed very little by variations in the inotropic state, so we come then to the oxygen cost of the physical activity of the heart, the mechanical activity, and this is most of the energy expenditure and oxygen utilization of the heart.

One of the reasons why so much attention has been paid over the years to a study of the determinants, particularly the mechanical determinants of myocardial oxygen consumption, is because they are so difficult to measure in man. One would like to have a way to estimate from readily measurable physical factors, such as the heart rate, the blood pressure, or even the ventricular pressure, the cardiac output or the rate of ejection, or some other handle to predict the myocardial oxygen consumption from something that you could measure in intact man. This would obviously relate to the kind of problems that one considers in designing or evaluating an exercise test.

This indirect measurement has challenged cardiac physiologists over the years. One of the first and very significant bits of experimentation done in Dr. Ernest Starling's laboratory in the period of 1912 to 1917 by Dr. Lovett Evans concerned the relationship between oxygen consumption of the heart muscle and the pressure-volume work of the ventricle—that is, the stroke work of the ventricle calculated as the product of the stroke volume and the pressure that the stroke volume is ejected against. One of the very first of the quantitative studies of the relationship of the mechanical activity of the heart to its oxygen consumption, the validity of which is still recognized, is that there is a relationship between the oxygen consumption and such a product, but it is not a simple relationship. They found that if one did the same amount of work and if the product of pressure times volume were plotted against the oxygen consumption, one could establish a nice relationship, if the pressure were kept constant and the stroke volume changed in an isolated heart-lung preparation. If, however, one got the same product of pressure and volume by a different combination of them, in other words, if one raised the pressure and lowered the stroke volume, a new relationship would be established such that the oxygen cost per unit work would be increased. In other words, it was more expensive to develop pressure than it was to shorten fibers against a lower pressure. One could not then conclude that stroke work *per se* was a fundamental determinant of oxygen consumption. These observations have been confirmed many times by many investigators since that work—the efficiency—of the ventricle depended on the relative contribution of pressure factors as compared to the volume factors of stroke work. In 1927 Dr. Visscher of the

University of Minnesota, then working with Dr. Starling, published a classic paper showing that there would be a very good relationship between the end-diastolic volume of the ventricle and the oxygen consumption of the ventricle, under wide conditions of varying pressures and volumes, so long as the biochemical state of the muscle did not change greatly and was not interfered with by the administration of epinephrine or catecholamines. This then was what was known, and what was accepted in its entirety for more than twenty years, until the late 1940's and early 1950's, when Dr. Louis Katz in Chicago began a series of investigations which have continued to this day. Dr. Katz, in a series of studies concerning the relationship of oxygen consumption to the mechanical activity of the heart under widely varying circumstances found that the best correlation he could establish was between the simple product of the blood pressure and the heart rate, without taking any other factors into account. However, he did find that if he gave calcium or digitalis, this whole curve would be shifted up to a new level, so that again one would have to conclude there were some other factors that would relate.

This work was soon followed by the reexamination of the question in the laboratories of Dr. Sarnoff at the National Institutes of Health, culminating in his publication in 1957 or 1958 of studies relating to the index of mechanical activities that he called the "tension-time index." This actually was the area under the ventricular pressure curve. He recognized the importance of the volume factor in the ventricle in relating tension to pressure, and therefore he used the pressure as an index to tension. What he said in essence was that if you had a ventricular pressure curve with a given area under it and you changed it in any way so that the area increased, the oxygen consumption of the ventricle would tend to parallel rather closely the area under the tension curve, and this relationship would be better than that obtained by the simple product of heart rate times blood pressure. This would also be better than any of the products of the calculations of stroke work, no matter how calculated. But he made a further reservation, and that was in relation to the steepness of rise of the ventricular pressure: if heart rate were allowed to change greatly, if the inotropic state of the muscle was changed by the administration of epinephrine or norephinephrine or calcium or digitalis that this relationship would be disturbed. He followed this clue up in a few years by other studies, in which he showed curves relating these two factors, that is, the oxygen consumption and the tension-time index which were very much like those shown for the relationship between blood pressure and heart rate from Dr. Katz's laboratory when he gave digitalis or calcium. In other words, we are back again, using different variables, to where we were at the time of Evans' studies. If one plotted the tension-time index of the pressure time integral, against the oxygen consumption in an isolated, metabolically supported heart one could establish a nice relationship. But if you gave digitalis, the relationship would be shifted, such that the oxygen consumption per unit tension-time index would be increased, and this seemed to have some relationship to the *rate* of tension development. These studies were published in 1963, I think. Subsequently, Dr. Braunwald and others in the cardiovascular laboratories at NIH have paid particular attention to the variable of the maximum *rate* of tension development, or the time derivative of the tension curve, and they have shown a very good relationship. If you leave everything else constant—if you keep the pressure constant, if you keep the volume of the ventricle constant and do nothing but introduce an inotropic intervention that causes the rate of tension development to change, the oxygen consumption of the ventricle will tend to vary in this direction. They have recently written a multifactorial equation in which they have attempted to put these things together and come up with a prediction. A few years ago Dr. Sheffield and others in our laboratory did a similar study in isolated, metabolically supported hearts, in which we measured and controlled the volume, measured the rate of tension development, the rate of pressure development, and also the rate of tension development directly and calculated. We looked at a series of comparisons under a wide variety of heart rate variations, change in end-diastolic volumes and changes in inotropic state introduced by a number of different drugs. We found that one could establish a highly significant correlation between oxygen consumption and three variables. One was the rate of tension development *per se*. In approximately one hundred observations we found a coefficient of correlation of about 0.6 between oxygen consumption and the rate of tension development, in a widely varying set of circumstances. We found essentially the same correlation for the time integral of tension, and we found essentially the same correlation for the peak tension that would be generated during a contraction. We could combine the rate of tension development with either one of the other two, and come up with a greatly improved correlation, but one which was still not sufficiently precise to allow us, in any given heart, to predict the oxygen consumption with the kind of precision that one is seeking. These studies are being continued in our laboratory now, using a different preparation, and one with which we can get a great many more samples of comparisons than we could then.

Dr. Blackburn: I am sure that all present recognize the interest in myocardial oxygen consumption in regard to our subject, the quantitation of the exercise ECG response, in any diagnostic or functional testing situation. We need to compare people under comparable work loads, that is, in the work done by the heart rather than external work, and the indirect measurement of this is what Dr. Reeves has very effectively reviewed for us. I wonder if one of you would give us the present status of any approaches to indirect measurements of myocardial oxygen consumption in office or field conditions, and how they might be used to find a more physiological standard testing procedure.

Dr. Blomqvist: I think that even though we can directly measure ventricular pressures and volumes and rate of pressure development in patients and some normal subjects or volunteers, it is so far not possible to do it under conditions of clinical exercise tests or in population studies, surveys, or diagnostic screening procedures. We have to supplement the information from detailed laboratory studies of hemodynamics by other and indirect studies. We simply go out and study patients with angina—patients with a stable level of angina—under various conditions and modifications of the exercise test, and measure what we can—heart rate and blood pressure—and in the same manner study apparently healthy subjects, along with electrocardiographic changes in the response to exercise—and in that way build up a bank of knowledge that we later can match with more detailed hemodynamic data.

Dr. Blackburn: How well, if at all, can we measure indirectly the rate of myocardial contraction, ejection or tension development?

Dr. Blomqvist: It might become possible, and it is worthwhile looking into. There is interest in this regard in carotid pulse wave analysis, upper thoracic impedance curves, chest wall displacement curves and even in ultrasound traces of ventricular action.

Dr. Burchell: Perhaps at this time it would be proper to introduce some of the problems that a physician might consider in exercising a patient, causing hypoxia to develop in parts of the myocardium. I was delighted to hear Dr. Reeves' comments about the relationship of the oxygen requirement of the myocardium in exercise. Years ago when I was with Dr. Visscher and he had just recently published his own legendary work on the relationship of the myocardial oxygen requirement and diastolic fiber length, I used to ask: "Well, isn't there more to it than this; doesn't the heart seem to work harder if one obstructs the aortic output?" Looking at isolated hearts at that time, there are a number of things that were rather interesting, and I have never been able to forget the questions that we discussed at that time. The heart really is the only organ in the body that kills itself; in other words, if one can put the heart at rest, then it doesn't need to have any coronary flow and then you can restart it at will, but if it works, then it kills itself, and it kills itself through two mechanisms. One is the mechanism of localized ischemia with arrhythmia and the other is illustrated by an isolated heart which is allowed to fail spontaneously. It becomes larger; the coronary flow increases tremendously, the heart gets larger and larger. With the cardiac enlargement, the actual amount of oxygen for the same external work increases tremendously in accord with the LaPlace law which has been particularly emphasized by Dr. Burton.

On the other hand, if one observes an isolated perfused heart in the laboratory, and adds epinephrine, adrenaline, one observes the heart to become pink and red, and the coronary sinus outflow, which has been dark red, becomes bright red. Despite the color of the heart, if one takes an electrocardiogram, one may see changes in the ST and T wave which we might regard as ischemic. This exemplifies the problem of the distribution of coronary flow within the coronary system. Could one have functional shunts analogous to those encountered in peripheral artery disease, whereby the peripheral area is robbed of its blood supply because of a proximal area with a lower resistance? Obvious question is, Does a short diastolic period and a noncompliant ventricle cause the flow in the subendocardial area to be grossly inadequate? In the ordinary exercise tests or other stress tests the gross changes in the electrocardiogram, which we would all agree as indicating that the myocardium is ischemic, follow a pattern of ST depression. This fits very nicely with the theory that there is a boundary zone in the mid-myocardium and that the endocardial area, as an internal shell, has become ischemic. There are instances of patients with such ST segment changes who have a structurally normal heart. Perhaps the greatest ST segment change that one can see in a normal heart is in infants with a very rapid tachycardia, and here one may have changes of two, three and four-tenths of a millivolt and for all the world it looks like a very ischemic heart, and indeed I believe it is. In addition we have patients with aortic stenosis who may show similar changes. Of interest in the last four or five years is the syndrome of obstructive or semi-obstructive hypertrophic cardiomyopathy in which there may be a very small end-diastolic ventricular volume. There are good coronary arteries and a good myocardium so far as we can tell from the ability of the person to exercise. Yet in certain instances, not necessarily during exercise but perhaps in the immediate postexercise period, when the patient is still standing and the heart is small, one can observe significant ST segment changes. I bring up these problems because they will continue to bother us, not only from the point of view of epicardial to endocardial distribution of flow, but from the possibility of shunts of a physiological type which could rob a peripheral area. Such phenomena would be accentuated if there were any localized coronary narrowing. At one time Dr. Visscher and I thought that the relative diastolic pressures in the two ventricles might influence the distribution of coronary flow in that, if we observed an isolated heart, causing it to fail by increasing the afterload on the left ventricle, in certain instances, if we increase the afterload on the *right* ventricle (increasing the Starling resistance in the pulmonary outflow tract), we found that the heart improved in its function with a decrease in size. We believed that there was perhaps redistribution of blood from the right coronary system into the left. It was a curious phenomenon, and we rather doubted that it would ever occur in the human, because the levels of pressure in the experimental situation were so artificial that one wouldn't think of it occurring in the human. Nevertheless, it was considered a possible explanation of why an individual with angina, developing congestive heart failure, lost his angina. I am sure that Dr. Brooks could add a great deal to and criticize and maybe destroy some of these suggestions that I have made.

Dr. Blackburn: Thank you, Dr. Burchell. Did you have a reply to that Dr. Reeves?

Dr. Reeves: I am intrigued by the last account but I would certainly agree that unless one knows the details of the distribution of coronary blood flow one cannot predict behavior. I think that was very clearly shown with some of the recent coronary vasodilators which greatly increase coronary blood flow and decrease coronary oxygen A-V difference, but do not relieve angina.

Dr. Blackburn: I can't think of a more appropriate summary of this question than we have had spontaneously this morning. I am very grateful to each of the members of this extemporaneous panel. We'll come back after coffee to start on bioengineering questions. Thank you all very much.

PART TWO

METHODS AND EARLY RESULTS OF AUTOMATED
COMPUTER PROGRAMS FOR EXERCISE
ELECTROCARDIOGRAPHY

4

Noise Reduction in Exercise Electrocardiograms by Digital Filter Techniques

Jobst von der Groeben, J. Gerald Toole, Charles S. Weaver, *and* John W. Fitzgerald

INTRODUCTION

THE PURPOSE of this report is to describe some of the digital filtering techniques which are presently used in our laboratory for the preparation of exercise ECG records for quantitative analysis. The electrocardiograms are recorded by the data acquisition system of Figure 4-1. Skin electrodes are placed in positions described by Frank. The circled letters A-F represent miniaturized amplifiers which are placed in close proximity to the electrode. These low-output-impedance amplifiers amplify the signals, and allow a low-noise, low-impedance transmission between the patient and the rest of the amplification system. The output of the preamplifiers feeds into differential amplifiers (1) through (6). The six potential differences of I-A, E-M, C-M, F-H, I-C, H-E are available as outputs. Weighting networks at the outputs of the differential amplifiers (WTG) provide the weighting of these potential differences according to the Frank System. The system therefore allows a choice between the six unweighted outputs or the three weighted X, Y and Z leads. We are presently comparing the amount of information contained in the six lead outputs with the amount of information contained in the X, Y and Z leads. The records presented in this discussion were all obtained from Frank weighted X, Y and Z leads.

ECG PROCESSING PROGRAM

Figure 4-2 is the schematic of the data processing system.

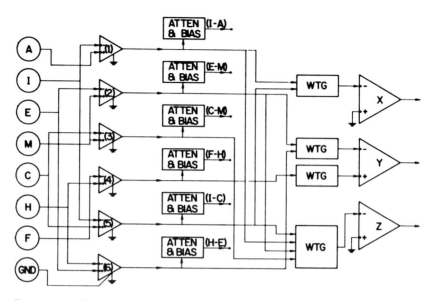

Figure 4-1. Data acquisition system. A, I, E, M, C, H, F (letters correspond to Frank electrode placement) represent preamplifiers located in the lead a few inches from the electrode. 1, 2, 3, 4, 5 and 6 are differential amplifiers using integrated-circuit operational amplifiers. Output of unweighted leads I-A, E-M, CM, FH, I-C, and H-E as well as weighted leads X, Y and Z are available. Weighting is done on the outputs of the six channels by an operational amplifier network.

Only the 60 cycle notched filter, the lowpass filter, the averaging program, and the muscle tremor adaptive filter will be discussed. Finally the filtered data will be presented as scalar leads and/or spherical coordinates as a function of time.

The use of any filter is optional and at the command of the teletype input. The data can be displayed either on the oscilloscope or on an incremental plotter. The display of digital raw data is important to the operator in choosing a particular filtering technique. Since this is strictly a research tool, we have not developed any fixed routine method for handling exercise data.

All of the individual blocks containing the digital filters, except averaging, are based on the same principle, namely, that successive samples of the signal are placed in an identical manner into a set of difference equations. The advantages of digital over analog filters are

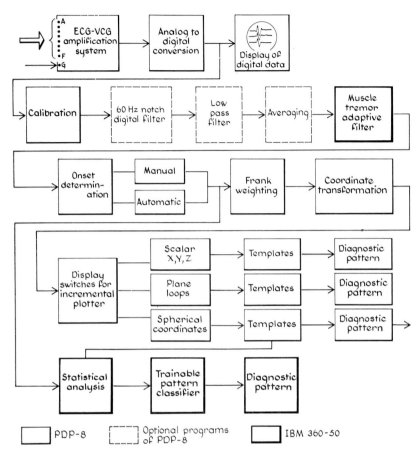

FIGURE 4-2. ECG Processing Schematic. All programs described in this report are carried out by a small general-purpose digital computer (PDP-8).

numerous. There is no drift in gain, bandwidth, or dc level; the shape of the frequency response curve stays constant; and the noise added during filtering is very low. The only practical realization of the sharp notch of the 60 cycle notched filter, for example, is with digital filtering techniques. The operator can select a filter parameter, such as cutoff frequency, by entering the instructions through the teletype.

The 60 cycle notched filter is used to remove ac pickup from the ECG data, and the filter's frequency response is shown in Figure 4-3. The notch is 1 cycle wide, and at 60 cycles the response is down 80 db. The bandpass regions are flat to six decimal places, and the phase

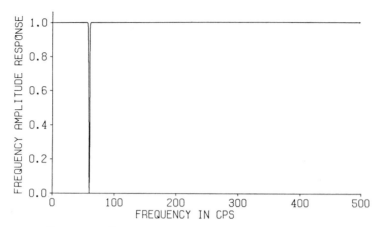

FIGURE 4-3. The 60 cps Notch Fliter Frequency Response.

shift away from 60 cycles is approximately zero with virtually no distortion of the ECG waveform. Figure 4-4 shows a single lead greatly contaminated with 60 cycles. After the ECG has been filtered by the notched filter, harmonics of 60 cycles and other noise components remain which are then removed by a lowpass filter.

The lowpass filtering also is done by solving a set of difference equations. The lowpass filter difference equations have been designed to have a sharp frequency cutoff, good rise time and no overshoot. Figure 4-5 shows the frequency response curves for filters with cutoff frequencies of 10 to 60 cps. The effect of successive lowpass filters on a single-lead ECG is shown in Figure 4-6. Some R wave attenuation but no drastic changes are seen down to 20 cycle cutoff, and there is a good reduction of the background noise.

As shown in the schematic (Fig. 4-2) a number of ECG beats may be averaged to reduce the background noise. The averaging algorithm operates on all three leads on real time data being digitized at a 1 kc rate, and it uses an arbitrarily selected lead as a reference for synchronization in processing multiple leads. The epoch is determined by slope measurements made on the incoming data; when the highest absolute slope averaged over a given period of time is recognized, 750 msec of data (centered about the epoch) are added point by point to the cumulative values previously obtained. The data are buffered to insure that P, QRS and T are included. After the desired number

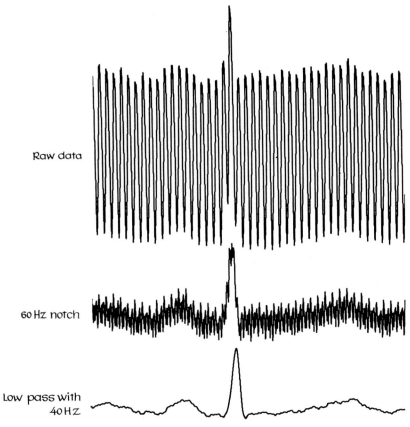

FIGURE 4-4. Effect of 60 cps filter on an electrocardiographic signal greatly contaminated with 60 cycle noise.

of beats have been processed, the averaged values are divided by the total number of beats in the average and then stored for further analysis. The program makes use of a digital oscilloscope display to show concurrently the ECG and the number of beats averaged. The data can be processed subsequently through a number of programs, including incremental plotting, filtering and coordinate transformation.

If the noise and the ECG spectra were known, a filter or difference equation could be described to maximize the ECG to tremor noise power ratio. Unfortunately every waveform represents a new set of circumstances with different spectra, and no fixed filter will maximize the ratio in all cases. For this reason it may be profitable

3 POLE LOWPASS FILTERS

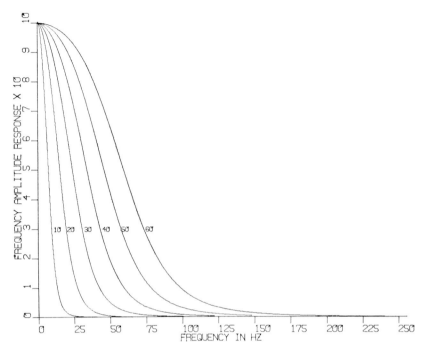

FIGURE 4-5. Frequency response curve of lowpass digital filters with cutoff at 10, 20, 30, 40, 50 and 60 cycles.

to use an adaptive or self-organizing filter. Such a filter takes measurements on the ECG and noise and adjusts a difference equation to give the best estimate of the ECG (in the least-mean-square-error sense), thus removing as much tremor as possible. (An adaptive filter has been programmed whose effect will be shown in Fig. 4-16.)

In one application of the filter techniques to the actual stress test procedure, the patient exercises on a bicycle ergometer. The test session is divided into seven consecutive periods of five minutes each with stepwise increase in work load, interrupted by rest periods. A continuous record is taken on magnetic tape throughout the entire session. The rest periods are spent sitting on the bicycle so that all data may be recorded with the same body position.

In order to demonstrate the various techniques of noise reduction, a record from a normal individual and one from the group with ab-

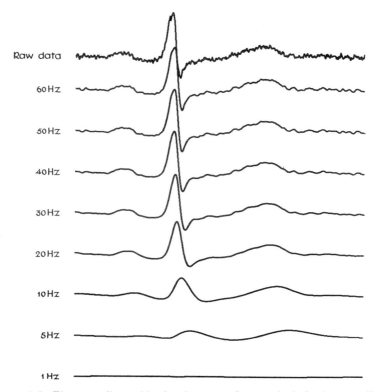

FIGURE 4-6. Electrocardiographic signal processed successively by lowpass filters 60 to 1 cycle.

normal exercise response was selected. The abnormal patient had to discontinue the test at the end of the 100 watt work load period because his maximal expected heart rate just barely exceeded 85 per cent of the limit set for a normal patient. His record was therefore taken at the peak of his maximal effort, that is, during the last minute of the 100 watt work load period.

Figure 4-7 shows the raw data obtained from the normal individual during the initial rest period and at the peak of exercise. The muscle tremor is naturally more pronounced in the Y lead than in the others. In the exercise record the tremor interferes seriously with recognition of the P wave and also to some extent of the ST segment. Figure 4-8 shows raw data from the abnormal patient at rest and at the peak of exercise. The muscle tremor is worse for this abnormal case than for

RAW DATA

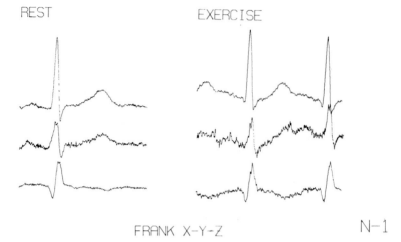

FIGURE 4-7. X, Y and Z leads (Frank system) of a normal individual, rest (*left*) and at the peak of exercise (*right*).

RAW DATA

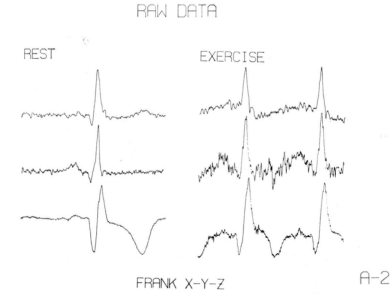

FIGURE 4-8. X, Y and Z leads of a patient demonstrating abnormal response.

30 CPS FILTER

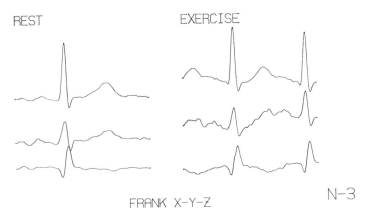

REST   EXERCISE

FRANK X-Y-Z   N-3

FIGURE 4-9. Record of a normal individual (raw data shown in Fig. 4-7) after 30 cps filter.

the normal. Low-frequency and high-frequency components are seen in the exercise noise pattern.

The normal record before and after exercise with a 30 cycle low-pass filter is shown in Figure 4-9. Although there is some improvement in the quality of the record, it is obvious that a considerable amount of noise is present in the filtered record. In Figure 4-10 the resting record in the abnormal case is well defined, showing clearly the shape of the P, QRS and ST-T segments. However, during exercise the low-frequency noise components severely interfere with the interpretation of the record.

Figure 4-11 shows the effect of a 10 cps filter on the resting and exercise ECG of a normal person. There is little noticeable distortion of the P and T waves. The resting and exercise records are also very similar. The effect of the 10 cps filter on the abnormal patient is shown in Figure 4-12. There is a striking difference between the resting and exercise records, especially during the terminal portion of QRS and in the ST-T segment.

Figure 4-13 shows an averaged record of 30 beats from a normal patient sampled at a rate of 1 kc/sec for each channel. Little differ-

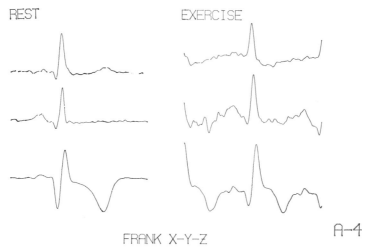

FIGURE 4-10. Record of a patient (raw data shown in Fig. 4-8) after 30 cps filter.

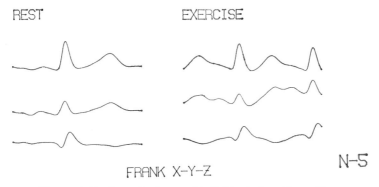

FIGURE 4-11. Record of normal individual after 10 cps filter.

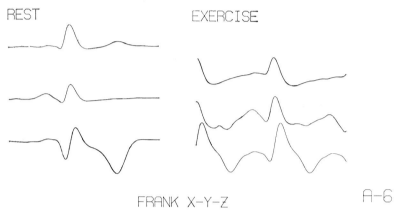

FIGURE 4-12. Record of patient after 10 cps filter.

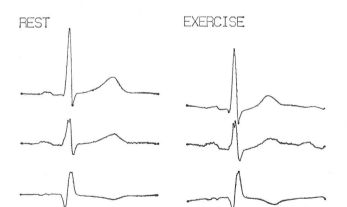

FIGURE 4-13. A 30-beat average at rest and at peak of exercise in a normal individual.

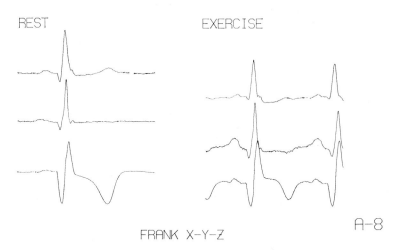

FIGURE 4-14. Thirty-beat average at rest and at peak of exercise in a patient with abnormal response.

ence is observed between the two records except for some flattening of T in lead X and some increase in magnitude of the negative T wave in lead Z. Lead Z is taken with plus polarity in the back, so the T wave in this individual is directed more anteriorly after exercise. The averaged data of the abnormal individual at rest and at the peak of exercise show striking differences (Fig. 4-14). Figure 4-15 is a plot of a recently developed program in which the 30-beat average before and after exercise is superimposed on one record. Note the height of the P wave before and after exercise and the change in the ST-T segment in lead X and Z, while the ST segment of lead Y remains unchanged. It should also be noted that the resting record shows an ST segment depression in Z which during exercise gradually developed into an ST elevation. In order to measure changes, therefore, emphasis should be placed not so much on the amount of depression or elevation but rather on the change in terms of millivolts.

The effect of the adaptive filter on the X, Y and Z leads, taken at the peak of exercise, is illustrated in Figure 4-16, where the left-hand diagram represents the raw data, and the right, the filter data. From limited experience it appears that adaptive filters function very sim-

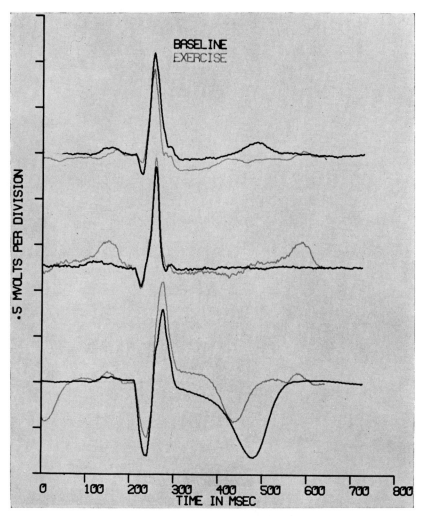

FIGURE 4-15. Baseline and peak exercise record (30-beat average) superimposed by digital plotter.

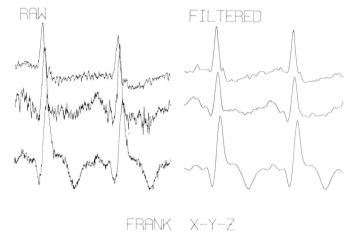

FIGURE 4-16. Raw data of patient with abnormal response during peak of exercise (*left*) processed through adaptive filter (*right*).

ilarly to lowpass filters. They automatically remove those frequency components from the signal which constitute the muscle tremor noise and they provide an optimal compromise on the basis of spectral analysis of noise and signal record.

POLAR COORDINATE DISPLAYS

In order to study quantitatively the instantaneous dipole vector position, the spherical angles are written as a function of time. The angles used to describe the spatial vector are seen in Figure 4-17. A sphere is projected into the chest with the vectors V_1 and V_2 to demonstrate the orientation of the coordinates. V_1 has an alpha value of $0°$ and a tilt value of $0°$. Alpha here corresponds to Einthoven's frontal plane angle. V_2 shows alpha at $+30°$ and a backward tilt of $+30°$. Alpha and tilt can also be understood as the longitude and latitude of a sphere which has the Z lead as the pole axis. The advantage of displaying spherical coordinates as a function of time over the loop display is that it combines the accurate time display of the scalar

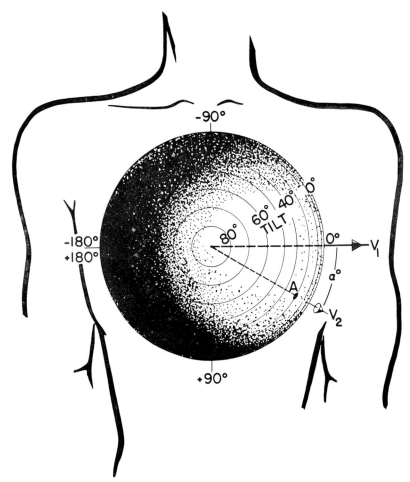

FIGURE 4-17. Orientation of heart vector within anatomical reference frame. Einthoven's angle alpha, the angle tilt, and the absolute vector magnitude are shown for two vectors. V_1 has $\alpha° = O°$, tilt $= O°$. V_2 has $\alpha° = +30°$, tilt $= +30°$ (posterior).

leads with the vectorial display of the Lissajous loop. Figures 4-18 and 4-19 are ST-T segment displays of alpha, tilt and spatial magnitude (SM) as a function of time. Since the ST-T segment is heart rate dependent, time normalization is necessary in order to arrive at comparable records of the rest and peak exercise periods. The program divides the ST-T segment into thirty equal parts. Figure 4-18 shows the record

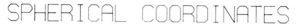

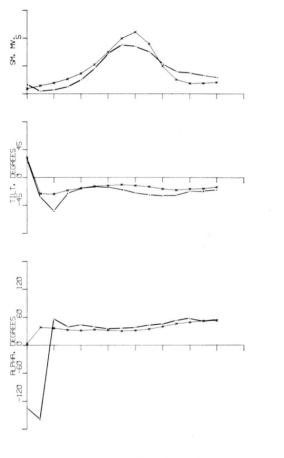

FIGURE 4-18. Spatial magnitude, tilt and alpha presented as a function of time. ST-T segment being time normalized, 30 averaged beats. This is the record of a normal individual.

SPHERICAL COORDINATES

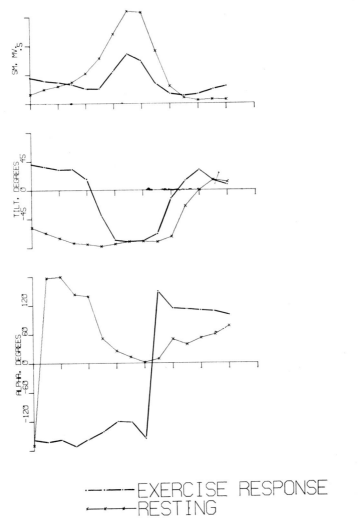

FIGURE 4-19. Same display of data as in Figure 4-18. Patient with abnormal response.

of the normal individual. The T wave at the time of maximal effort shows (a) a slight reduction in amplitude; (b) a slight vertical displacement of alpha, and (c) moderate anterior tilting. The abnormal response is shown in Figure 4-19. The T amplitude of the exercise record falls to 50 per cent of normal value, the ST segment shows an increase of more than 100 per cent of the resting value, and the ST and T segments demonstrate marked changes in alpha and in tilt.

A word of caution must be added to the spherical angle display. First of all, large angular changes can be produced by minute changes in the rectangular coordinates if both contributing coordinates have small values. It seems advisable to introduce threshold values into the program to avoid a meaningless display.

SUMMARY

Preliminary conclusions from our studies of stress test data are these:
1. With the use of small electrodes and miniaturized amplifiers in close proximity to the electrodes, excellent records were obtained even during the peak of exercise on the bicycle ergometer. Naturally these records had a large amount of muscle tremor, but they had little or no drift and, therefore, stayed within the assigned dynamic range of the magnetic tape recorder or the analog-to-digital (A-D) system.
2. Four kinds of digital data manipulation were used to improve the quality of the records.
   a. A notched digital filter for records containing 60 cycles.
   b. Lowpass digital filters equivalent to three-pole analog filters. These filters, although they severely disturb the QRS complex when inside the 30 and 20 cycle range, demonstrate the ST-T wave changes characteristic of ischemic changes.
   c. Adaptive filter techniques in the initial stage of developments. From limited experience it appears that adaptive filters function very similarly to lowpass filters.
   d. Averaging appears to be the method of choice if the signal is stable and the diagnostic changes are not lost. Averaging of 20 beats with heart rates in excess of 120 provides a window width of less than ten seconds. This should be a sufficiently small interval for most diagnostic procedures. The simultaneous dis-

plays of baseline and peak exercise records of X, Y and Z, as well as the time function values of the spherical angles, appear to be of great value for establishing diagnostic decision regions.

DISCUSSION

Dr. Schmitt: Dr. von der Groeben, you have said nothing about the aliasing interaction between your sample data and the digital filter. Now how do you escape that problem? I mean that the data you present to the system is sample data, isn't it?

Dr. von der Groeben: Right.

Dr. Schmitt: It is digitized at intervals.

Dr. von der Groeben: It comes in at 1 kc frequency or 1 msec intervals.

Dr. Schmitt: And it is then processed in a digital filter which must do it in quantized fashion.

Dr. von der Groeben: Right.

Dr. Schmitt: Therefore the aliasing phase relationship between the digital sampling and digital filter repetition rate will inevitably give a phase distortion? If you do it a dozen times you get a dozen different answers, not negligibly different. You take exactly the same data and present it to the same digital filter at microsecond shifting intervals you'll get different filter characteristics.

Dr. von der Groeben: The records which we have seen and which we have used have shown insignificant variation on repeat processing.

Dr. Schmitt: Not enough to bother you?

Dr. von der Groeben: Not enough to bother us in clinical interpretation.

Dr. Schmitt: This usually comes up sharply when someone talks about a one-cycle-wide filter, for example.

Dr. Weaver commented: Digital filtering is a well-founded and rigorous engineering discipline, and its results can be predicted with the same degree of accuracy as for analog filtering. However, it is possible to design digital filters much more accurately than analog filters, and digital filtering probably will become quite common in several branches of medical data processing.

Our sampling rate of 1 kc is well above the Nyquist sampling rate and no significant or even measurable aliasing is present. Careful measurements have shown that usually there is very little energy above 150 cps in an ECG. Nyquist's well-known spectrum sampling theorem shows, among other things, that there is no aliasing if the sampling rate is twice greater than the maximum frequency (the Nyquist sampling rate) of the energy that is present. So a sampling rate as low as 300 samples per second would be sufficient.

It is unclear to me what you mean by aliasing. The spectrum of a sampled signal is periodic with a period equal to the sampling frequency. The spectrum shape in each period is identical to the shape of the spectrum of the unsampled signal if the sampling rate is greater than the Nyquist rate. If the sampling rate is less the spectra in successive periods merge; and if the sampled signal is then filtered by a lowpass filter with a bandwidth equal to the sampling rate, the filtered spectrum will be similar to the unsampled spectrum with the ends folded back toward zero frequency. This is the condition that is commonly known as aliasing. It is impossible to reproduce faithfully the continuous (or unsampled) signal from the sampled signal if aliasing is present.

In our filters and in almost all digital filters each signal sample is entered into the filter and a new output is calculated, and there is no difference in the sampling rate and filter output rate. This has nothing to do with aliasing. There is a small but fixed time required for the computer to make the calculations, but this is easily calibrated out if the need arises. Dr. Schmitt apparently is assuming that a small shift in the phase of the sampler (the A to D converter) will cause large changes in the filter output. It is well known and quite easy to prove that this is not true when the sampling rate is greater than the Nyquist rate. An input sampling rate greater than the Nyquist rate guarantees that the *continuous* signal (e.g., the filtered ECG) obtained from the digital filter output is independent of the phase of the sampler. There will be no change in filter characteristics.

The final point you raise concerned signal and filter quantization. The theory of error due to quantization is well developed, and the distortion is exactly equivalent to that caused by addition of a small amount of white noise to the filter input. Error calculations were made and this distortion was found to be negligibly small with the quantization levels used. We feel that quantization distortion will rarely be significant in digital ECG processing systems.

5

Computer Quantitation of the ST Segment Response to Maximal Treadmill Exercise

Paul L. McHenry

THE SCHOOL OF Aerospace Medicine (SAM) is presently utilizing a totally computerized program for quantitation of the ST segment response to maximal treadmill exercise. The following is a description of our methods of data collection and analysis.

The importance of the slope as well as the depression of the ST segment is well recognized in the quantitation of postexercise electro-cardiographic responses. In designing our program we felt that computation of the slope of the ST segment might prove equally as important in defining early abnormalities during maximal or near-maximal treadmill exercise. Since even minor degrees of artifact or noise in the final averaged QRS-T complex can lead to a significant error in the slope determination of the ST segment, our methods of data collection have evolved after considerable efforts to obtain maximal noise reduction at its source.

The use of special electrodes designed and manufactured by the SAM Instrumentation Section has greatly enhanced our ability to obtain relatively noise free signals. These electrodes are shown in Figure 5-1. They are silver-silver chloride electrodes, 12 mm in diameter, encased in a lightweight plastic. Direct physical contact of the electrode with the skin is avoided by embedding the electrode within the plastic holder so as to maintain a constant 2 mm distance between the skin and the contact surface of the electrode. In this way electrical conduction is accomplished solely by the electrode paste. This type of electrode design is especially important in eliminating excessive baseline drift.

[61]

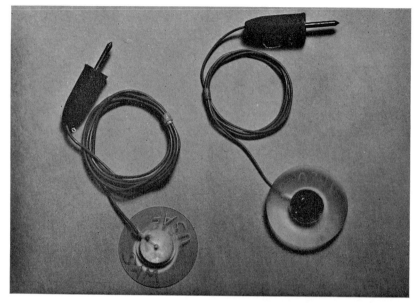

FIGURE 5-1. Silver-silver chloride electrodes used for data collection.

Prior to electrode placement the skin is carefully cleansed with alcohol and acetone and the superficial horny layer is removed by means of a high speed drill fitted with a small, oval dental burr. This procedure has proven superior to manual techniques of skin preparation and it is painless when care is taken to remove only the very superficial layer. For electrode placement we have found that optimal noise reduction can be obtained by placing the X axis electrodes in a right and left chest V5 position. This electrode placement avoids large muscle masses which can be a source of considerable noise and artifact. Data collected simultaneously from this electrode placement and a standard V_5 lead postexercise have revealed no significant discrepancies in the ST segment response.

Before each recording the resistance across the electrodes, the wires and the skin contact points are carefully checked by means of a volt-ohm meter. The electrode position on the skin is firmly maintained by use of adhesive discs and the terminals of the ohm meter are connected to the two electrode wires. The electrode circuitry is deemed satisfactory only if the resistance is less than 1000 ohms.

21st Min.T.M.Exercise
Rate 200/min

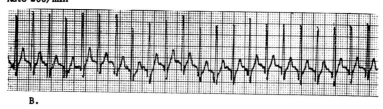

B.

16th Min.T.M.Exercise
Rate 192/min

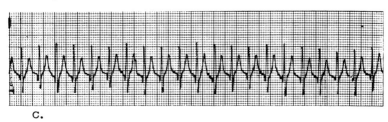

C.

20th Min.T.M.Exercise
Rate 196/min

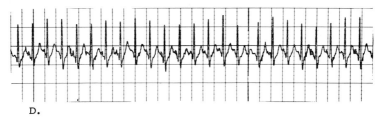

D.

16th Min.T.M.Exercise
Rate 188/min

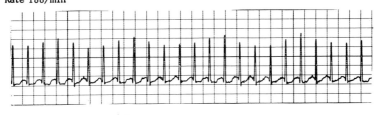

FIGURE 5-2. Electrocardiographic recordings collected during the last minute of treadmill exercise. The top two records are direct Sanborn write-outs. The bottom two are oscillographic write-outs reproduced from the magnetic tape at a paper speed of 20 mm per second.

Our treadmill program utilizes a constant speed of 3.3 mph and a 1 per cent (2/3 degree) elevation per minute. The majority of subjects reach maximal exercise levels, as determined by oxygen consumption, after a period of fifteen to twenty minutes. This program has considerable advantage in terms of noise reduction over programs which increment the treadmill speed, since sudden increments in muscular and mechanical activity are avoided.

The output from the preamplifier of a Sanborn 964 electrocardiograph is recorded on a single track of magnetic tape by means of an Ampex FR-1300 frequency modulation analog data recorder. Figure 5-2 represents typical data obtained with this approach.

Computer quantitation of the taped data involves the generation of square wave triggers corresponding to the negative slope of the R waves and analog to digital (A/D) conversion. This is accomplished by feeding the data in parallel into a TR-20 Analog Computer (Electronics Associates, Inc.) and a CSC Micro-Sadic A/D Converter (Consolidated Systems, Corp.). A trigger is generated for one hun-

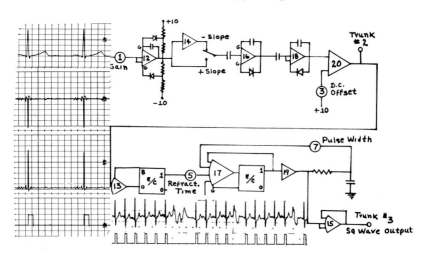

FIGURE 5-3. Block diagram of the analog computer circuit. The pen records to the left represent from top to bottom (1) the magnetic tape ECG input; (2) the negative time derivative input into amplifier 20; (3) the offset and inverted time derivative used to generate the trigger pulse in the comparator trigger (E/C), and (4) the trigger pulse generated at the time the magnitude of the time derivative exceeds the zero baseline.

The ECG recording at the bottom is explained in the text.

dred consecutive QRS complexes from each of several preselected time intervals before, during and after exercise. These intervals are identified on the magnetic tape by means of a time code. Figure 5-3 is a block diagram of the analog computer circuit. The output from amplifier 14, an upright QRS complex, is passed through bandpass filters set at a frequency-amplitude range best suited for the down slope of the R wave in amplifiers 16 and 18. The time derivative of the QRS is then formed and the positive derivative of the R is clipped off by means of diodes. The resultant negative derivative is passed into amplifier 20 where it is inverted and the baseline is biased down to a negative value. As this point the derivative can be projected upon an oscilloscope (Trunk #2) and its magnitude adjusted by means of Gain 1. Only derivatives with magnitudes exceeding the zero baseline will result in a square wave being generated by the comparator trigger (EC). Proper adjustment at this stage can prevent triggering on any excessive baseline noise as well as on the majority of premature ventricular contractions. Triggering on premature ventricular contractions is further eliminated by means of a refractory time programmed into the circuit during which time no additional trigger pulses can be generated (amplifiers 17 and 19). The ECG strip at the bottom of the circuit diagram illustrates this selective rejection of premature or ectopic ventricular complexes by the trigger generator.

The parallel inputs into the A/D converter are digitized at a rate of 500 samples per channel per second for computer analysis. A series of one hundred 1 mv standardization waves are also digitized.

Computer averages of the digitized data of one hundred complexes from the resting and maximal exercise ECG of fifty subjects were analyzed to select intervals in the PQ and ST segment for programmed identification and quantitation. The addresses corresponding to the first positive derivative of the QRS and the peak of the R wave were found to maintain the most consistent time relationships to the terminal PQ and the initial ST segments respectively (Fig. 5-4). Starting at a point 30 msec before the first positive derivative of the QRS, a 10 msec interval within the terminal portion of the PQ segment could be identified in every instance without overlapping into the Q wave. A point 50 msec from the peak of the R wave fell within the first 10 msec of the ST segment in the majority of subjects. A 10 msec interval

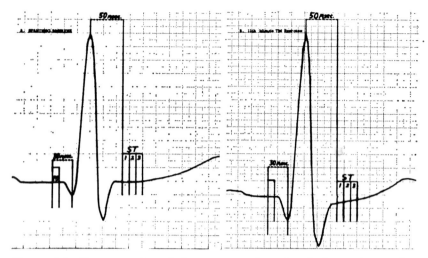

FIGURE 5-4. Computer plots of the averages of one-hundred complexes taken from the baseline and the last minute of exercise. The location of the PQ segment and the ST segments 1, 2 and 3 in relation to the QRS are illustrated.

starting at this point was designated as ST_1 for quantitation of ST depression. In the occasional subject with a minor delay in terminal intraventricular conduction, a second 10 msec interval (ST_2) starting at 60 msec after the R peak provided a comparable area in the ST segment for quantitation (Fig. 5-5). This latter interval along with a third 10 msec interval ST_3 were chosen for the ST segment slope determination.

The digital computer, a Philco 2000, is programmed to locate the square wave and find the corresponding point in time on the negative side of the R wave. Starting at 150 msec before this trigger point, the computer stores the voltages of 200 consecutive addresses over a 400 msec period for each QRS-T complex. Corresponding addresses for four groups of twenty-five complexes are then averaged using every fourth QRS-T from a series of one hundred. The four groups of twenty-five complexes are used to determine the statistical variability of the data.

On each group of twenty-five averaged complexes the fifteenth address before the first positive derivative of the QRS is located, and the mean voltage of the first five addresses beyond this point is computed for the PQ segment. The address 50 msec beyond the R peak

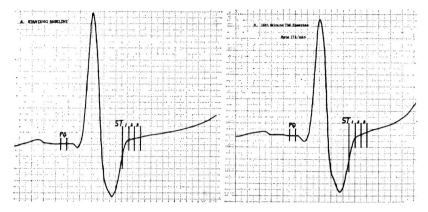

FIGURE 5-5. Computer plots of the averages of one-hundred complexes in a subject with a terminal delay in intraventricular conduction. ST_2 occupies a comparable area in the ST segment to ST_1 in the subject with normal intraventricular conduction (Fig. 5-4).

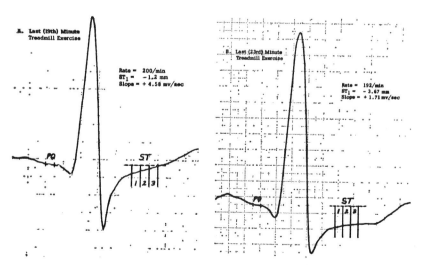

FIGURE 5-6. Computer plots of the averages of one-hundred complexes from the last minute of exercise for two subjects. The computed ST_1 depression and ST slope values are also listed. *A* represents data from a normal subject and *B* the data from a subject with arteriosclerotic heart disease.

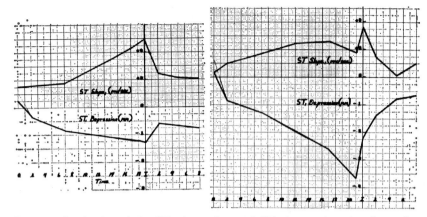

FIGURE 5-7. A plot of the ST_1 depression and ST slope values for the entire exercise and postexercise periods for the two subjects in Figure 5-6. Time is on the abscissa in minutes, ST depression in mm and ST slope in mv/sec is on the ordinate.

is then located and a mean voltage for each of two consecutive 10 msec intervals, ST_1 and ST_2, is computed. ST segment depression relative to the PQ segment is then computed in millivolts as follows:

$$ST \text{ depression} = \frac{\text{mean ST - mean PQ}}{\text{mean millivolt calibration}}$$

The ten address voltages of the ST_2-ST_3 segments are then combined to compute the slope by means of a least squares fit. A computer plot of the average of one hundred complexes from the last minute of exercise is shown for two subjects in Figure 5-6. The ST_1 segment depression and the ST slope computed for the last minute are also listed. A linear plot of the ST_1 depression and the ST slope for the entire exercise period and the postexercise period is shown for these same two subjects in Figure 5-7.

Table 5-I shows the final computer printout which gives the computed ST depression and slope for each time interval. These values represent the means of the four groups of twenty-five complexes for the same interval. The standard error or a measure of deviation about the mean of the four groups is also given.

A graph giving the ST_1 depression and ST slope values for the last minute of exercise on the first forty-eight subjects studied by this

TABLE 5-I

COMPUTER PRINTOUT OF THE ST DEPRESSION AND ST SLOPE VALUES FOR EACH SELECTED
TIME INTERVAL BEFORE, DURING AND AFTER EXERCISE

Data recorded prior to exercise includes a reclining and a standing baseline. Immediate postexercise data is recorded with the subject standing, while the 2, 5 and 7 minute postexercise periods are recorded with the subject reclining.

Period	Lead	Heart Rate	ST1		ST2		Slope (mv/sec)	
			Deprs.	St. Err.	Deprs.	St. Err.	Slope	St. Err.
Recline	X	61.	0.01198	0.00225	0.03717	0.00108	2.31721	0.10732
Baseline	X	87.	0.04266	0.00310	0.06974	0.00231	2.47576	0.18567
2- 3	X	116.	—0.05432	0.00592	—0.01101	0.00472	2.94271	0.42633
7- 8	X	140.	—0.09672	0.00699	—0.05206	0.00611	2.52221	0.35853
12-13	X	163.	—0.12661	0.00232	—0.07857	0.00370	3.15694	0.62225
17-18	X	184.	—0.13985	0.00185	—0.08697	0.00370	5.74454	0.35095
Last Min.	X	197.	—0.16140	0.00493	—0.08667	0.00697	6.44463	0.31466
Immediate	X	190.	—0.07944	0.01076	0.04226	0.00998	7.82755	0.46550
2 min.	X	116.	—0.09597	0.00275	—0.04266	0.00262	2.70945	0.21103
5 min.	X	116.	—0.09096	0.04255	—0.06161	0.03368	2.86485	1.71810
7 min.	X	104.	—0.05556	0.01208	—0.03856	0.00386	1.73931	0.17866

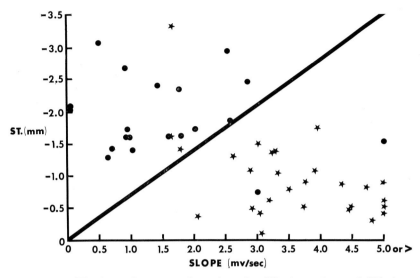

Figure 5-8. The last minute exercise values for ST$_1$ depression and ST slope are plotted for forty-eight subjects with ST depression on the ordinate and ST slope on the abscissa. The dots represent subjects with clinically suspected cardiac disease, the stars, subjects with no clinical evidence of cardiac disease (*see text*).

method is shown in Figure 5-8. The dots represent flying personnel who underwent evaluation at the School of Aerospace Medicine primarily to determine their cardiovascular status. The majority of these were asymptomatic individuals who were found to have labile nonspecific T wave changes or borderline responses to the double Masters test during routine annual electrocardiographic testing. Their average age was forty-three years. The subjects represented by the stars were mostly asymptomatic individuals being evaluated for some special Air Force project. Their average age was thirty-six years.

As can be noted, a clear separation of these two groups is obtained using both ST segment and slope values while considerably more overlap exists if only one of these parameters is used. Of those subjects with suspected cardiac disease, a final clinical diagnosis of arteriosclerotic heart disease was made in nine. All of these subjects fall above the line dividing the graph in Figure 5-8. This line has been drawn on the graph only as a visual aid and as such has no statistical derivation. In those subjects with a diagnosis of arteriosclerotic heart disease, the ST segment response to treadmill exercise was not used to arrive at this diagnosis.

Three of the apparently normal subjects were found to have values more closely approximating those in the suspect group. Likewise, several subjects in the suspect group in whom no definite clinical diagnosis of heart disease could be made had responses which more closely grouped them with the clinically abnormal subjects.

Only time and follow-up evaluation will determine if this apparent greater separation of groups utilizing ST slope as well as ST depression turns out to have a predictive value in detecting early coronary artery disease.

DISCUSSION

Dr. Schmitt: Thank you very much Dr. McHenry. Does anyone have an immediate question or two? I was going to ask Mr. Berson if he has ever done these calculations on the capacitant integration slopes in the ST time region? Do you remember how those numbers compare with the slopes that Dr. McHenry is reporting here? It is my memory that these are smaller but not a different order of magnitude. I was wondering whether you would consider those as a partial cause of the slope.

In other words, Dr. McHenry, you are undoubtedly using amplifiers that are as nonresponsive at low frequencies as is decent for exercise work, and there Mr. Berson has shown to demonstrate a slope shift in this region, an electrogenic slope. Now I wonder how much a part of your response was that as against the honest physiological part, and was this a complicating factor or not?

It would be an easy thing to check and to see. I suspect that it would be at most about 10 per cent of the amplitude and consequently not important, but it is certainly something worth checking.

Dr. Blackburn: I want to confirm Dr. McHenry's success in use of a dental drill in the skin preparation. It is faster and more effective in reducing skin impedance and less painful than rubbing or scratching the skin. The tiny concavity produced on removing the horny skin layer requires a week or so to heal, however, and frequent repetitive tests would give a problem.

I also want to emphasize the danger, both in lesser reliability of point recognition and in diagnostic interpretation, from using ST-T sampling points at fixed intervals from a fiducial point in the QRS, and especially in single lead analysis. Should we not be working toward identification and sampling of points on a spatial magnitude curve and points in the ST-T region chosen in relation to length of the cardiac cycle rather than tied by a fixed interval to QRS?

6

Noise Reduction and Representative Complex Selection in the Computer Analyzed Exercise Electrocardiogram

Larry K. Jackson, Roger Simmons, Robert C. Leinbach,
Stuart W. Rosner, Andrew J. Presto, Anna Lea Weihrer
and Cesar A. Caceres

The electrocardiographic response of the heart to stress induced by exercise has been studied as a tool for identifying individuals at greater risk of developing clinical coronary heart disease (1,2) as well as those coronary patients with greater risk of early death (3). While questions regarding the clinical value of this tool have been raised (4), innovations in stress techniques, lead systems and instrumentation promise to increase the sensitivity and specificity of exercise electrocardiography. With these innovations, new problems are created by numerous differences among investigative groups in test techniques and instrumentation. Answers to important epidemiologic questions are impeded by difficulties in comparing experiences among investigative groups.

One problem contributing to this confusion is the presence of wide differences both among and within groups in the interpretation of the exercise electrocardiogram (EECG), as was recently demonstrated by Blackburn and others (5). It was against this background that our group became interested in the development of a digital computer program to analyze and interpret the EECG. It was hoped that by providing a method for standardized and objective interpretation, the value of the tool both for epidemiologic and clinical use might be enhanced. An anticipated large-scale exercise intervention study employing the EECG, sponsored by the U.S. Public Health Service Heart Disease Control Program, provided impetus to this work.

[73]

It is the purpose of this paper to describe a first-generation computer program for analyzing the EECG that is experimentally operational now, give some data on its accuracy, and to discuss means we are developing to deal with noise, a major problem area in the analysis of signals recorded under stress.

The system which has been described in detail in earlier publications (6,7) employs a data acquisition console equipped with a quarter-inch magnetic tape recorder and an encoder, an analog tape transport with a Krohn-Hite variable bandpass filter and various switches necessary to play analog data into the computer, a CDC 160-A computer, one tape unit, and a line printer. Although this system can be used for on-line real-time analysis, off-line batch-type processing has proved most practical.

The program is capable of analyzing any lead or series of non-simultaneous leads and by preceding the EECG signal with a recorded code, it will ultimately be able to print out the exercise regimen of the particular type of exercise test being recorded. Although initial efforts have been to identify patterns of ECG change presently accorded clinical significance, further development will in addition provide a means of identifying new perhaps more discriminating diagnostic items in the signal and give a statistical interpretation of ECG changes. Figure 6-1 illustrates a sample of the present printout format. Amplitudes and durations of major waveforms are given, along with heart rate, amplitude values along the PPR and STT segments, segments, and elapsed time from the beginning of the test for each set of measurements. With a more recent development, a descriptive statement is printed out when the above data describes either an ischemic or junctional ST depression. Modifications in the present printout format in Figure 6-1 are being studied. In order to make the program general purpose, two types of printout are contemplated; one detailed enough to meet research needs and a more concise form for clinical use. Two versions under consideration are pictured in Figures 6-2 and 6-3.

Figure 6-2 illustrates a page from the research form, which represents a detailed analysis of eighteen seconds of ECG data. By means of the encoder on the data acquisition console, a limited amount of clinical information along with a patient identification number is

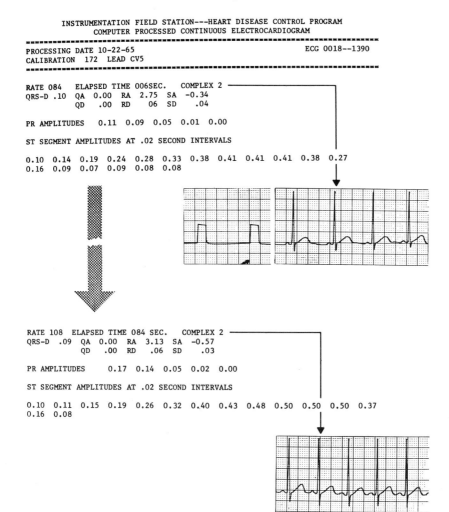

INSTRUMENTATION FIELD STATION---HEART DISEASE CONTROL PROGRAM
COMPUTER PROCESSED CONTINUOUS ELECTROCARDIOGRAM

PROCESSING DATE 10-22-65   ECG 0018--1390
CALIBRATION 172 LEAD CV5

RATE 084   ELAPSED TIME 006SEC.   COMPLEX 2
QRS-D .10   QA 0.00 RA 2.75 SA -0.34
            QD   .00 RD   06 SD   .04

PR AMPLITUDES   0.11 0.09 0.05 0.01 0.00

ST SEGMENT AMPLITUDES AT .02 SECOND INTERVALS

0.10 0.14 0.19 0.24 0.28 0.33 0.38 0.41 0.41 0.41 0.38 0.27
0.16 0.09 0.07 0.09 0.08 0.08

RATE 108 ELAPSED TIME 084 SEC.   COMPLEX 2
QRS-D .09 QA 0.00 RA 3.13 SA -0.57
            QD   .00 RD   .06 SD   .03

PR AMPLITUDES   0.17 0.14 0.05 0.02 0.00

ST SEGMENT AMPLITUDES AT .02 SECOND INTERVALS

0.10 0.11 0.15 0.19 0.26 0.32 0.40 0.43 0.48 0.50 0.50 0.50 0.37
0.16 0.08

FIGURE 6-1. Sample of current printout format.

recorded in coded form preceding the ECG data and appears at the beginning of the printout. Also recorded in this manner is a code which will identify the type of exercise test being recorded, the leads used, and the lead sequence. As shown in Figure 6-2, the current test phase appears above the ECG data along with the work load, expressed, in the case of treadmill tests, as treadmill speed and

PAT NO. 0067 HT 70 WT 180 AGE 39 SEX M MEDS ANTIHYPERTEN, THIAZ

CLINICAL DX HEART DIS SUSPECTED, CLASS UNKNOWN, CHRON LUNG DIS BP H

GRADED TREADMILL TEST CALIB 0.90 CM/MV TAPE E018 PROC DATE 10-23-66

TEST PHASE 4 - 3 MPH. 7% GRADE

	ELPSD TIME 081(MIN)				ELPSD TIME 082(MIN)				ELPSD TIME 083(MIN)			
	Val	Chng 1	Chng 2	Slp	Val	Chng 1	Chng 2	Slp	Val	Chng 1	Chng 2	Slp
PO1	.00	-.10	.00	00	.02	-.08	.02	00	-.02	-.12	-.04	00
PA	.13	-.02	.00	00	.09	-.06	-.04	00	.11	-.04	.02	00
PD	.10	.02	.00	00	.10	.02	.00	00	.10	.02	.00	00
P'A	.00	.00	.00	00	.00	.00	.00	00	.00	.00	.00	00
P'D	.00	.00	.00	00	.00	.00	.00	00	.00	.00	.00	00
PR	.16	.01	.00	00	.17	.02	.01	00	.16	.01	-.01	00
PR/R-R	.26	.01	.00	00	.27	.02	.01	00	.24	-.01	-.03	00
QA	.00	.00	.00	00	.00	.00	.00	00	.00	.00	.00	00
QD	.00	.00	.00	00	.00	.00	.00	00	.00	.00	.00	00
QA/RA	.00	.00	.00	00	.00	.00	.00	00	.00	.00	.00	00
RA	.63	-.10	.00	00	.60	-.13	-.03	00	.64	-.09	.04	00
RD	.03	-.01	.00	00	.03	-.01	.00	00	.03	-.01	.00	00
RAR	.10	-.05	.00	00	.10	-.05	.00	00	.10	-.05	.00	00
SA	1.00	.50	.00	00	1.01	.51	.01	00	.98	.48	-.03	00
SD	.05	.00	.00	00	.05	.00	.00	00	.05	.00	.00	00
SAR	.25	.12	.00	00	.25	.12	.00	00	.25	.12	.00	00
QRSD	.08	-.01	.00	00	.08	-.01	.00	00	.08	-.01	.00	00
STT0	-.30	-.28	.00	45	-.29	-.27	.01	43	-.23	-.21	.06	45
STT1	-.28	-.26	.00	17	-.23	-.21	.05	22	-.23	-.21	.00	00
STT2	-.27	-.22	.00	11	-.25	-.20	.02	-11	-.23	-.18	.02	00
STT3	-.26	-.21	.00	22	-.25	-.20	.01	11	-.23	-.18	.02	00
STT4	-.23	-.21	.00	56	-.23	-.21	.00	48	-.23	-.21	.00	62
STT5	-.11	-.21	.00	74	-.14	-.24	-.03	71	-.04	-.14	.10	77
STT6	.13	-.12	.00	77	.06	-.19	-.07	77	.19	-.06	.13	76
STT7	.31	-.07	.00	50	.28	-.10	-.03	66	.35	-.03	.07	42
STT8	.25	-.15	.00	-11	.31	-.09	.06	-48	.28	-.12	-.03	-65
STT9	.11	-.21	.00	-64	.17	-.05	.06	-65	.14	-.18	-.03	-64
STT10	.05	-.15	.00	-35	.10	-.10	.05	-50	.08	-.12	-.02	-39
STT11	.04	-.16	.00	00	.05	-.15	.01	-27	.06	-.14	.01	-11
STT12	.05	-.11	.00	-06	.05	-.11	.00	00	.06	-.10	.01	00
STT13	.03	-.13	.00	-11	.05	-.11	.02	-06	.06	-.10	.01	-06
STT14	.03	-.08	.00	-11	.04	-.07	.01	-11	.05	-.06	.01	-11
STT15	.01	-.07	.00	-11	.03	-.05	.02	-17	.04	-.04	.01	-17
STT16	.01	-.04	.00	00	.01	-.04	.00	-11	.02	-.03	.01	-11
JTD	.20	.00	.00	00	.22	.02	.02	00	.20	.00	-.02	00
JTD/R-R	.33	-.01	.00	00	.36	-.02	.03	00	.34	.00	-.02	00
QTD	.28	-.01	.00	00	.30	.01	.02	00	.28	-.01	-.02	00
QTD/R-R	.46	-.03	.00	00	.50	.01	.04	00	.47	-.02	-.02	00
UA	.05	.02	.00	00	.03	.00	-.02	00	.03	.00	.00	00
PO2	.00	-.05	.00	00	.02	-.03	.03	00	.00	-.05	-.02	00
R-R	.61	.02	.00	00	.60	.00	-.01	00	.59	.00	-.01	00
RATE	98	-03	00	00	100	-01	02	00	101	00	01	00
COMPLEX ANALYZED	02				02				03			
LEAD	CV5				CV5				CV5			
NOISE CODE(STT/PPR)	2/1				1/0				0/0			
PLOT NUMBER	2441				2442				2443			
DX CODE	J3C2				J2A1				I2B0			

FIGURE 6-2. Basic data sheet from proposed modification of printout format.

elevation. For each data block analyzed, the elapsed time between it and the beginning of exercise is given. Parameters are listed at the right. P01 and P02 are amplitude values at the onset of P waves on either end of the complex measured and are referenced to the QRS onset baseline. Amplitudes and durations of P, P′, Q, R, S and U waves are included. Units of measurement are seconds and millivolts. Durations of PR, JT and QT intervals are given, along with their rate-corrected values. R and S wave areas are given along with Q wave amplitude adjusted for R wave amplitude. The STT segment is represented by an amplitude at its onset and sixteen time-normalized amplitude values referenced to a QRS-QRS onset baseline. Four vertical columns contain measurements from one four-second time block of data. Column 1 lists the values of the various parameters measured from a single complex picked to represent the time block. Column 2 entitled Chng 1, lists the change in these parameters from pre-exercise resting values. Column 3 entitled Chng 2 lists the change in these parameters from the values of the preceding time block as an index of rate of change of parameters with exercise. Column 4 entitled slp lists slope values expressed in degrees for points on the STT segment. The complex analyzed, the lead being recorded, a code representing the quality of data in the STT and PPR segments, and a data storage or plot number is listed for each time block. The data in these four columns is interpreted, and a diagnostic code representing this interpretation appears below the data.

Figure 6-3 illustrates a more concise form with data from the entire test summarized on a single sheet. Clinical information coded into the record appears at the top. Test data is grouped into that reflecting heart rate response to the test and ECG response. An interpretation is given at the bottom of the page followed by a blank for the reviewing physician's signature. Data under the heart rate response section appears in columns according to the phase of the test in which it occurs. Phase length is given in minutes. Activity is described for each test phase. In the case of the graded treadmill test this consists of rest or treadmill work at certain speeds in miles per hour and treadmill elevation in percent grade. In the case of a bicycle test, activity would be expressed in KPM, and in step tests, in steps per minute. Maximal heart rate is given for the pre-exercise rest phase

MEDICAL SYSTEMS DEVELOPMENT LAB --- HEART DISEASE & STROKE CONTROL PROGRAM
COMPUTER PROCESSED EXERCISE ELECTROCARDIOGRAM
UNIVERSITY OF MINNESOTA

PAT NO. 0067 HT 70 WT 180 AGE 39 SEX M MEDS ANTIHYPERTEN, THIAZ

CLINICAL DX HEART DIS SUSPECTED, CLASS UNKNOWN, CHRON LUNG DIS   BP H

GRADED TREADMILL TEST   CALIB 0.90 **CM/MV** TAPE E018 PROC DATE 10-23-66

HEART RATE RESPONSE

TEST PHASE	0	1	2	3	4	5	6	7	8
PHASE LENGTH (MIN)		1	2	2	3	6			
ACTIVITY (MPH/GRADE)		REST 2/7		R 3/7		R 4/7		R 5/7	R
MAXIMAL HEART RATE		102	111		127				
MAX ACCEL (BEATS/MIN)			60		102				
ACCEL AT MAX HEART RATE (BEATS/MIN)			60		50				
MIN HEART RATE		90		94		98			
MAX DECEL (BEATS/MIN)				30		60			
HEART RATE TWO MIN POST EX						104			
HEART RATE FOUR MIN POST EX						100			
HEART RATE AT 85% OF PREDICTED MAX		162							
PREDICTED OXY CONSUMP (L/MIN)		1.2		2.0					
TREADMILL WORK CAPACITY 85%			NOT REACHED						

ECG RESPONSE

RESPONSE	PHASE	DURATION(MIN)	LEAD	PLOT NO.
0.1 MV J DEPRESSION	1	0.5	CV5	2367
TYPE B-2	2	0.3	CV5	2372
	3	1.4	CV5	2411
0.2 MV J DEPRESSION	3	1.0	CV5	2423
TYPE A-1	4	0.6	CV5	2431
0.3 MV J DEPRESSION	4	0.7	CV5	2440
TYPE C-2				
0.2 MV ISCHEMIC	4	2.0	CV5	2464
DEPRESSION TYPE B				
QT PROLONGATION	4	0.8	CV5	2474
TYPE B				

INTERPRETATION (MATTINGLY CRITERIA)
                2306 POSITIVE TEST _____ M.D.

FIGURE 6-3. Summary sheet from proposed modification of printout format.

and for each phase of exercise. Maximum acceleration of heart rate in beats per minute, to be used as an index of stress, is given for each phase of exercise. Acceleration at maximal heart rate in beats per minute for each exercise phase is given to indicate proximity to steady state conditions needed for valid ancillary measurements such as oxygen consumption. Minimum heart rate is given for each rest period. Cardiovascular function is further indexed by the maximum deceleration of heart rate during recovery in beats per minute and heart rate at two and four minutes post exercise. Heart rate at 85 per cent of predicted maximum is listed for the subject, in accordance with, the coded clinical information described above and Robinson's data (8). As an index of treadmill work, predicted oxygen consumption in liters per minute is listed for each phase of exercise. This data is from measurements made on normals at various treadmill settings (9), and is listed for the subject according to the exercise regimen coded into the record and the number of phases of this regimen he begins. Treadmill work capacity 85 is a gauge of cardiovascular function similar to the WL150 designed by Hellerstein (10). It is simply the predicted oxygen consumption data described above at 85 per cent of predicted maximal heart rate. Descriptive items, under ECG response include various types and magnitudes of STT change as well as some types of conduction delay and ectopic beats. Items reflecting STT change correspond to items in the Minnesota code (11) and to some additional items of experimental interest. The test phase in which each item occurs is given, along with the length of time this change persists, the lead in which it occurs, and the data storage or plot number for the last time block in each phase reflecting the change. These types of data display represent those under consideration and have not yet been incorporated into the program.

A simplified version of the program logic is presented in flow diagram form in Figure 6-4. In brief, data is input in four-second blocks after A-D conversion, and a derivative value is immediately computed for each digital amplitude value. The program orients itself by identifying locations of all QRS complexes in the data block. This is done by finding maximum negative slopes in the block. Arrhythmic areas are next identified by assessing R-R interval regularity. If nonarrhythmic areas can be found in the data block, QRS onsets and ends are identi-

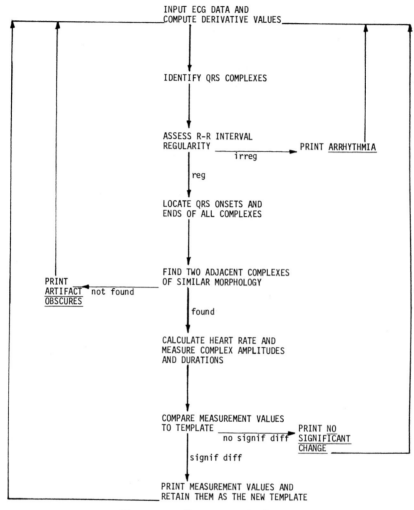

INPUT ECG DATA AND
COMPUTE DERIVATIVE VALUES

IDENTIFY QRS COMPLEXES

ASSESS R-R INTERVAL
REGULARITY _____ irreg → PRINT ARRHYTHMIA

reg

LOCATE QRS ONSETS AND
ENDS OF ALL COMPLEXES

FIND TWO ADJACENT COMPLEXES
PRINT   OF SIMILAR MORPHOLOGY
ARTIFACT ← not found
OBSCURES

found

CALCULATE HEART RATE AND
MEASURE COMPLEX AMPLITUDES
AND DURATIONS

COMPARE MEASUREMENT VALUES   PRINT NO
TO TEMPLATE _____ no signif diff → SIGNIFICANT
                                                                    CHANGE

signif diff

PRINT MEASUREMENT VALUES AND
RETAIN THEM AS THE NEW TEMPLATE

FIGURE 6-4. Program logic diagram.

fied for complexes in these nonarrhythmic areas. The next step involves
identifying a complex for measurement that is relatively undistorted
by baseline shift, random noise, or aberrant conduction. This is done
by finding two adjacent complexes with similar STT and PPR morphologies. When a suitable complex is identified, the previously mentioned amplitude and duration measurements are made. Before these
measurements are printed out, however, they are compared to meas-

TABLE 6-I

COMPARISON OF COMPUTER WITH MANUAL MEASUREMENTS
OF TWELVE ECG VARIABLES FROM 84 CARDIAC CYCLES

ECG Variable	Mean Difference	95% Confidence Limits
Q amp	0.010 mv	+.0004 to +.019
R amp	0.031 mv	—.011 to +.073*
S amp	0.010 mv	—.004 to +.024*
Q dur	0.003 sec.	+.002 to +.004
R dur	0.002 sec.	—.0009 to +.001*
S dur	0.008 sec.	+.003 to +.013
Amplitude at:		
ST onset	0.033 mv	—.003 to +.068*
40 msec after onset	0.034 mv	+.006 to +.062
80 msec after onset	0.016 mv	+.003 to +.029
160 msec after onset	0.025 mv	+.004 to +.047
PR Amplitude at:		
20 msec before QRS onset	0.004 mv	—.002 to +.009*
40 msec before QRS onset	0.017 mv	+.008 to +.026

*Comparisons are not significant when confidence limits include zero.

urements made on previous time blocks and printed out only if they represent a significant change. When nonarrhythmic and undistorted areas cannot be found in a time block, statements to these effects are printed in place of data. This cycle is repeated then with the input of another block of data. The program is described in greater detail in a previous publication (12).

The results of a small accuracy study are shown in Table 6-I. Eighty-four cardiac cycles were selected randomly from the ECGs of ten normal subjects exercising on a bicycle ergometer. Lead CV5 was used and recordings were continued during exercise. A comparison was made between computer and physician measurements of twelve ECG variables from enlarged ECG plots. Mean differences and 95 per cent confidence limits are listed. Several differences are statistically significant, particularly amplitudes at the beginning and end of the STT segment. The overall result is regarded as reasonable for a first-generation program, but indicates need for improvement. One of the problems contributing to errors is difficulty in locating accurate wave onsets and ends at high heart rates. This is correctable by having various program constants vary with R-R interval length. A far more challenging problem is that of noise related error, a discussion of which forms the body of this report.

TECHNIQUES FOR NOISE REDUCTION

Special problems exist in extracting meaningful data from the exercise or other monitoring ECGs which often contain considerable noise. These problems are accentuated by a trend in exercise electrocardiography toward recording continuously during the exercise period (13) and increasing the severity of exercise (14). Factors responsible for the noise thereby recorded have been discussed by Blackburn (15). Although some noise reduction may be accomplished with proper care in electrode application and grounding, extraction of representative data from the EECG remains an ever-present problem— both for the physician reader and for computer analysis programs.

Several points need emphasis before we discuss techniques for "extraction of meaningful data" or "noise reduction" in ECG processing. The electrocardiogram is at best only an index to the electrical activity of the heart. It is well known that our recording and display devices have a great and often poorly standardized influence on the representation of the heart's electrical activity. Furthermore, our understanding of the physiology involved in producing the signal is limited. Therefore, distinction between what is signal and what is noise is necessarily poor. The physician probably attempts to make the distinction by relating a particular segment of the cycle in question to corresponding segments in adjacent cycles. The relationships thus made are in turn related to his mental library of relationships compiled from previous experience in viewing other curves as well as to incomplete knowledge of the physiology responsible for the signal. Distinctions thus made are necessarily based on a consideration of probabilities and may not be accurate. It is important to realize these basic limitations in electrocardiography when one considers techniques for noise reduction or extraction of signals from noisy records.

For purposes of discussion, noise as previously described may be provisionally classified into three types. Figure 6-5 represents cyclic noise of 60 cps frequency, which is commonly encountered, but uncommonly of the amplitude shown in the Figure. Figures 6-6 and 6-7 represent random noise of differing average amplitude. Figure 6-8 also shows random noise but is included to illustrate baseline shift, a cyclic or noncyclic type of low-frequency noise.

There are many possible approaches to coping with the problem of

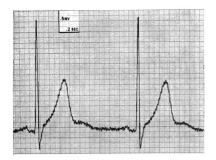

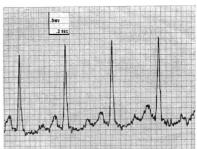

FIGURE 6-5. Example of 60 cps noise.

FIGURE 6-6. Example of low amplitude random noise.

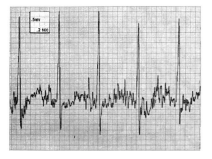

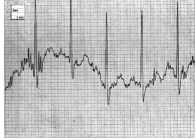

FIGURE 6-7. Example of high amplitude random noise.

FIGURE 6-8. Example of baseline shift with random noise.

noise. Since noise does not always fit a nice mathematical description, empirical techniques as well as mathematical ones may be applicable. We have been considering analog filtering, digital computer mathematical smoothing, analog averaging, digital computer averaging, and digital computer routines for noise identification and avoidance.

ANALOG FILTERING

Baseline shift can be eliminated by filtering out low frequencies in the area of 1 to 2 cps, but not without distorting data significantly, as was recently demonstrated by Berson and Pipberger (16). Certain ECG morphologies predispose to the creation of false ST depression when low frequencies above 0.05 cps are filtered out. Lowering the high-frequency limit of an analog filter can eliminate some random and cyclic noise from the PPR and STT segment regions. Although several

authors including Kerwin (17), Langner (18), Gilford (19) and
Dower (20) describe ECG distortion, at least below 75 cps, it is tempting to wonder if the practical advantages for exercise electrocardiography of filtering frequencies even down to 20 cps as suggested by
Freiman (13) might outweigh the ECG complex distortion tendencies
of the technique. Such a judgment can reasonably be made only when
weighed against the advantages and disadvantages of other noise
reduction techniques, as will be demonstrated later. An example of
the effect of analog filtering on the ECG is illustrated in Figures 6-9
through 6-12. These ECGs, as all of those in the following illustrations,
are computer plots from digital data.

ECG data distorted by cyclic noise is shown in Figure 6-9. This was
recorded on magnetic tape with our data acquisition console which
contains an amplifier with an effective frequency range of 0.05 to
160 cps. With the aid of a marker on the magnetic tape the same
data was played through a Krohn-Hite variable bandpass filter successively with the high-frequency filter limit at 80 cps (Fig. 6-10),

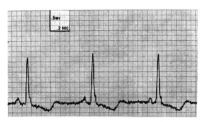

FIGURE 6-9. Noisy data recorded with
an effective system frequency range of
0.05 to 160 cps (3 db points).

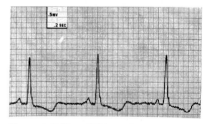

FIGURE 6-10. Noisy data recorded
with an effective system frequency
range of 0.05 to 80 cps (3 db points).

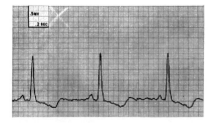

FIGURE 6-11. Noisy data recorded with
an effective system frequency range
of 0.05 to 40 cps (3 db points).

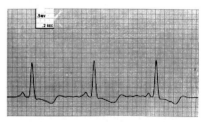

FIGURE 6-12. Noisy data recorded with
an effective system frequency range
of 0.05 to 20 cps (3 db points).

40 cps (Fig. 6-11), and 20 (Fig. 6-12). Low-frequency limit was kept at DC. It will be noted that there is progressive attenuation of the noise with a fairly smooth curve appearing at 20 cps (Fig. 6-12). There is concurrently some attenuation of both the P and R waves, removal of a real notch on the downslope of the R wave, but little change in the STT segment in this example. The advantages of this technique are that it is simple, requires no program development, and sacrifices no processing time. The disadvantage is that it is capable of data distortion and when applied to data must be applied indiscriminately whether noise is present or not. There is no opportunity to test data for the presence of noise to determine whether the filtering technique is applicable.

DIGITAL COMPUTER SMOOTHING

Several mathematical techniques for smoothing data are available. These have been used primarily in representing economic statistics, but two (the moving point average, MVAT, and the parabolic smoothing technique, PST, have been suggested for use in smoothing exercise ECG data by Rautaharju (21) among others. We have had experience with these and also a median point smoothing technique (MPT). The MVAT is a method by which a number of consecutive data points representing a segment of curve are averaged. This averaged value is used to replace the central data point in the segment of the curve. This process is repeated after the curve segment is moved forward one data point, resulting in an attenuation of small noise spikes. The MPT is similar except that the central data point is replaced by the median value of all the data points in the curve segment rather than the mean of these points. The PST involves fitting a segment of the curve to a parabola using a least squares method. The central value in this curve segment is replaced by the C value (constant) of the parabola chosen. The more time consuming process of finding other coefficients for the parabola in the curve fitting process is not necessary. As with the other techniques, this cycle is repeated as the curve segment moves forward through the ECG complex. Smoothing effect increases with the length of the curve segment or the number of points in the curve segments.

Figures 6-13 through 6-19 illustrate and compare the effects of these techniques on ECG data. A short segment of ECG data re-

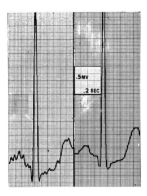

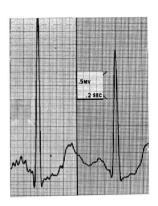

FIGURE 6-13. Smoothing with the 15-point median point technique (MPT).

FIGURE 6-14. Smoothing with the 15-point moving average technique (MVAT).

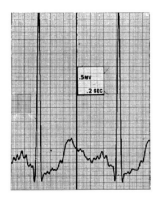

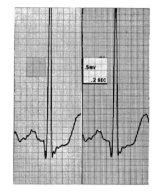

FIGURE 6-15. Smoothing with the 15-point parabolic smoothing technique (PST).

FIGURE 6-16. Smoothing with the 9-point moving average technique (MVAT).

corded in digital form on magnetic tape was subjected to the smoothing techniques mentioned. A complex from this segment of ECG before it was smoothed is shown on the left in Figures 6-13, 6-14 and 6-15. In Figure 6-13 the same complex smoothed with the 15-point MPT is shown on the right. Since the A-D conversion rate is 500 samples per second, making data points 0.002 seconds apart, this means that a single data point is smoothed or corrected by replacement with the median value of the 14 surrounding points, representing a segment of ECG curve 0.030 seconds in length. In Figure 6-14 the

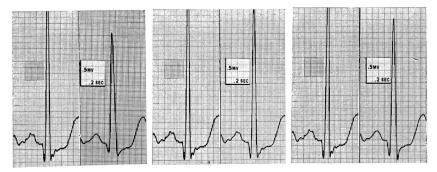

FIGURE 6-17. (*left*) Smoothing with the 15-point moving average technique (MVAT).

FIGURE 6-18. (*middle*) Smoothing with the 15-point parabolic smoothing technique (PST).

FIGURE 6-19. (*right*) Smoothing with the 27-point parabolic smoothing technique (PST).

15-point MVAT and in Figure 6-15 the 15-point PST modify the same complex. The gross distortion of the complex by the MPT (Fig. 6-13) excludes it from further consideration. Smoothing effect is noted with the MVAT (Fig. 6-14), and although not totally clear from these illustrations the points of P wave onset as well as QRS and ST onset are made more obvious.

Considerable attenuation of peaks and nadirs of true components of the signal such as Q, R and S waves is a drawback of the technique. There is less distortion of the true components of the complex with the PST (Fig. 6-15), but also less smoothing effect as compared to the MVAT when the number of points used to smooth a single data point are equal. However, by varying the number of these points one can hope to find a method that reduces the data distortion and retains the noise reduction tendencies of these techniques as is illustrated in Figures 6-16 through 6-19. This series of illustrations has in common with the previous series the same unsmoothed complex on the left compared to its smoothed form on the right. In Figure 6-16, in an attempt to see if the data distortion tendencies of the MVAT can be reduced, the number of points used (which determines degree of smoothing effect) is decreased from 15 to 9. This indeed reduces data distortion but reduces smoothing effect as well. Figure 6-17 shows smoothing effect but also distortion effect increased by increas-

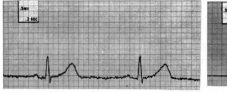

FIGURE 6-20. Noisy data recorded with an effective system frequency range of 0.05 to 160 cps (3 db points).

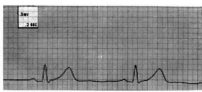

FIGURE 6-23. Noisy data recorded with with an effective system frequency range of 0.05 to 20 cps (3 db points).

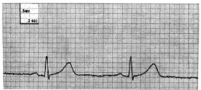

FIGURE 6-21. Noisy data recorded with an effective system frequency range of 0.05 to 80 cps (3 db points).

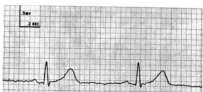

FIGURE 6-24. Noisy data recorded with an effective system frequency range of 0.05 to 160 cps (3 db points) and smoothed with a 15-point parabolic smoothing technique (PST).

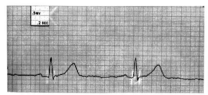

FIGURE 6-22. Noisy data recorded with an effective system frequency range of 0.05 to 40 cps (3 db points).

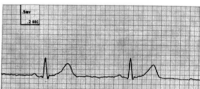

FIGURE 6-25. Noisy data recorded with an effective system frequency range of 0.05 to 160 cps (3 db points) and smoothed with a 21-point parabolic smoothing technique (PST).

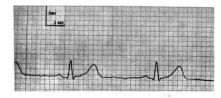

FIGURE 6-26. Noisy data recorded with an effective system frequency range of 0.05 to 160 cps (3 db points) and smoothed with a 27-point parabolic smoothing technique (PST).

ing the number of points to 15 for the MVAT. Figure 6-18 shows the 15-point-PST effect, and again it can be noted to have less smoothing effect than the MVAT when a comparable number of points is used, but the data distortion is also less. The inference from this series of figures is illustrated in Figure 6-19, which shows the effect of the PST when the number of points used is increased to 27. Here we see a good smoothing effect comparable to that obtained with the 15-point MVAT but with less data distortion effect. It will be noted that a peculiarity of both the MVAT and the PST is that while they attenuate Q and R waves they may increase the amplitude of S waves. In summary, then, of the three mathematical smoothing techniques, PST seems to give the best noise reduction effect with the least data distortion or the best signal-to-noise ratio, provided a large enough number of points is used.

PST is compared to analog filtering in Figures 6-20 through 6-26. Figure 6-20 pictures a computer plot of a block of ECG data played into the computer through a Krohn-Hite filter with the low-frequency limit at DC and the high-frequency limit set at 2000 cps. The frequency limits of this system are effectively 0.05 to 160 cps, as dictated by the amplifier of the data acquisition console. Figures 6-21, 6-22 and 6-23 represent plots of the same data played from analog tape through the same filter with the high-frequency limit moved down to 80 cps (Fig. 6-21), 40 cps (Fig. 6-22), and 20 cps (Fig. 6-23). Figures 6-24, 6-25 and 6-26 show plots of the same block of data after it has been processed from digital tape with the 15-point (Fig. 6-24), 21-point (Fig. 6-25), and 27-point (Fig. 6-26) PST. It can be seen by comparing Figure 6-23 (analog filter at 20 cps) and Figure 6-26 (27-point PST) that although data distortion is present with both techniques, when smoothing effect is similar, there is less data distortion with the 27-point PST. This is evidenced by preservation of the small Q wave, less widening of the R wave, less shortening of the ST segment, and less distortion of the S wave, as is shown in tabular form in Table 6-II.

Disadvantages of the mathematical smoothing techniques are that they increase processing time and are responsible for some data distortion. Their advantages are that they allow one to reclaim data that is otherwise not analyzable, data that may be occurring at a crucial

TABLE 6-II

COMPARISON OF ANALOG FILTERING AND PARABOLIC
SMOOTHING TECHNIQUES ON NOISY DATA

Parameters	Raw Data	Analog Filtering	Parabolic Smoothing
PA	.09	.05	.05
PD	.07	.07	.10
QA	.04	.00	.04
QD	.01	.00	.02
RA	.50	.40	.43
RD	.04	.06	.05
SA	.13	.03	.06
SD	.02	.03	.02
QRSD	.07	.09	.09
STO	.02	.03	.02
STD	.10	.06	.09
TA	.33	.33	.33
TD	.17	.20	.19
PR	.13	.12	.13
QT	.34	.35	.37

Parameters are measured in seconds and millivolts. Analog filtering is accomplished with a Krohn-Hite variable bandpass filter set at dc and 20 cps. Parabolic smoothing is accomplished by fitting data to 27-point parabolas.

point in the test, and data that can be judged by manual methods to contain significant diagnostic information. Data distortion and processing time problems can be greatly minimized by employing the smoothing technique discriminatingly to noisy data that has been detected, typed and located by a noise test. We can thus avoid processing the QRS complex, an area relatively infrequently distorted by noise, most apt to be distorted by the smoothing technique, and long enough to contribute significantly to smoothing processing time. This flexibility is not possible with presently conceived analog methods such as analog filtering. The mathematical smoothing discussed here is best suited to smoothing relatively low amplitude random and cyclic noise with short cycle length. Noise with cycle length approximating the length of ECG segments and waves is smoothed relatively poorly with these mathematical techniques and is more amenable to other techniques to be discussed.

Since some data distortion by the smoothing technique is unavoidable, interpretation of the smoothed complex with present diagnostic criteria needs further study. However, at present, qualitative changes in the smoothed complex can be predicted, and with more experience it may be possible to predict these changes quantitatively with some degree of reliability so that diagnostic criteria may be corrected for smoothing effect. We are trying to obtain this type of data on a variety of different ECG morphologies. For the present, data that is analyzed only after smoothing will be so identified for the user.

ANALOG AVERAGING

Analog averaging has been used extensively by several groups. Its advantage is that it requires little increase in processing time and is less expensive than digital systems. It is effective in smoothing low-noise deflections with long cycle length since it smooths by relating a particular curve segment to corresponding segments in adjacent cycles rather than to surrounding points in the same cycle. Its disadvantages have been discussed by Rautaharju (22) and include difficulty in dealing with baseline shift and nonrandom noise, averaging of non-homogeneous transients and obscuring diagnostically important waveform change. Requirement for physician editing is a major disadvantage when automatic analysis of large amounts of data is contemplated.

DIGITAL COMPUTER AVERAGING

Digital computer averaging has an advantage over analog averaging in that it can be applied to data after it has been tested and found to be noisy. Complexes with large noise transients that would distort the averaged complex can be screened out. Also some of the baseline shift areas can be corrected by a linear correction technique, especially if used with a noise test routine. Its disadvantages are ones it shares with analog averaging and the considerable sacrifice in processing time. It also shares with the analog averaging technique an ability to deal with low noise deflections of long cycle length better than the mathematical smoothing techniques. We are developing a routine for complex averaging with the digital computer for experimental use.

DIGITAL COMPUTER PROGRAM ROUTINE FOR NOISE RECOGNITION AND AVOIDANCE

The ECG is a repetitive signal, although not strictly so; and although items of interest in the EECG may be transient changes in this signal, these changes must persist at least for several complexes to be reliably distinguishable from noise. These observations are the basis for a computer program routine for recognizing distorted complexes and excluding them from analysis. It is a type of noise test and is essentially logic that looks for a complex that has close agreement in morphology to an adjacent complex as determined by sampling both complexes at fixed intervals from fiducial points in each complex and determining agreement between amplitudes in each of these two cycles at each of these sampling points. Disagreement at any set of sampling points identifies one of these complexes as not representative of the time block. This routine, termed the Parallel Check, is detained in a previous publication (12). We have observed that noise complicating pattern recognition is usually of relatively low amplitude and often comes in transient bursts. Noisy time blocks at times contain good complexes undistorted by noise. The testing of data with this technique and the selection of a single undistorted complex for measurement seems to be the most valid way to represent the data in a time block. The problem is that there are at times no undistorted data to select. For this reason, modification of this technique and combination with one of the discussed noise reduction techniques in an analysis program routine seems necessary.

In summing up the problem of noise, varied types and magnitudes of noise may be encountered, and there are differences in the applicability of various techniques for dealing with noise which depend on its type and magnitude. One can guess that the cardiologist himself unconsciously employs differing mental mechanisms for extracting data when interpreting ECGs that contain noise or exhibit much beat-to-beat morphologic variation, mechanisms which probably vary according to the type and magnitude of noise.

In summing up early experience with some of these techniques, it appears that (a) analog filtering is inferior to some of the mathematical smoothing methods in improving the signal-to-noise ratio; (b) of three mathematical smoothing techniques tested, the PST gives the best improvement in signal-to-noise ratio; (c) ECG complex averaging methods work better than mathematical smoothing when noise deflections are of cycle length approximating that of the ECG segment or wave it distorts; (d) routines for testing data and avoiding noise are most valid where applicable, and finally (e) more quantitative data gauging signal-to-noise ratio effects of these techniques is necessary. On the basis of these impressions, an approach to dealing with the problem of noise in EECG signal processing has been outlined in the form of a program routine which is being tested and which is detailed below.

NOISE REDUCTION AND REPRESENTATIVE COMPLEX SELECTION ROUTINE

This routine is applied to each four-second time block of data analyzed, begins with data input, and ends with the selection of a single representative complex from the time block for measurement. Its purpose is to test the data block for noise content and type, select the most representative complex in the block for measurement, and to identify the quality of the complex analyzed. On the basis of the noise test or representability assessment, a time block or segments of a time block are either (a) excluded entirely from analysis; (b) analyzed after mathematical smoothing; (c) analyzed after complex averaging; (d) analyzed without noise reduction, or (e) analyzed with or without noise reduction with certain of the less important parameters of the complex going unmeasured. In brief, all five are accomplished by assessing agreement between up to thirty-one measured characteristics of a complex and standards for these measurements for the time block and tagging each complex with a grade label reflecting its representability of the time block. This routine is shown in diagrammatic form in Figures 6-27 through 6-30 and outlined in stepwise form below.

Step 1—Defective Data Check

This step is designed to identify the absence of ECG signal or the presence of grossly distorted data. When a time block fails this check the statement, *Defective Data,* is printed out.

Step 2—Arrhythmia Check

This step is designed to identify the presence of arrhythmic complexes and to exclude them from further analysis. All nonarrhythmic complexes are tagged with a grade label A. If there are two adjacent A complexes in a time block it passes this check. When the check is failed, the time block is not further analyzed and the statement,

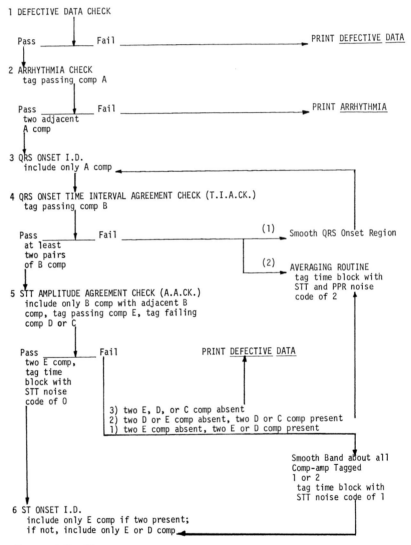

FIGURE 6-27. Noise reduction and representative complex selection routine.

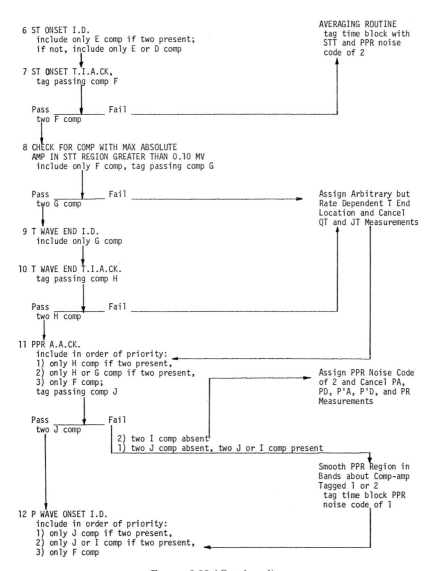

6 ST ONSET I.D.
   include only E comp if two present;
   if not, include only E or D comp

AVERAGING ROUTINE
   tag time block with
   STT and PPR noise
   code of 2

7 ST ONSET T.I.A.CK,
   tag passing comp F

Pass _____ Fail
 two F comp

8 CHECK FOR COMP WITH MAX ABSOLUTE
AMP IN STT REGION GREATER THAN 0.10 MV
   include only F comp, tag passing comp G

Pass _____ Fail
 two G comp

Assign Arbitrary but
Rate Dependent T End
Location and Cancel
QT and JT Measurements

9 T WAVE END I.D.
   include only G comp

10 T WAVE END T.I.A.CK.
   tag passing comp H

Pass _____ Fail
 two H comp

11 PPR A.A.CK.
   include in order of priority:
   1) only H comp if two present,
   2) only H or G comp if two present,
   3) only F comp;
   tag passing comp J

Assign PPR Noise Code
of 2 and Cancel PA,
PD, P'A, P'D, and PR
Measurements

Pass _____ Fail
 two J comp

   2) two I comp absent
   1) two J comp absent, two J or I comp present

Smooth PPR Region in
Bands about Comp-amp
Tagged 1 or 2
   tag time block PPR
   noise code of 1

12 P WAVE ONSET I.D.
   include in order of priority:
   1) only J comp if two present,
   2) only J or I comp if two present,
   3) only F comp

FIGURE 6-28 (*Continued*).

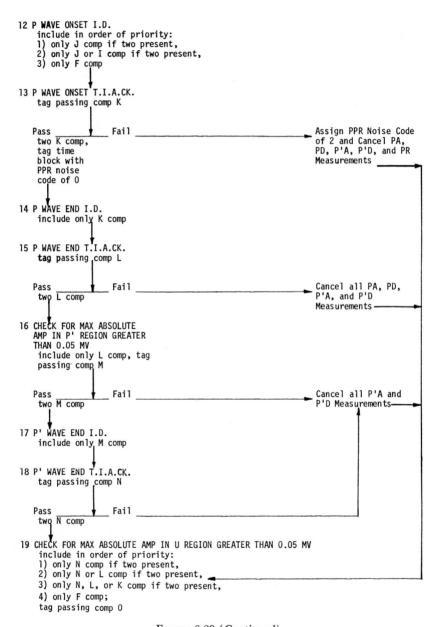

12 P WAVE ONSET I.D.
   include in order of priority:
   1) only J comp if two present,
   2) only J or I comp if two present,
   3) only F comp

13 P WAVE ONSET T.I.A.CK.
   tag passing comp K

   Pass _____ Fail _____ Assign PPR Noise Code
   two K̄ comp,   of 2 and Cancel PA,
   tag time   PD, P'A, P'D, and PR
   block with   Measurements
   PPR noise
   code of 0

14 P WAVE END I.D.
   include only K comp

15 P WAVE END T.I.A.CK.
   tag passing comp L

   Pass _____ Fail _____ Cancel all PA, PD,
   two L̄ comp   P'A, and P'D
                                                               Measurements

16 CHECK FOR MAX ABSOLUTE
   AMP IN P' REGION GREATER
   THAN 0.05 MV
   include only L comp, tag
   passing comp M

   Pass _____ Fail _____ Cancel all P'A and
   two M̄ comp   P'D Measurements

17 P' WAVE END I.D.
   include only M comp

18 P' WAVE END T.I.A.CK.
   tag passing comp N

   Pass _____ Fail
   two N̄ comp

19 CHECK FOR MAX ABSOLUTE AMP IN U REGION GREATER THAN 0.05 MV
   include in order of priority:
   1) only N comp if two present,
   2) only N or L comp if two present,
   3) only N, L, or K comp if two present,
   4) only F comp;
   tag passing comp O

FIGURE 6-29 (*Continued*).

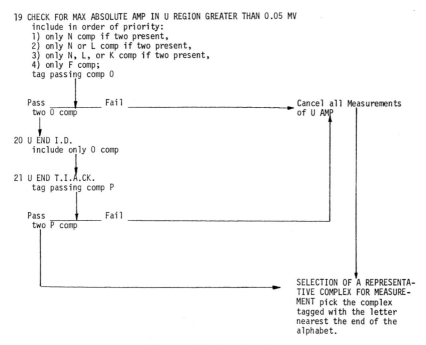

19 CHECK FOR MAX ABSOLUTE AMP IN U REGION GREATER THAN 0.05 MV
   include in order of priority:
   1) only N comp if two present,
   2) only N or L comp if two present,
   3) only N, L, or K comp if two present,
   4) only F comp;
   tag passing comp O

Pass _____ Fail _____ Cancel all Measurements
   two O comp   of U AMP

20 U END I.D.
   include only O comp

21 U END T.I.A.CK.
   tag passing comp P

Pass _____ Fail _____
   two P comp

SELECTION OF A REPRESENTA-
TIVE COMPLEX FOR MEASURE-
MENT pick the complex
tagged with the letter
nearest the end of the
alphabet.

FIGURE 6-30 (*Continued*).

Arrhythmia, is printed out. When the check is passed but there are some complexes without a grade label, the block proceeds along the analysis routine but measurements on it are printed out along with the statement, *Arrhythmia.*

Step 3—QRS Onset Identification

QRS onsets are identified for all complexes in the block labeled A.

Step 4—QRS Onset Time Interval Agreement Check (T.I.A.CK.)

This step includes a subroutine that is used to evaluate the validity of various wave or segment onset and end locations which may be initially mislocated due to noise distortion. In this step it is used to evaluate the QRS onset locations in the time block. In general, this is done by comparing time intervals between these locations and fiducial points in the cycle such as the point of the maximum negative derivative or the R peak with corresponding time intervals in the time block. Onset locations are judged valid and labeled to this effect if these time intervals agree closely with a standard value for the time block. The subroutine is outlined in stepwise form below.

1. Measure time intervals between QRS onset location and R peak for all A complexes in the time block.
2. If the range of values for these intervals in the time block is equal to or less than 2K, where K is a constant which assumes a different value for each different type of wave or segment onset or end location being evaluated, all the A complexes in the block are also labeled B.
3. If the range of values for these intervals is greater than 2K, find a standard value for the time block. This is done by dividing the range into three equal subunits, finding the subunit containing the largest number of time interval values, and identifying the central value of this modal subunit of the range as the standard.
4. Compare each of these intervals to the standard. If the *difference* is equal to or less than K label the complex with a B. If the difference is greater than K the complex does not receive a grade label.

This check is passed if at least two pairs of adjacent B complexes are found. If this check is failed, the PST is applied to the QRS onset region and the time block proceeds through step 3 again. If this check is failed for the second time, the time block is labeled with a STT and PPR noise code of 2 and enters the complex averaging routine.

Step 5—STT Amplitude Agreement Check (A.A.CK.)

This step is a modification of a technique referred to earlier as the Parallel Check routine. It is a subroutine that evaluates agreement between amplitudes at a specific set of locations on each complex to amplitudes at corresponding locations on other complexes in the time block. Its purpose is to detect, type and locate noise in the STT and PPR segments as well as assign the time block to appropriate noise reduction techniques. In this step the STT region is being evaluated. Only B complexes with B complexes following are included. The subroutine is outlined in stepwise form below.

1. Define regions of each complex for amplitude comparison. For the STT regions, this begins with the maximum negative deriva-

tive and ends at a point 75 per cent of the interval between consecutive complex maximum negative derivatives.

2. Define locations in these regions for amplitude comparison by identifying locations of sixteen equally spaced points covering the region.

3. Find amplitudes at these points measuring from QRS onset to QRS onset baselines. This will result in the production of individual values to be subsequently referred to as complex-amplitudes that equal in number the number of B complexes in the time block multiplied by 16.

4. Arrange this group of complex-amplitudes into a matrix with sixteen columns and a row for each B complex in the block. Each column contains amplitude values from similar locations on STT segments. Each row contains amplitude values from the same complex.

5. Evaluate the range of values in each column. If the range is equal to or less than 2C, where C is a constant that assumes a different value for each column, label each complex-amplitude in that column with a grade 0.

6. For column ranges greater than 2C, find standard values for the column. This is done by dividing the range into three equal subunits, finding the interval that contains the largest number of complex-amplitude values, and identifying the central value in this subunit as the standard value.

7. Evaluate the representability of each complex-amplitude by comparing it to the standards for the columns that contain them and apply a grade label to each complex-amplitude reflecting its representability.

   a. If the difference between complex-amplitude and the standard for its column is equal to or less than C1, label the complex-amplitude 0.

   b. If the difference is greater than C1 but equal to or less than C2, label the complex-amplitude 1.

   c. If the difference is greater than C2 but equal to or less than C3, label the complex-amplitude 2.

   d. If the difference is greater than C3, label complex-amplitude 3.

8. This results in the STT region of each complex having a six-

teen digit code reflecting its noise content, type and location; the validity of its linear baseline, and in general its ability to represent the time block. Read the sixteen digit codes and assign a single grade to each complex according to the representability of its STT region.

   a. Label all complexes having only 0's in their sixteen digit codes with an E.

   b. Label all complexes having only 0's or 1's and having not more than three consecutive 1s in their codes with a D.

   c. Label all complexes having only 0's, 1's, or 2's in their codes with aC.

   d. Complexes with 3's in their codes are not labeled.

This check is passed if two E complexes are found, the time block being labeled with an STT noise code of 0. If this check is failed, three possible alternative pathways in the analysis scheme are available for the time block depending on its noise content. If at least two D complexes or a D and E complex are found in the time block, it is smoothed with the PST being directed to small bands about complex-amplitudes labeled 1 or 2. The time block is then labeled with an STT noise code of 1 and proceeds to step 6. If 2 D or E complexes are not found, but 2 D or C complexes are found, the time block proceeds to the complex averaging routine where it is assigned STT and PPR noise codes of 2. If 2 E, D, or C complexes are not found the time block is not further analyzed and the printout displays the statement, *Defective Data*.

Step 6—ST Onset Identification

ST onset is identified on E complexes only if at least two are present. If two are not present only E or D complexes are included in this identification.

Step 7—ST Onset Time Interval Agreement Check

This step is an evaluation of the validity of ST onset locations using the same logic used in step 4 to validate QRS onset locations. The differences are that only E or D complexes are included in the check, the K value is different, and the passing complexes are labeled F instead of B. The check is passed if two F complexes are found. If it is failed, the time block proceeds to the complex averaging routine.

Step 8—Check for Complexes with Maximum Absolute Amplitudes in the STT Region Greater than 0.10mv

This check is in preparation for the location of T wave ends and attempts to test for the presence of a measurable T wave. Only F complexes are included in the check and passing complexes are labeled G. The time block passes the check if two G complexes are found. If it is failed, T wave ends are not located, arbitrary but rate dependent T wave ends are assigned, and the time block proceeds to step 11. Tags are placed so that no QT or JT measurements are made on this time block.

Step 9—T Wave End Identification

T wave ends are located on G complexes only.

Step 10—T Wave End Time Interval Agreement Check

This is an evaluation of T wave end locations using the techniques outlined in step 3. Differences are that only G complexes are included, the K value is different, and passing complexes are labeled H. The time block is passed if two H complexes are found. If the check is failed, as in step 8 rate dependent T wave ends are assigned and QT and JT measurements are prohibited.

Step 11—PPR Amplitude Agreement Check

This step is an evaluation of the noise content and representability of the PPR segment which is essentially the same as the STT segment technique outlined in step 5. If two H complexes are present only these are included in this check. If these are not present, and two H or G complexes are present, only these are included. If two H or G complexes are not present only F complexes are included. Passing complexes are labeled J and the time block passes the check if two J complexes are found. Failing complexes are labeled I. If the check is failed by the time block, and two J or I complexes are present, the PPR region is smoothed with the PST directed to small bands about complex-amplitudes labeled 1 or 2. The time block is then labeled with a PPR noise code of 1. If the time block fails the check and two I complexes are absent, a PPR noise code of 2 is assigned, the measurements of P and P′ wave as well as PR segment are prohibited, and the time block proceeds to step 19.

Step 12—P Wave Onset Identification

P wave onset is identified on J complexes only if two are present. If two J complexes are not present and two J or I complexes are present, only these are included. If these are not present, only F complexes are included.

Step 13—P Wave Onset Time Interval Agreement Check

This is an evaluation of the validity of P wave onset locations according to the technique described in step 3. The order of priority of complexes to be included in this check appears in step 12. Passing complexes are labeled K. The time block passes the check and is assigned a PPR noise code of 0 if two K complexes are found. If it is failed, a PPR noise code of 2 is assigned and P wave measurements are prohibited as outlined in step 11. The time block then proceeds to step 19.

Step 14—P Wave End Identification

P wave ends are located only on K complexes.

Step 15—P Wave End Time Interval Agreement Check

The validity of P wave end locations is determined according to technique previously outlined in step 3. Only K complexes are included in the check and passing complexes are labeled L. The time block passes the check if two L complexes are found. If the check is failed, all measurements of P and P′ waves are prohibited and the time block proceeds to step 19.

Step 16—Check for Maximum Absolute Amplitude in the P′ Wave Region Greater than 0.05 mv

This step is in preparation for the location of P′ wave ends and attempts to determine if a P' wave is present. Only L complexes are included and passing complexes are labeled M. The time block passes if two M complexes are found. If the check is failed, P' wave measurements are prohibited and the time block proceeds to step 19.

Step 17—P' Wave End Identification

P' wave ends are located only on M complexes.

Step 18—P' Wave End Time Interval Agreement Check

The validity of P' wave end locations is determined by previously outlined techniques. Only M complexes are included in the check and passing complexes are labeled N. The time block passes the check if two N complexes are located. If it is failed, P' wave measurements are prohibited.

Step 19—Check for Maximum Absolute Amplitude in the U Region Greater than 0.05 mv

This step is in preparation for the location of U wave end and attempts to determine if a measurable wave is present. The order of priority for inclusion of complexes in this check is as follows: only N complexes if two present; only two N or L complexes if two present; only N, L, or K complexes if two present, and only F complexes. Passing complexes are labeled 0 and the time block is passed if two 0 complexes are found. If it is failed, the measurement of U wave is prohibited.

Step 20—U Wave End Identification

U wave ends are located only on 0 complexes.

Step 21—U Wave Time Interval Agreement Check

The validity of U wave end locations is determined according to previously outlined techniques. Only 0 complexes are included in this check and passing complexes are labeled P. The time block passes if two P complexes are located. If it is failed, U wave measurement is prohibited.

Step 22—Selection of a Representative Complex for Measurement

This is the final step in this routine. In it a single complex is picked for measurement that has been determined to best represent the time block. The complex labeled with the letter nearest the end of the alphabet is that complex.

The workability of this routine remains to be proved, but initial inspection of tracings, applying the routine manually, is encouraging.

SUMMARY

A description of a computer program for analyzing the exercise electrocardiogram has been presented along with some accuracy data. The problem of noise in the signal has been related to various techniques for noise detection and reduction. An experimental routine has been presented which attempts to deal with noise and the problem of choosing a representative complex for measurement.

ACKNOWLEDGMENT

The authors wish to acknowledge their appreciation for invaluable assistance in the preparation of this manuscript from Sidney Abraham, Chief Statistician, Mort Gilbert, Information Officer, and Barbara Jordan, Secretary; all are members of the Medical Systems Development Laboratory, Public Health Service.

REFERENCES

1. MASTER, A.M., and ROSENFELD, I.: Criteria for the clinical application of the "two-step" exercise test. *JAMA, 178*:283, 1961.
2. ROBB, G.P., and MARKS, H.H.; Evaluation of type and degree of change in postexercise electrocardiogram in detecting coronary artery disease. *Proc Soc Exp Biol Med, 103*:450, 1960.
3. MATTINGLY, T.W.: The postexercise electrocardiogram: its value in the diagnosis and prognosis of coronary arterial disease. *Amer J Cardiol, 9*:395, 1962.
4. FRIEDBERG, C.K.; JAFFEE, H.L.; PORDY, L., and CHESKY, K.: The two-step exercise electrocardiogram: a double-blind evaluation of its use in the diagnosis of angina pectoris. *Circulation, 26*:1254, 1962.
5. BLACKBURN, H.: The exercise electrocardiogram. I. Differences in interpretation. Report of a technical group on exercise electrocardiography. *Amer J Cardiol 21*:871, 1968.

6. Specifications of Physiological Data Acquisition System. Available through James Landoll, Medical Systems Development Laboratory, PHS, 2121 "K" St., N.W., Washington, D.C., 20037.

7. CACERES, C.A., *et al.*: *Diagnostic Computers.* Springfield, Thomas (in press).

8. ROBINSON, S.: Cited by Sheffield in Graded exercise in the diagnosis of angina pectoris. *Mod Conc Cardiovasc Disc, 34*:1, 1965.

9. WORKMAN, J.M., and ARMSTRONG, B.W.: A nomogram for predicting treadmill walking oxygen consumption. *J Appl Physiol, 19*:150, 1964.

10. HELLERSTEIN, H.K.; HORNSTEN, T.R.; GOLDBERG, A.; BURLUNDO, A.G.; FRIEDMAN, E.H.; HIRSCH, E.Z., and MARK, S.: The influence of active conditioning upon subjects with coronary artery disease. Cardiorespiratory changes during training in 67 patients. *Canad Med Assoc J, 96*: 758, 1967.

11. BLACKBURN, H.; KEYS, A.; SIMONSON, E.; RAUTAHARJU, P., and PUNSAR, S.: The electrocardiogram in population studies. A classification system. *Circulation, 21*:1160, 1960.

12. ROSNER, S.W.; LEINBACH, R.C.; PRESTO, A.J.; JACKSON, L.K.; WEIHRER, A.L., and CACERES, C.A.: Computer analysis of the exercise electrocardiogram. *Amer J Cardiol, 20*:356, 1967.

13. FREIMAN, A.H.; TOLLES, W.; CARBERY, W.J.; RUEGSEGGER, P.; ABARQUEZ, R.F., and LaDUE, J.S.: The electrocardiogram during exercise. *Amer J Cardiol, 5*:506, 1960.

14. DOAN, A.E.; PETERSON, D.R.; BLACKMON, J.R., and BRUCE, R.A.: Myocardial ischemia after maximal exercise in healthy men. *Amer Heart J, 69*:11, 1965.

15. BLACKBURN, H.: The electrocardiogram in cardiovascular epidemiology. Problems in standardized application. *Ann NY Acad Sci, 126*:882, 1965.

16. BERSON, A.S., and PIPBERGER, H.V.: The low frequency response of electrocardiographs, a frequent source of recording errors. *Amer Heart J, 71*: 779, 1966.

17. KERWIN, A.J.: The effect of the frequency response of electrocardiographs on the vectorcardiographs. *Circulation, 8*:98, 1953.

18. LANGNER, P.H., and GESELOWITZ, D.B.: Characteristics of the frequency spectrum in the normal electrocardiogram and in subjects following myocardial infarction. *Circ Res, 8*:577, 1960.

19. GILFORD, S.R.: Cited by Kerwin (17).

20. DOWER, G.E.; MOORE, A.D.; ZIEGLER, W.G., and OSBORNE, J.A.: On QRS amplitude and other errors produced by direct-writing electrocardiographs. *Amer Heart J, 65*:307, 1963.

21. RAUTAHARJU, P.M.: Deterministic type waveform analysis in electrocardiography. *Ann NY Acad Sci, 128*:939, 1966.

22. RAUTAHARJU, P.M., and BLACKBURN, H.: The exercise electrocardiogram. Experience in analysis of "noisy" cardiograms with a small computer. *Amer Heart J, 69*:515, 1965.

DISCUSSION

Dr. Freiman: Dr. Jackson, if you handle noise by different techniques from complex to complex, how do you determine whether the change in the complex is due to the method of manipulation of the signal, or an actual change in the signal?

Dr. Jackson: Very important. When you test this datum, you label it, and when you apply a smoothing or an averaging routine to it, you have to indicate this, it has to be labeled. Right now, we can only guess at what change this should make diagnostically. It will take a long time to know for sure. The only thing we can do now is to label it and study it against clinical correlates. In the instance of a markedly positive test that is distorted by noise, you couldn't analyze it unless you smoothed it. You can't apply recognized clinical data for interpreting it. However, there is diagnostic information there, likely; and there is a possibility that you can say something about this person, so the only approach is to get it into the program, to smooth it, to label what you've done, and then you have to apply a different set of criteria to interpret these records. Obviously we don't have yet the background to do it, but we have to develop an approach to this data.

Dr. Schmitt: Dr. Jackson, in doing parabolic smoothing you have apparently used just one particular pattern of parabolic smoothing, haven't you? That is, you used various elements and various numbers of sample points in it. Does it not grossly influence your results as to which particular parabolic smoothing you use.

Dr. Jackson: Well, what I showed was different points, this was just an experiment as to what it would do. If you use parabolic smoothing routinely, you just pick one set of points.

Dr. Schmitt: No, this is not what I mean. I mean that the effective frequency smoothing effect of a parabolic filter is dependent on the curvature and the loading of the parabolic filtering. You've not really pointed out all the potentialities and dangers of it. You've simply taken a representative one, haven't you.

Dr. Jackson: That's quite right.

Dr. Schmitt: This is what I wanted to make sure of—this doesn't necessarily represent all parabolic smoothing.

Dr. Jackson: That's right—you have related a given point that is out of line to other points in the area; this has potentialities for distortion, and it's an inconstant treatment of an area, but it can provide some diagnostic information.

Dr. Schmitt: Now the logical extension of this that your laboratory has the hardware to do, and that I don't happen to have available, is using a modulated parabolic smoothing, which appears to be a composite answer that's useful, in which these two parabolic parameters are modulated in terms of where you are in the complex that you know—this is the technique.

Dr. Jackson: Oh yes—you would vary the number of points according to the region.

Dr. Schmitt: Not the number of points necessarily, but the time separation of the points, which is the other parameter, so that you do, in the fast complex, a narrow-gauge smoothing, and in the slow complex, a gross smoothing. You just "know" there isn't going to be a spike in the T wave, and if there is you just don't *want* to know it anyhow!

Dr. Jackson: Right. The other approach is just to apply this in specific areas best suited to the particular technique you decide on.

Dr. Schmitt: Yes, so that the computer doesn't really mind changing its bag of tricks in mid-flow.

Dr. Jackson: Right.

Dr. Schmitt: Except that our programmers are reluctant, the computers aren't.

7

Electrocardiographic Signal Analysis Without Averaging of Complexes

L. T. Sheffield, M. D. Perry, L. N. Larkin
J. A. Burdeshaw, D. V. Conroy, *and* T. Joseph Reeves

The aim of our project in developing computer analysis of the exercise electrocardiogram was to achieve accuracy of measurement free of the interobserver variations shown to exist in electrocardiographic interpretation; to realize pertinent measurements, particularly relating to heart rate and ST segment changes, and to have these available to the physician almost instantaneously in easily applicable form.

PROCEDURE

What followed was a series of steering conferences of clinicians, mathematicians, engineers and programmers. Single complexes were to be measured rather than the average of many superimposed heart cycles, because of our experience in seeing occasionally a positive response which was so transient as to be lost if averaged in with many others. Then, too, the difficulty of preventing premature beats or other transient changes from degrading an averaged result deterred us from using an averaging technique as we began. We defined an electrocardiographic sampling period of two seconds, permitting the finding of two successive QRS complexes even at slow heart rates.

The maximum value of the R wave downslope was taken as the landmark for detection of QRS complexes because of the favorable ratio between it and other parts of the electrocardiogram and its ac-

Note: This work was supported by NIH Grants HE-10885 and HE-11310, grant from Ayerst Laboratories and by Clinical Research Center Grant 2MO1 FR-32-07.

[108]

companying noise. Correction of baseline shift was recognized as necessary for accurate amplitude measurements. Filtration of the signal, or smoothing, while not particularly desirable, was agreed necessary and tolerable. Rather than attempt to measure every possible characteristic of the electrocardiogram, it was agreed to measure at least the heart rate, J point amplitude, ST segment slope, ST area and T wave amplitude. If feasible, other measurements were to be added. A delay of thirty seconds from sampling to reporting was set as maximal, with a goal of fifteen seconds or less cycling time.

The program was to consist of discrete subroutines each of which performed a single major function.

Output features of the program were defined: Measurements were to be communicated by teletypewriter in the exercise laboratory. An analog output was chosen depicting the complex actually measured for comparison with the original.

DESCRIPTION OF ACTUAL PROGRAM
FIGURE 7-1

Start

Subject identification is performed.

Calibrate

One mv square wave is applied at amplifier input; all subsequent measurements divided by this value.

Examine

During a two-second interval the first time derivative is examined and maximal negative value taken as QRS complex landmark. When this value, $\pm$ 25 per cent, recurs, data storage begins and continues for 2000 points (2 seconds).

Parabolic Filter

A 29-point filter subroutine smooths data array, reducing muscle artifact and other noise.

First Derivative

Differences between successive points are stored in another 2000-

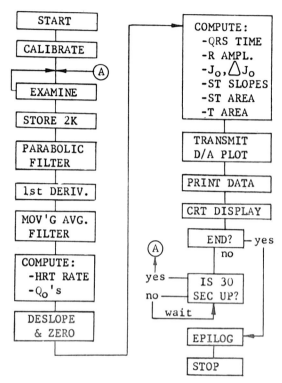

FIGURE 7-1. ECG Analysis Program. Refer to text for description.

point array (changed to 5-point derivative calculation in October, 1967 to improve signal-to-noise ratio) (Fig. 7-2).

Moving Average Filter

The first derivative array, which is not subjected to amplitude analysis, is smoothed by a 17-point moving average filter which removes 60 cycle power line noise and reduces noise of biological and interface origin. Successive point differences are taken from this array to form the second time derivative (d^2/dt) of the electrocardiogram.

Compute Heart Rate

The time intervals between three successive d_{max} (maximum negative derivative) detections are averaged, divided by 3600 and stored

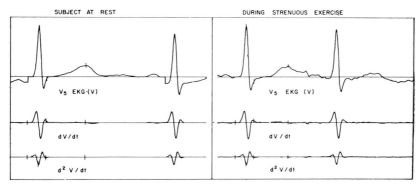

ELECTROCARDIOGRAPHIC SIGNALS
TRACED BY DIGITAL PLOTTER AFTER
PROCESSING BY PDP-7 COMPUTER

VERTICAL MARKS IDENTIFY COMPUTER-RECOGNIZED: Q_0, R peak, J_0, T peak

FIGURE 7-2. Note the first derivative (*middle trace*) and the second derivative (*lower trace*). The nadir of the first derivative is an excellent landmark for recognizing the occurrence of a QRS complex. The second derivative is used for finding QRS onset and termination.

as heart rate. To find Q_0 the d^2/dt signal is examined, moving backward from d_{max} for the last significant deflection which is followed by an electrically quiet zone, i.e., $< 5\mu v$, peak to peak within the region of 40 to 60 msec preceding d_{max}.

Deslope and Zero

Two consecutive Q_0 events are identified and the amplitude difference between them is used to find slope of the existing "baseline shift" or ultra low frequency distortion component. This slope is subtracted from every point of the signal under analysis, which effectively removes any linear component of baseline wander. The measured amplitude value of Q_0 is then subtracted from every point in the signal, establishing Q_0 at a zero value baseline from which other amplitudes are measured. The effect of this process may be seen in the resting record of Figure 7-2, and in Figure 7-3.

Compute QRS Time

J_0 is identified from d^2/dt as the last significant deflection following d_{max}, after which a quiet zone is encountered. Q_0 to J_0 time is stored as QRS time.

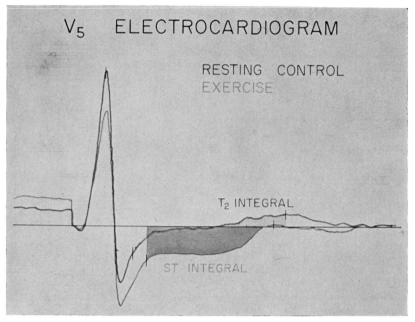

FIGURE 7-3. Rest and exercise records are superimposed. The darkly shaded area is the ST integral, expressed in microvolt-seconds. The lightly shaded area is the "T_2" integral (from the X-point to the peak of the T wave). Records are from a subject with angina pectoris.

R Amplitude

The maximum signal value occurring between Q_0 and d_{max}, confirmed by similar preceding and following values and by zero crossing of d^1/dt, is stored as R amplitude.

J_0, $\triangle J_0$

The initial amplitude of J_0 with respect to baseline is stored. It is subtracted from subsequent J_0 values and the value of change in J_0 is stored for reporting.

ST Slopes

The amplitude of J_0 is subtracted from signal amplitude at $J_0 +$ 80 msec and $J_0 +$ 120 msec, divided by $\triangle t$ and stored as ST slopes 1 and 2. Since this program has been put into actual use, it has been recognized that these values could be improved by computing the mean slopes between these points.

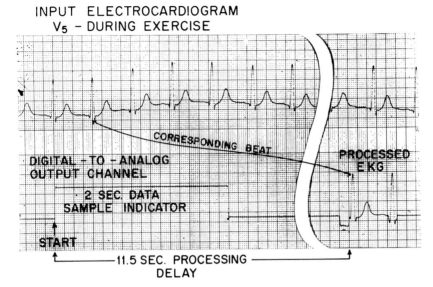

INPUT ELECTROCARDIOGRAM
V_5 – DURING EXERCISE

FIGURE 7-4. The first beat after beginning of data sampling, as indicated on the lower trace, is the one which is analyzed. The computer transmits this signal for comparison with the original, after a brief processing delay.

ST Area

As a single overall figure representing induced ST changes, the area between the baseline and the ST segment is calculated as the time-voltage integral from J_0 to the X point or zero crossing of the ST segment, or to rate-predicted T peak time, whichever occurs earlier (Fig. 7-3).

T Area

The area or integral from X point to the peak of the T wave is calculated and stored, for correlation with ST measurements (Fig. 7-3).

Transmit D/A Plot

After the above computation, the corrected signal array is transmitted sequentially at real-time rate to the test laboratory (Fig. 7-4). Just preceding transmission a recorder control impulse is generated by the computer for starting the recorder. This impulse is terminated after the end of signal transmission. These signals may be used for display

DR. L.T. SHEFFIELD EXERCISE SCALAR-ECG EXPERIMENT
PATIENT NAME & DATE: WM. GALLAWAY
EXERCISE LEVELS & COMMENTS: REEL 5 TEST 18
APPLY CALIBRATE SIGNAL AT ECG LEADS, THEN PRESS CONTINUE
WHEN READY TO START EXPERIMENT, PRESS CONTINUE AND SET
AC SWITCH 0 UP TO STOP EXPERIMENT

TIME MIN	HEART RATE	QRS-T MSEC	JO MV	ST-INT UVS	T-INT UVS	ST-1 MV/S	ST-2 MV/S	R-AMP MV
.02	79	80	−.16	−1.1	26.0	3.1	2.6	.87
1.46	77	80	.01	−1.0	27.1	3.0	2.5	.92
2.45	110	95	−.01	−1.8	19.5	2.9	2.8	.79
2.84	110	90	.11	−.3	23.1	2.0	2.1	.81
3.29	116	85	.01	−.7	29.2	3.4	3.2	.87
3.70	115	95	−.13	−3.2	20.9	4.8	3.9	.83
4.06	113	105	−.05	−1.8	12.8	3.7	3.4	1.00
4.46	113	105	.01	−2.0	16.2	2.3	3.3	.89
4.93	116	80	−.13	−3.0	23.0	4.7	4.0	.92
5.41	117	95	.02	−2.0	10.2	2.5	2.9	.97
7.01	132	105	−.00	−2.1	12.7	3.7	3.1	.95
6.69	132	110	−.08	−8.4	35.6	2.3	2.3	.94
7.14	135	95	−.30	−10.3	11.4	5.6	4.9	.82
7.51	145	80	−.21	−4.2	4.9	5.6	3.0	.95
7.88	79	105	−.01	−4.6	117.0	4.5	3.6	.69
8.35	153	120	.13	−2.2	1.7	1.7	−.1	1.07

FIGURE 7-5. Specimen computer report teletyped in the exercise laboratory during the exercise test.

on a storage oscilloscope, with the start-stop impulses used for control of the storage screen.

Print Data

The most time consuming portion of the operation is the tele-typing of a line of measurements in the test laboratory (Fig. 7-5). At ten spaces per second this requires over seven seconds. It may be reduced to less than one second by presentation cn one-half of the screen of a split screen storage oscilloscope, to be followed by a complete teletyped report at the end of the test.

CRT Display

This option, which may be deleted by an input register switch on the computer, displays on an oscilloscope the corrected signal array for a predetermined interval of six seconds, or as another option, indefinitely, for examination of the array by the computer operator. This is a programmer option and not used during "live" testing. The CRT display subroutine is also used to stop the program and bridge from the measured data array to the digital plotter to produce large-size traces of the electrocardiogram, the first time derivative and the second time derivative of the tape recorded signals (Fig. 7-2).

Is Thirty Seconds Up?

Is a program option causing the analyses to be begun at exactly thirty-second intervals if this is desired. The alternative is a free running mode in which a new analysis is begun as soon as the preceding one is completed. In either case the exact time of analysis relative to beginning of the test is printed on each line of measurement.

Epilog

When depression of the appropriate key of the teletypewriter signals the computer that the test is completed, the calculated Q_0 - T_{peak} times are all printed in order at the bottom of the page and "end of test" is typed.

EXPERIENCE WITH THE PROGRAM

Clinical experience began with the very pleasant surprise that this program processed live electrocardiographic signals from resting normals without omitting a single measurement cycle. Traces from processed cardiograms resembled the originals in every important aspect except for the smoothing of nonelectrocardiographic noise and straightening of the baseline. The filtration reduced R wave peak amplitude by about 10 per cent; so the filter was made removable whenever accurate QRS amplitude measurements were desired. It was found that electrocardiograms during moderate exercise of normals and patients could be processed with only an occasional lapse. Submaximal exercise electrocardiograms could be analyzed provided scrupulous attention was given to obtaining the best possible electrode to skin contact, including dermabrasion of the electrode sites.

It is not at all surprising that older tape recordings of maximal exercise tests proved only partially measurable by this program, just as we are not surprised when we are not able visually to analyze a portion of a high performance exercise electrocardiogram.

We have analyzed records from over one-hundred normals and about twenty-four ischemic heart disease patients, and our two main conclusions are that the basic elements of the program function properly, suggesting that the method of approach is sound; and that retrospective analysis of pre-computer-era tapes may be fairly limited.

Reported measurements from beats judged technically satisfactory by visual observation have appeared to be accurate and useful. Numerical values for ST integral and ST slopes have paralleled the degree of their apparent normality or abnormality. The only real limitation in the use of the program for clinical diagnosis would appear to be that of furnishing the computer with a usable electrocardiogram.

Minor technical improvements we have found desirable would include self-checking features which would signal whenever the electrocardiographic quality becomes too low, whenever predetermined limits for any parameter are exceeded, and a subroutine which would signal a significant change in rhythm.

Major technical considerations include the continual search for better means of improving electrocardiographic signal quality during submaximal exercise, including the possible use of different lead configurations and artificial means of reducing electrical and biological interference. A combination of the present program with selective signal averaging over short time periods is one approach we are currently examining.

In summary we have developed a program for the automatic measurement of the exercise V_5 electrocardiogram and have established its operability at moderate work levels. Ways to extend the degree of its operability have been proposed and are under development. Signal averaging is a tempting method for eliciting measurable signals; but before use in a clinical setting, means should be found to prevent atypical beats from being included and to avoid averaging over significant electrocardiographic changes of state, whether in rhythm, IV conduction or ST segment alteration.

ACKNOWLEDGMENT

The authors wish gratefully to acknowledge the assistance of Mrs. Linda Stephens, Research Technician, Mrs. Juanita Brasher, Project Secretary, Mrs. Myrnie Driskill, Research Assistant, Technicians of University Hospital Electrocardiographic Laboratory and Mr. Mark Goldberg, Electronics Technician.

8

Arrhythmia and Waveform Analysis Programs

Alvin H. Freiman

Theoretically, the full capability of the digital computer would be realized if electrocardiographic signals recorded continuously during exercise were obtained from those leads containing maximal information and then subjected to detailed analysis for each beat. This ideal arrangement assumes that we could delineate those leads containing the maximum amount of information and continuously record these leads with a noise level sufficiently low to permit automatic analysis. One step backward from this ideal approach would be to utilize these same leads and either decrease the artifact to a level consistent with continuous analysis, or subject the signal to an averaging technique in which there would be no distortion of the resultant average and which would contain all of the information present in each component beat. Another approach, and one that has been commonly used, would be to select the lead system containing minimal noise which is felt to contain some, if not all, of the desired information. This latter approach has consisted basically of finding electrode locations resulting in minimal muscle potentials during exercise, and using electrodes and electrode binding techniques to minimize baseline shift. This approach has, unfortunately, resulted in the proliferation of lead systems bearing little quantitative relationship to each other, the results of which cannot be easily compared. Despite this multitude of lead systems and varying types of electrodes resulting in significant decrease in the artifact present in the electrocardiographic signals, it is usually true that the level of noise during strenuous physical activity is such as to severely impair continuous electrocardiographic

Note: This work was supported in part by NCI Grant CA-08748.

analysis by computer methods. It is improbable, on the basis of our past experience, that future development in electrode technology and in lead placement would result in signals sufficiently free from artifact to permit such detailed analysis. This is especially true in view of the fact that one component of the artifact, namely baseline shift, probably originates not only from the electrode skin interface but also from deeper tissues.

Another approach involves manipulation of the electrocardiographic signal by either filtering or smoothing techniques. Such techniques, while they may result in a signal which is suitable for analysis, do involve some degradation of the signal from its original status, resulting in possible loss of information. The applicability of this technique, therefore, depends to a large extent on the type of information desired from the signal and how seriously this information would be distorted by the method employed.

Another technique involves average transient computing in which a group of sequential complexes are averaged and then analyzed. This technique is based on certain assumptions which must be kept in mind in terms of its effect. It assumes that the signal is basically repetitive and that the signal resulting from averaging will, therefore, contain all of the data present in each of the component complexes. While it is probably true that some of the changes which occur do so at a gradual rate and that variation from one beat to the next would not, therefore, be particularly troublesome, it must be recognized that certain portions of the complex are not repetitive even at rest and that some of these changes will be partially repressed by averaging. Another problem, inherent in average transient computing, results from any variation in the point of triggering at which averaging starts. A third point relative to average transient computing is the assumption, which is inherent in the use of the technique, that the noise which is present is essentially random. If, however, the noise is not random but is repetitive throughout the signal, then average transient computing cannot be expected to be effective. A final point is the necessity to exclude inhomogeneous transients, especially arrhythmias, from average transient computing. With the onset of an arrhythmia, sequential averaging would not only be useless but would, in fact, yield totally misleading information. It would seem desirable, therefore, to be able to preprocess the electrocardiographic signal and to pick out those areas where an arrhythmia exists. The goal of such preprocessing would depend upon the information which is desired from the signal. The first use would be to exclude arrhythmias from sequential averaging, and the second use of such preprocessing would be to detect arrhythmias for immediate detailed analysis. Conceivably, such preprocessing could serve one or both functions, depending upon the needs of the investigator or the clinical situation. In situations involving the continuous recording of the electrocardiogram during exercise, continuous average transient computing could proceed unless the preprocessing technique indicated the presence of an arrhythmia which would interdict analysis of the resulting signal complex. In other situations, such as during continuous monitoring in either intensive care or coronary care units, one could conceive of periodic average transient computing and digital analysis at preset intervals, provided that no arrhythmia were present during the signal to be analyzed. This preprocessing would, in addition, designate the presence of an arrhythmia to allow for digital analysis of this portion of the signal.

Functions of Analog Preprocessing:
      1. Exclude Arrhythmias from Sequental Averaging
      2. Initiate Digital Arrhythmia Analysis
Functions of Digital:
      1. Analyze Averaged Signals
          a) Continuously
          b) Intermittently
      2. Analyze Arrhythmias on Signal

FIGURE 8-1. Functions of preprocessing of electrocardiographic data.

Figure 8-1, then, summarizes the possible functions of preprocessing of electrocardiographic data, possibly by analog technique, together with its interaction with the digital method. It must be pointed out that one must define the requirements for rhythm analysis in such a system because it is important under most circumstances that we know more than whether or not an arrhythmia exists. In addition to this basic knowledge, we would usually want to know the type of arrhythmia, the frequency with which any given arrhythmia occurs over a period of time, whether the frequency of arrhythmia is increasing or decreasing and the relationship of the ectopic to the normal complexes and to themselves. We are currently studying and testing such preprocessing by analog means, attempting thereby to simulate the human method for recognizing arrhythmias. During exercise, this analog preprocessing would serve to interrupt the digital analysis of the average transient computed electrocardiographic signal and allow certain conclusions to be drawn concerning the arrhythmia, then initiate digital analysis of the arrhythmia if feasible. The technique involves, first, the establishment of a normal template of rate together with an estimate of whether the basic rhythm falls within normal levels or is itself an arrhythmia. If the basic rhythm is regular and a subsequent beat falls outside of a preset percentage of template values, then an arrhythmia probably exists and can be recognized by one of several criteria. An abnormal beat under these circumstances, would occur either well prior to its expected time of arrival or well after it should have arrived. If this difference is sufficiently large, then we can be sure that the origin is from a different pacemaker or represents a variation in conduction from the same pacemaker. The next criterion involves the analysis of the configuration of the complex itself, namely, the amplitude and duration of the aberrant complex. This second criterion, including both amplitude and duration, will apply equally well if the beat arises in the expected interval or relatively close to it. If the basic rhythm is irregular, as in atrial fibrillation, then we cannot establish a template and cannot, therefore, expect to recognize aberrant rhythm on the basis of timing. Under these circumstances we must rely on the configuration of the aberrant complex itself. By the use of such analog preprocessing we can, therefore, specify the characteristics of any given complex, indicating that the complex represents in all probability an arrhythmia and can use this data in two ways. We can, first of all, indicate the necessity for detailed analysis of this segment for precise definition of the arrhythmia by digital means, as well as indicating that the complex cannot be included in the sequential averaging technique. We can, in addition, set absolute levels of bradycardia or tachycardia above or below which digital analysis would be indicated. Such a system, of course, involves a memory loop to allow sufficient time for subsequent digital analysis. The overall data flow of the signal would then be as follows: The signal would proceed through analog preprocessing for determination of arrhythmia. The signal would proceed on magnetic tape through a memory loop circuit after the analog preselection. The analog portion would determine the basic rate, amplitude and duration of the QRS complexes as well as the absolute rate at which the QRS complexes occur. If all of these criteria remain within preset levels, then the resultant signal would proceed to average transient computing and digital analysis or, under other circumstances, to storage and periodic average analysis. In the event of significant deviation of the rate, amplitude or duration, the analog computer would signal the digital computer to proceed with arrhythmia analysis of the signal for a period of time prior to the appearance of the arrhythmia. It would also indicate that no signal averaging was to proceed during this period of time.

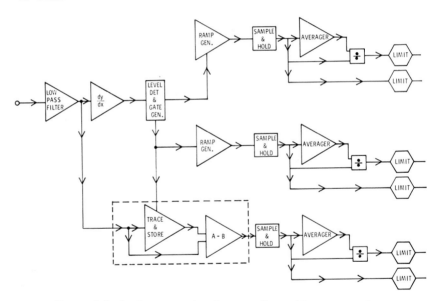

FIGURE 8-2. Analog system for electrocardiographic preprocessing.

Figure 8-2 represents a system with which we are now working to accomplish this end. The signal enters through a lowpass filter to remove high frequency noise from the signal, then passes through a differentiator with resultant first derivative of the signal. The signal then enters into a level detector which picks discrete points on the QRS derivative, the output of which is used for timing. The signal then proceeds to a ramp generator, the peak output voltage of which is analogous to the RR interval, and into a sample and hold circuit in which the dc output representing the peak voltage from the ramp generator is analogous to the RR interval. The signal then passes to the averaging circuit, the lowpass filter in which the dc is analogous to the average RR interval, then to the divider circuit computing the average between the RR interval and the instantaneous RR interval, the output from this circuit flagging if the ratio or the absolute level of rate exceeds preset limits. Similar processing is indicated for the QRS duration and QRS amplitude circuits. It should be noted that while we are proceeding with an analog configuration, future developments, especially of small digital equipment, may show that it is more desirable to do all analysis in digital mode.

We are also attempting to present the results of arrhythmia analysis in a form which would be easily readable over a period of time. For this purpose we plot on the ordinate the RR interval, while on the abscissa we plot starting from an arbitrarily set zero point the increment of both amplitude and duration, both expressed as positive values. With this technique, sinus rhythm with a steady RR interval and no change in amplitude or duration would be represented by a single point; constant RR interval with change in either amplitude or duration would be expressed as a vertical line. Variation in the RR interval with no change in amplitude or duration would be represented by a horizontal line. Supraventricular premature contractions would have a shorter RR interval but the amplitude and duration of the complex would be usually unchanged. Ventricular premature contractions or supraventricular premature contractions with aberrant conduction would have both a short RR interval and a different location on the Y axis. One shortcoming of such a method of display is that it does not differentiate between changes in amplitude and duration. Despite this, such a method of display may have clinical usefulness to summarize the presence or absence of arrhythmias and their type. Other methods of graphically displaying significant information appear to be necessary.

DISCUSSION

Dr. Schmitt: Dr. Freiman, I think you didn't tell us what the nature of the display was—whether this was a memory scope or otherwise?

Dr. Freiman: It was a memory scope. You're perfectly correct.

This is the first crude effort, and the question now comes up of a different type of display, possibly numerical. A second possibility would be a representation, on request, of aberrant beats as a function of time, and this is not intended as a fixed mode. This is really our first attempt to compress a large amount of data taken over a long period of time into something that might be useful clinically in the situations I have mentioned.

Question: Other people spoke today about averaging. One of the methods that was brought out was averaging over a large number of cycles and coming up with one complex that is representative. Another idea is looking at a small group of complexes, comparing certain parameters of these complexes, and on that basis deciding that these are typical, and selecting one of them and making all measurements on it. Then there could be the method of taking a number of complexes and deciding whether or not these are typical and taking measurements then from each of these complexes and coming up with numbers that are averages or means of all of the eight or ten or so complexes. There probably are other methods, too, and I was wondering if someone would like to comment on the applicability of the different averaging methods.

Dr. Schmitt: I think that a number of people have been commenting on these for the last three hours or so.

Question: I would like to have some sort of summary.

Dr. Schmitt: Well, we have about ten or so minutes left. You've asked a question that I think pertains to the whole.

The triggering question I was thinking of was this:

Suppose we did have all the gadgetry we wanted and it could really do what we wished it could do—what would we like it to do in processing this exercise data particularly? What is the goal, what is the idea of this analysis we'd like to have it make? Can we verbalize this? Do we want an epitome of the representative electrocardiogram, or isn't that what we want? Do we want the representative repetition rate, or isn't that what we want? Do we care about the form, or are we more interested in the contrast of differences?

Dr. Jackson: Yes, I would say the best thing possible is to get a representative complex, and you have to resort to other techniques if that's not possible.

Dr. Schmitt: You say you would like to pick a representative complex?

Dr. Jackson: Right. I like to look, as Mr. Berson said, for typical complexes, and if I can find them, I like to make a measure on one. If I find a string of typical complexes, I don't see the value of wasting time summing these. If I judge that they are typical, then I think the measurement of one would be the first need. But since we do have some beat-to-beat variation in noise, it seems to me that you have to resort to other techniques when your perhaps best technique fails.

Dr. Schmitt: I think you don't mean what you say.

I could go through, let's say, 1000 complexes and pick the most representative one. This would be guaranteed to have quite a bit of noise on it, because they generally do, and so your representative complex would be a pretty noisy one. It would be of some particular duration—not reflecting the before and after aspect of exercise, but something in between, more like the average segment of the population.

Dr. Jackson: What I'm suggesting is that when we pick a representative complex, this would be more representative of a very short block of data, and therefore, would be many complexes representing before and after exercise.

Dr. Schmitt: But wouldn't you like to have as much clean of noise as possible? If you really want a representative complex, you want it to be representative of the physiological activity underlying the record, deprived of as much extraneous as possible.

Dr. Jackson: I don't know if we commonly have that much noise. We've gotten a lot of stuff from Minnesota, where they've given a good deal of care to their recording of stress cardiograms, and it's been my experience that the most common problem we have is a rather small, low-amplitude random noise, which we might be willing to sort out all smooth and take a reading on ourself, but which would complicate pattern recognition. The noise is not that big a problem, most of the time.

Dr. Schmitt: I didn't mean that noise was necessarily a problem, but I think that the study of noise is only a very trivial part of our interest, so I think we'd much rather have a complex free of noise if we can get it.

Dr. Freiman: I seem to have much more trouble with noise than other people, even under the most exacting of circumstances. During heavy exercise the amount of noise that we get is more than I think one could tolerate, in terms of any detailed analysis.

Secondly, I can't help wondering sometimes, whether in the attempt to carry out detailed digital analysis, we are not getting ourselves in the situation where we have to begin to manipulate the signal, distort it, and come out with something which may not be very representative of the underlying signal at its source, and attempt to carry out detailed analysis of a partial artifact.

Comment: I would like to make a comment on the analogy of the average sex, which is binary. I think in the ST segments in which we see gradual changes, as far as averaging is concerned, we find it almost ideal, providing things are stable. Now this isn't always the case. For instance, we do see a shift from depression to elevation, and this shift may occur over a period of fifteen to twenty or thirty seconds, gradual changes. Certainly if you average you are not going to see the maximum change and you're losing very significant information. That, I think, is the disadvantage and I think one point that hasn't been worked out is that we're just in the initial stages—how does the whole pattern behave through the procedure of stress, and how much do we have to stress the patient, when is the peak when we can expect the best data. I don't think that any of us really has that answer, but I think averaging has turned out to be sort of a happy compromise, and not an average sex.

Dr. Schmitt: You sensed what I was driving at; because of the exigencies of the day-by-day difficulties of doing it, we tend to make our analyses in terms of two things; the arithmetic in the computers we know, and the hardware we know, and within the suppressed physiology we're after.

I'm inclined a little bit to look for what we're trying to find out physiologically, and invent if necessary the hardware we need and get after it. The kind of analysis that appeals to me especially is something loosely called the "unwrapping" analysis, where you essentially say, "Here is a mess—well, we know something about that. We know the heart generally beats or doesn't beat. All right now, that tells us something. Now unwrap these beats. Let us say that insofar as these are all beats, they are representative of a beat; and insofar as they are different, they represent an arrhythmia."

Now we know that exercise modifies the electrocardiogram. Tell me what doesn't? As knowledgeable physiologists and knowledgeable data processors, we should seek—not what we can show, with the greatest floss, smoothing technique or something-or-other, but what we can squeeze out, even dirty, valuable juice.

Question: I think that one of the things we are trying to look at that hasn't been looked at before in the light of classical cardiology and mentioned before today, is the duration of the QRS complex. This is nearly as possible the depolarization time, from the first significant groups of the fibers to the last significant group of them. Do you think the exercise response here might possibly show a differentiation?

Dr. Schmitt: I think you would find a definition of this that was operationally measurable; that there is something that relates to excitation of depolarization, region by region, into voltage measurements somewhere.

Comment: Yes, and it might have discriminatory value from a diagnostic standpoint.

Dr. Schmitt: This points, for example, to other than simple, quiet resting electrode placements, doesn't it?

Comment: Yes, I think it would require three-dimensional segments.

Dr. Schmitt: I was going to suggest that it might require more than three—I suspect that it's at least four-dimensional, in order to find more than a spatial dipole, which will not show regional timing. You were saying by implication we should go at least four components, which is contradictory to our tidy tradition. Perhaps we'll want to carry the discussion in some other direction—I was just trying to stimulate it a little.

Dr. McHenry: I just wanted to make one comment. I think I detect a note of defeatism here. You say you take that dirty old tracing and try to clean it up. It's really not been our experience that data cannot be cleaned up at the source. I detect today that most people take an attitude that there is nothing that you can do about all this artifact and all this noise; of course we have to define noise as various types. I think our finding with data collection is that the majority of the tracings can be—some information can be gotten from them without computer analysis, and we found that if great care is taken in collecting data, that the analysis of twenty-five complexes is sufficient. I would say that we got very little statistical variation between the four groups of twenty-five in any given segment. I don't think we should give up in trying to clean up the dirty records and the noise at the source. I still think it's possible to get relatively good records that do not require high-low pass filters and various types of filtering aspects. I'm not yet ready to admit this is all necessary.

Dr. Schmitt: Maybe you are taking out the responsibility for some of the noise, but I worry that probably you would have a complex that comes through beautifully with no obvious noise on it, that is stylized and perfectly reproduced both time and again, that represents something other than what you think it represents—but in fact, is noisy. Let's say, for example, what we are sensing in a lead. If we are not sensing parts that you think we are—do you consider this as noise or not? In other words, is distortion a noise in your book, or not? When you get a signal that does not represent what you think it should be representing, is this not a noisy signal, or do you consider it just a distortion and not a distortion from noise?

Comment: Well, I'm sure they all have the same meaning. I have a tendency to think of this as distortion rather than noise, but do we know whether the resting electrocardiogram represents what we think it does?

Dr. Schmitt: We know it doesn't.

Comment: It seems to me we've been satisfied with this for years, at least most people have, and the aim of exercise electrocardiography, as I see it, is to be able to get the same information from the data during exercise that we're getting after. Now maybe we want to go deeper, but at least this would be my first aim in trying to interpret and get data from the exercise electrocardiogram. I don't think that we can assume that the best signals we obtain from the body surface can be the ones that are the cleanest looking. I think we must strive for getting the maximum information from the body and find some way of extracting the maximum information, and I don't think we can assume they're clean. They can be cleaned up at the source.

Dr. Schmitt: You are saying then, that perhaps we should take somewhat less convenient signals in order to have them meaningful or more feasibly important.

Comment: Right.

Dr. Schmitt: Is there someone in the audience who would like to question this information?

Comment: I wonder if you could comment on the adequacy of wave recognition programs in determining beginnings and ends of waves.

Dr. Schmitt: You are asking about beginnings and ends of waves in which terms—of cleaning up so that you can see beginnings and ends clearly?

Comment: No, I am talking about the ability of your particular mathematical alphabets to perform this job of identifying the beginnings and ends of the waves. In talking about the use of the ST area, you make some differential diagnosis, and we want to be able to identify J point with some sort of consistency. I am just wondering how your computer programs do this kind of thing.

Dr. Schmitt: I would like to ask you first, how do you define a J point?

Comment: That is essentially the question I am asking you. How do you instruct your computer system?

Dr. Schmitt: I think the question of how you tell the computer is begging the question of how we tell ourselves, other than, "You know what I mean when I point it this way." And really, when you get down to the details of it, it turns out this is pretty ambiguous and tends to be an arbitrary thing slipped in by computer programmers, sometimes without very much regard to physiology.

Comment: What happens in offset procedures, for instance in averaging, is something remarkably similar to what the human eye does, and I think the averaging and cleaning up the record does something that the human eye of an experienced ECG reader does. For instance, if an experienced ECG reader wants to determine whether there is a small R wave in lead V_1, and the record is superimposed with muscle tremor noise, he looks at a number of beats and finds whether this R peak occurs at the same time. In averaging actually we are cleaning up the record in the same manner, and in determining onsets we found that averaging, I think, has improved the quality of the record. Of course, if you have a clean record from the source, then there is no need in doing this, but I think that averaging improves greatly the onset and offset determinations of the record.

Dr. Brooks: I have a question, very generally, three questions that bother me when I hear you folks talk about things I don't understand very well. I do agree with Dr. Schmitt that this, what you call noise, is extremely important to recognition. I am wondering if noise is something that has nothing to do with the heart—what the eye definition of noise is. That's point number one—I am wondering what noise is.

Number two is that it seems to me that rather than endeavor to get that constant, that we ought to know the degree of change in this heart in the various components as this heart goes under stress, so that the common denominator may be nothing but the degree of fluctuation, but our comrades say there is more significance. Therefore we might find out by averaging or random sampling the most important thing that can be learned about the heart from the physiological point of view.

Number three—it might be that the problem here is that it is highly dangerous to categorize an area where fluctuation exists in time situations by a divergence or by varied spacing. It is all on a relationship, and this tends to be one of the major problems you are talking about, this misinformation of phase. It may be varied by 100 per cent—it may skip by 100 msec and be an entirely different order of magnitude, and if it forms generally we have no proper meaning of it. I do want to congratulate you all on defining the problem.

Dr. Schmitt: Yes, I think you point very sharply at this strange problem, the transformation of the physiological and anatomically related things that we want to know about into their electric equivalents, that do not have a uniform personality. I think particularly tiny changes that are measurable and may look like noise may be very sensitive to the physiological things we care about, whereas gross things may be almost unrelated, and it may be sort of a disciplinary problem in saying these are the things that I care about, exercise probably influences these, and how they manifest themselves. We are overcomputerizing some certain aspects of it, and forgetting some simple things that might give us some very important answers.

Well, it isn't so much that we want to have the last word—though I think you might suspect that.

9

Quantitative Exercise Stress Testing in the Naval Aviator Population and in the Projected Apollo Spacecraft Experiment MO-18

RAPHAEL F. SMITH

I SHOULD LIKE to describe a system of exercise stress testing which has proved to be useful in the cardiac evaluation of naval aviators. I shall also describe an experiment in the Apollo spaceflight series in which this method is to be utilized.

THE PROBLEM

In the naval aviator population, especially with pilots of high performance aircraft, there is a greater demand for diagnostic accuracy than there is in the population at large. The disastrous consequences of a coronary incident in flight can easily be imagined, and, indeed, some twenty accidents have been caused by sudden incapacitation due to coronary heart disease (1). Our paramount need, therefore, is a sensitive test to detect imminent functional impairment due to coronary arteriosclerosis.

On the other hand, it is also exceedingly expensive to train a military pilot. The cost of the training syllabus for a student aviator is approximately $100,000, and after he receives his wings, costs for operational training in high performance aircraft increase in exponential fashion. Thus a false negative diagnosis places the aviator and

Note: Opinions or conclusions contained in this report are those of the author and do not necessarily reflect the views or endorsement of the Navy Department.

This study was supported in part by NASA Defense Purchase Request T-23237(G).

crewmen at tremendous risk while a false positive diagnosis is a costly error in terms of replacing the pilot lost to operational flying.

It is not necessary to review critically the diagnostic error rates of the conventional exercise stress test that have been found in longitudinal studies (2, 3) since the need for improvement of exercise stress testing is generally recognized and, indeed, is the theme of this conference. We became convinced that the ratio of incorrect diagnoses to correct diagnoses could not be improved to the degree needed in aviation by merely juggling the amount of ST segment depression that could be accepted as a normal limit. For this reason we have approached the problem of exercise stress testing in a somewhat different manner.

THE APPROACH

Standardization of the Exercise Load

We subscribe to the concept that the type of exercise used in electrocardiographic exercise tests is not important as long as it is adequate to stress the individual. We compared external work performed on the bicycle ergometer, Harvard step device (single 20-inch step), and the Master two-step device by measuring net oxygen consumption in a group of young volunteers (4). In Figure 9-1 net oxygen consumption is plotted against duration of exercise on the three devices. The rates of work were 150 watts on the ergometer and twenty steps per minute on the Harvard step device. For the Master step device the work load was varied according to Master's recommendations. In our cardiac clinic we have used the Harvard step device for many years and have found that it is often necessary to assign a heavier work load to a well-conditioned man in order to elicit the electrocardiographic pattern of coronary insufficiency (5). It can be seen from Figure 9-1 that the net oxygen consumption on the ergometer roughly corresponds to that on the Harvard step device. We finally selected the bicycle ergometer to supply the work load because with this device the electrodes stay in place better and the work load can be precisely controlled. Since the naval aviator population is very homogeneous in that men are selected by anthropometric standards and are

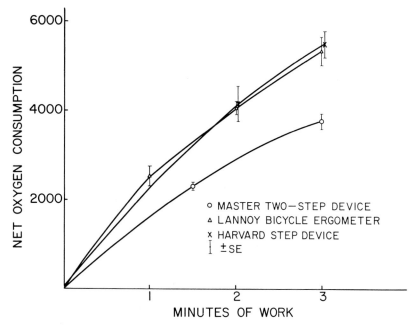

FIGURE 9-1. A graph comparing net oxygen consumption for exercise on the bicycle ergometer (150 watt load), Harvard step device (20 steps per minute) and Master two-step device. (By permission of the American Heart Association, Inc.)[8]

required to maintain their weight within certain limits, we believe that the question is not critical of whether to provide a fixed exercise load or a load that is dependent on the weight of the patient such as exercise against gravity on the step device. Thus our population, as well as the external work load, can be considered partially "standardized." In random samples of our population we have observed that for a fixed load of 150 watts for two minutes on the ergometer, the variance of pulse rate response in the ECG immediately after exercise was less than that of the resting control tracing. With this exercise load there was a negative correlation ($r = -.33$, $p < .001$) between the size of the patient and the pulse rate after exercise. This suggested that the larger men were stressed less with the fixed exercise load than were the smaller men. The correlation between subject size and resting pulse was not significant.

Lead System

Silver-silver chloride electrodes, diameter 1.5 cm, were applied with moleskin in the Frank lead configuration (6). The Frank normalizing resistor network was utilized with the base resistance value 100,000 ohms.

Analysis of Exercise Response

It was evident from previous clinical experience with exercise tests that the electrocardiographic manifestations of early coronary heart

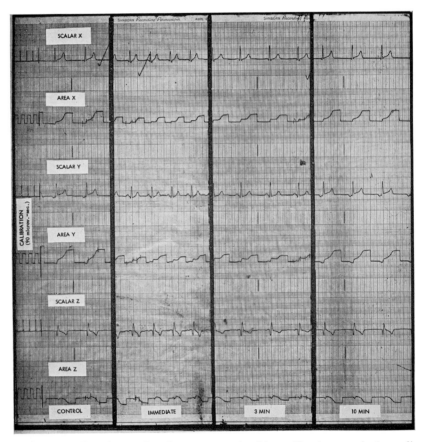

FIGURE 9-2. Exercise tracing from a normal subject. Tracings made immediately, three minutes and ten minutes after exercise. (By permission of the American Heart Association, Inc.)[8]

disease would appear in the repolarization process. Since these potentials are of relatively low magnitude but of long persistence, we hypothesized that an area analysis such as mean vector analysis would be particularly sensitive to changes in the repolarization process. To measure electrocardiographic area a special purpose analog computer was designed to integrate the ECG wave form (7). In addition to carrying out the operation of integration, the device automatically adjusted the period of integration for changes in heart rate. Figure 9-2 shows a normal exercise sequence. The scalar ECG appears above its area trace for leads X, Y and Z. A calibration signal is shown in the far left side of the photograph. In testing an individual a control

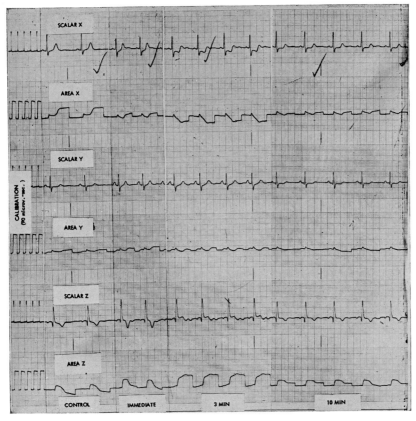

FIGURE 9-3. Exercise tracing from a patient with angina pectoris. (By permission of the American Heart Association, Inc.)[8]

tracing is run, the patient is given two minutes of exercise at an ergometer load of 150 watts, and the electrocardiogram is recorded on FM magnetic tape for a ten-minute period after exercise. A recording from a patient with mild angina pectoris is shown in Figure 9-3. The QRS area, early repolarization area, T area and ventricular gradient area are measured from the integral trace. Figure 9-4 is a diagram showing how these items are measured from the time integral of the electrocardiogram. Since we could not precisely define the ST segment, initial repolarization (TI) was chosen to approximate the ST segment. The area from the end of QRS (J point) to the mid-point in the T wave is used as a measure of TI.

After studying exercise stress tests done in this manner in patients with angina pectoris we began to note that vector direction rather than magnitude offered the best possibility of differentiating normals from abnormals. Our analysis consists of expressing four areas of the

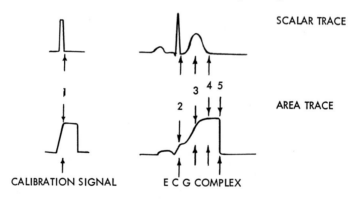

MEASURED:

1 Height of calibration integral
2 Height of QRS integral
3 Height of TI integral
4 Height of T integral
5 Height of QRST integral (ventricular gradient)

CALCULATED:

$$\text{Area of ECG deflection (microvolt-seconds)} = \frac{\text{Height of deflection (mm)} \times \text{Calibration Area (microv.sec.)}}{\text{Height of calibration signal (mm)}}$$

FIGURE 9-4. Method of area analysis. (By permission of the American Heart Association, Inc.)[8]

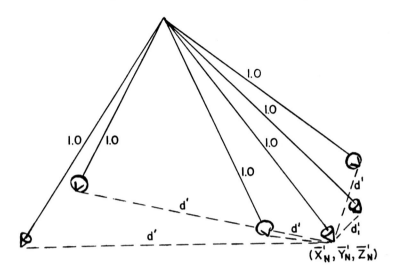

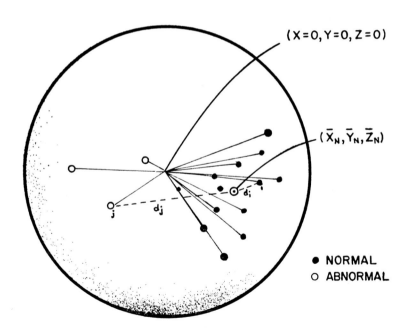

FIGURE 9-5. (*above*) A graphic concept of unity vectors and the relative distance (d′) from the average unity vector. (*below*) The projection of terminus-points on the surface of a sphere. j is a hypothetical abnormal point; i is a hypothetical normal point; X_n, Y_n and Z_n is the average normal point. (By permission of the American Heart Association, Inc.)[8]

electrocardiogram (QRS, TI, T and G) as spatial mean vectors; normalizing these vectors so that each vector magnitude is the same but the original vector direction is preserved; measuring the dispersion of the vectors about a central value in a carefully studied normal population; and comparing an individual's mean vector direction with the cluster of normal vectors. The diagnostic parameter which is used to make this comparison is the relative distance of the terminus of an individual vector from the terminus of the average vector of the normal group. In a normal population these distance values (d') will have a normal distribution for each period after exercise. A derivation of Student's *t* test is used to compute a score that is an index of the individual's position in the distribution of normal values. Figure 9-5A shows the d' measurement and Figure 9-5B shows that the vector termini can be considered as a cluster of points on the surface of a sphere with a radius of 1.0. The statistical proof of this analysis appears in Appendix 1 and Appendix 2 of a recent publication (8). The calculation of spatial mean vectors and the statistical analysis were done with a Univac 418 digital computer.

Study Populations

We have carefully studied two normal groups. One hundred and forty asymptomatic men from the survivors of the 1000 aviator longitudinal study (9) were selected as potential control subjects if they were free from angina pectoris in the opinion of a separate medical team assigned to the project. Since our study proposed to compare persons with a low probability of significant coronary disease with a group of patients with a high probability of coronary disease, subjects were eliminated from the group of 140 men if they exhibited abnormal values of epidemiologically proven risk factors for coronary disease. In the 1000 aviator longitudinal study frequency distributions of blood pressure, cholesterol, serum lipoproteins and postprandial blood sugar are known (10). The 80th percentile was the value chosen as the upper limit of normal for each of these cardiovascular risk factors. As a result of these stringent criteria, ninety-six asymptomatic men were eliminated from the normal group and the remaining forty-four constituted one control group for our study. The ages of this control group ranged from forty-three to fifty-five years with a mean age of forty-seven years. A second normal control group was made up of fifty-five young men ordered to have a comprehensive medical examination because of special conditions of their military duty. Included in this group were astronaut candidates, Navy test pilots, and volunteer research subjects. The mean age of the group was twenty-nine years. This group is used for comparison with younger patients. The third study group was made up of patients with angina pectoris. These men were referred for study if they had a definite history of angina pectoris, normal or essentially normal resting electro-cardiograms with no evidence of a previous myocardial infarction, and enough cardiac reserve by history to enable the patient to undergo exercise stress slightly greater than that of the Master two-step test. Eleven patients were included in this group. They were all naval officers or naval petty officers with a mean age of forty-six years.

RESULTS

The clinical group of patients with angina pectoris was compared with the normal control population of similar mean age. The t scores for QRS, TI, T and G resulting from this analysis are shown in Table 9-I. Somewhat to our surprise the VCG item which con-sistently provided diagnostic information was the T wave direction in the three-minute postexercise period. The t scores were greater than 1.85 ($p < .05$) for the 11 patients with angina pectoris and greater than 2.76 ($p < .01$) for ten of the eleven patients. These data indi-cate that the test is a sensitive one since there were no false-negative errors when the p .05-level is taken as a rejection level. To consider false-positive errors a similar analysis of the T vector three minutes after exercise was done for each member of the normal control group. Five of the forty-four normal control subjects had a d' score that was significantly different from that of the other forty-three men. Each of these five men was carefully studied and no cardiovascular disease was apparent.

Cumulative percentage curves showing the distribution of d' scores for the normal group (N = 44), the group with positive risk factors (N = 96), and the angina pectoris group (N = 11) are shown in Figure 9-6. We realize fully that in order to validate this test method we must follow these subjects and patients to determine the incidence

TABLE 9-I

THE t-TEST SCORES OF d' VALUES OF SPATIAL VECTOR DIRECTIONS
FOR ELEVEN PATIENTS WITH CORONARY HEART DISEASE
MEASURED PRIOR TO EXERCISE, AND IMMEDIATELY, THREE
MINUTES, AND TEN MINUTES AFTER EXERCISE ($P_{0.005}$ = 1.68;
$P_{0.01}$ = 2.42; $P_{0.001}$ = 3.55)

Patient	Resting and time after exercise	QRS	TI	T	G
46	Resting	—0.696	—1.621	0.106	—0.229
	Immediate	—0.489	—0.653	1.297	1.074
	3 min	—0.575	0.477	3.735	2.538
	10 min	—0.358	—0.844	1.669	1.492
50	Resting	0.789	0.894	2.879	—1.244
	Immediate	—0.102	0.841	3.941	1.252
	3 min	0.583	1.466	4.555	1.441
	10 min	0.944	0.984	3.529	—1.254
68	Resting	0.049	—1.368	—0.552	0.062
	Immediate	0.498	—0.660	0.553	1.724
	3 min	—0.487	1.087	3.384	1.684
	10 min	—0.338	—0.260	—0.774	0.286
70	Resting	0.227	0.695	0.519	—1.528
	Immediate	—1.066	0.568	—0.169	—0.393
	3 min	—0.420	1.001	4.713	0.316
	10 min	0.122	—1.215	0.294	—1.465
78	Resting	—0.785	2.816	2.476	0.360
	Immediate	0.913	0.229	1.862	2.858
	3 min	0.737	0.909	4.242	4.043
	10 min	—1.475	2.129	4.479	1.511
85	Resting	0.108	—0.615	1.605	—0.700
	Immediate	0.702	1.133	3.930	3.655
	3 min	—0.264	1.524	4.824	3.129
	10 min	0.420	1.034	4.822	0.873
97	Resting	—1.264	—1.406	—0.478	—0.317
	Immediate	0.368	—0.090	—0.314	1.172
	3 min	0.521	1.958	4.318	3.322
	10 min	—0.513	0.604	1.772	1.870
113	Resting	1.148	1.054	2.415	—0.506
	Immediate	—0.073	0.455	3.378	—0.085
	3 min	—0.239	0.592	3.662	2.081
	10 min	0.094	0.694	3.808	0.856
118	Resting	—1.296	—0.223	—0.720	—1.172
	Immediate	—0.417	—0.979	0.068	0.065
	3 min	—0.094	1.145	4.283	3.316
	10 min	—0.866	—0.909	1.141	0.851
168	Resting	1.885	—0.173	—0.571	0.008
	Immediate	1.849	1.310	0.791	0.231
	3 min	1.572	1.384	1.850	0.457
	10 min	1.723	—0.244	—0.035	—0.512
296	Resting	0.797	—1.017	—0.219	0.175
	Immediate	0.624	1.327	1.302	0.921
	3 min	0.357	2.304	2.769	0.774
	10 min	0.029	2.340	3.673	0.803

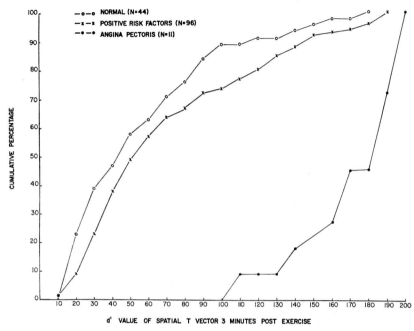

d' VALUE OF SPATIAL T VECTOR 3 MINUTES POST EXERCISE

FIGURE 9-6. Cumulative-percentage curves for normal group, group with positive risk factors, and angina pectoris group.

of symptomatic coronary heart disease and that our study will be incomplete without this longitudinal follow-up. However, within the scope of this study, this method of exercise stress testing shows promise of improving diagnostic accuracy in electrocardiographic stress testing.

MO-18 APOLLO SPACEFLIGHT EXPERIMENT

We have a unique opportunity to apply the methods described above in the Apollo Applications Program. This National Aeronautics and Space Administration project is a complex series of space flights (Fig. 9-7) that involves initial rendezvous with a spent stage of the Saturn rocket, the establishment of an orbiting laboratory, return of the crew to Earth, and a second series of flights and rendezvous with the orbiting laboratory at a later date. A series of scientific and medical experiments will be carried out during the project. The time available for medical experiments on the first portion of the flight will be approximately eleven days; in the second phase of the flight

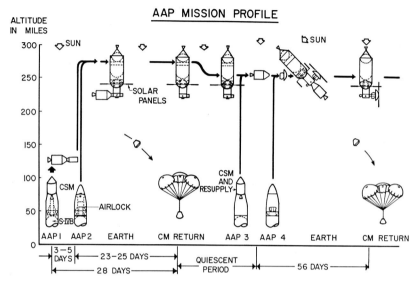

FIGURE 9-7. Profile of Apollo Applications Project. (Reprinted with permission from *Circulation,* Vol. 34:1044, 1966.)

there will be thirty-eight days available for medical experiments. The orbiting laboratory is quite roomy and consists of several compartments. Experiments will be carried out in a "shirt sleeves" environment (without pressure suits) at 100 per cent oxygen at 5 psia.

In experiment MO-18 we plan to utilize the Frank lead system and serially record vectorcardiograms. In addition, a bicycle ergometer will be used to furnish a standardized work load, and postexercise electrocardiograms will be relayed to receiving stations by a digital telemetry system. We will have access to the astronaut crewmembers prior to the flight for multiple control studies and we will retest the crewmembers after their return to Earth. During the flight we will test each astronaut at intervals of three days. The electrocardiographic recording systems used in the previous space flights have not been adequate for quantitative interpretations. Since electrocardiographic changes have been observed in simulated weightless states such as prolonged water immersion and prolonged bed rest, quantitative electrocardiographic analysis should yield interesting findings in space flights of long duration.

REFERENCES

1. MASON, J.K.; TOWNSEND, F.M., and JACKSON, J.R.: Death from coronary disease while at the controls of an aircraft. *Aerospace Med, 34*:858, 1963.

2. MATTINGLY, T.W.; ROBB, G.P., and MARKS, H.H.: Electrocardiographic stress tests in suspected coronary disease: Long-term statistical evaluation of the types of response to the double standard two-step exercise test and the anoxemia test. WRAIR-75-57. Washington, D.C., Walter Reed Army Institute of Research, Walter Reed Army Medical Center, 1957.

3. RUMBALL, A., and ACHESON, E.D.: Latent coronary heart disease detected by electrocardiogram before and after exercise. *Brit Med J, 1*:423, 1963.

4. SMITH, R.F.: Comparison of three exercise devices for the electrocardiographic stress test. NSAM-906, Pensacola, Fla., U.S. Naval School of Aviation Medicine, 1964.

5. GRAYBIEL, A., and ALLEBACH, N.W.: Work electrocardiogram. *Amer J Cardiol, 3*:430, 1959.

6. FRANK, E.: An accurate clinically practical system for spatial vectorcardiography. *Circulation, 13*:737, 1956.

7. ARNOLD, T.G., and SMITH, R.F.: Instrument for electrocardiographic area measurements. NSAM-895, Pensacola, Fla., U.S. Naval School of Aviation Medicine, 1964.

8. SMITH, R.F., and WHERRY, R.J. JR.: Quantitative interpretation of the exercise electrocardiogram. *Circulation, 34*:1044, 1966.

9. GRAYBIEL, A.; PACKARD, J.M., and GRAETTINGER, J.S.: Twelve year follow-up study of 1056 U.S. Naval flyers. *Milit Surg, 112*:328, 1953.

10. OBERMAN, A.; LANE, N.E.; MITCHELL, R.E., and GRAYBIEL, A.: The thousand aviator study: Distribution and intercorrelation of selected variables. Monograph 12. NASA R-136 and U.S. Public Health Service. Pensacola, Fla., Naval Aerospace Medical Institute, 1965.

DISCUSSION

Dr. Smith: Doctor Otto Schmitt asks in essence whether we used a curvilinear expression of the difference between an individual vector terminus and the mean vector terminus of the normal group, or whether a linear measurement was made.

The curvilinear measurement could be considered as the arc of our hypothetical sphere with unity radius and the linear measure as the chord. For small differences between the individual vector terminus and the terminus of the central value there would be very little difference in the arc length and the chord length. The relationship between arc and chord can be appreciated from the following two equations:

$$\text{Arc} \quad = \frac{\pi r \theta}{180}$$

$$\text{Chord} = 2r \sin \tfrac{1}{2}\theta$$

where r is the radius of the sphere, and θ is the central angle. For the extreme case when angle θ is 180°, the d′ value in our method of analysis would be 2.0 and the length of the arc would be 3.1. We have compared curvilinear d′ values (arc length) in our analysis and have found that they are not as discriminating as linear d′ values (chord length).

10

Fourier Analysis of Exercise Electrocardiograms

L. H. Dworetzky, R. I. Bristow, J. M. Endres,
G. J. Haupt, *and* N. C. Birkhead

INTRODUCTION

THE FOURIER SERIES is perhaps the most powerful mathematical method in existence for the description and analysis of periodic wave forms. Since the Exercise Electrocardiogram (EECG) is essentially periodic in time, it is natural to employ a Fourier series to describe it; that is to describe it by an infinite, linear sum of harmonic terms in the form

$$y(t) = \frac{A_o}{2} + \sum_{n=1}^{\infty} A_n \cos (2\pi n f_o t - \varnothing_n) \qquad (1)$$

where:

$$
\begin{aligned}
y(t) &= \text{Potential of the EECG at any instant} \\
n &= \text{Index of summation} \\
A_n &= \text{Amplitude of the } n^{th} \text{ harmonic} \\
f_o &= \text{Heart rate} = \text{frequency of first harmonic} \\
\varnothing_n &= \text{Phase of the } n^{th} \text{ harmonic}
\end{aligned}
$$

Among the advantages of this representation is the ability to look at the wave as a function of frequency. Information which is not readily visible in the time domain is often apparent in the frequency domain.

Although the Fourier series has been available for over 150 years to describe periodic functions, this method has been applied to the electrocardiogram only very recently. Scher and Young (1) utilized a Fourier series to study the QRS complex in seventeen normal persons and eight patients. The basic objective of their study was to

[145]

determine the frequency components of these electrocardiograms to evaluate the frequency bandwidth requirements for ECG recorders. The QRS complex can be expected to contain the highest frequencies in the ECG. In part, they determined that frequencies of 100 cycles per second or higher make up less than 10 per cent of the amplitude of the fundamental of the QRS complex. Cady and associates (2) utilized the amplitude relationships of certain selected harmonics of a Fourier series to separate left ventricular hypertrophy from normal electrocardiograms. They also found that a very close fit to the original electrocardiograms could be reconstructed from the first thirty-four Fourier terms. In 1962, Thompson (3) published a study of Fourier analysis of normal cardiograms and on the basis of this study, he believed that further use of this technique might be very valuable in providing clinically useful information. In particular, he suggested that a correlation between variation of the amplitude of certain harmonics and various clinical states might be evolved.

The present study deals with the application of the Fourier analysis technique to electrocardiograms obtained at rest and during two levels of exercise in a group of eleven normal subjects and twelve patients with abnormal exercise cardiograms. This preliminary study is part of a long-term effort undertaken to characterize the exercise electrocardiogram and to search for new discriminants between normal and abnormal records, which are not obvious by inspection of the tracing.

METHODS

Exercise electrocardiographic recordings were analyzed of eleven normal subjects and twelve patients studied in the Ergocardiographic Laboratory of the Division of Research, Lankenau Hospital. The eleven normal subjects ranged in age from eighteen to twenty-two years and were previously shown to be free from cardiovascular disease by history, physical examination, chest x-ray and rest electrocardiograms. They also had normal peripheral and central arterial pressure pulses directly recorded, normal arterial indicator dilution curves, and normal hemodynamic responses to a 70° head-up tilt test and the Valsalva maneuver.

The twelve patient records were selected from the files of the Ergocardiographic Laboratory. The ages of these patients were as follows:

forty to forty-nine years—two patients; fifty to fifty-nine years—three patients; sixty to sixty-nine years—five patients; and seventy to seventy-nine years—two patients. Although all twelve patients were ambulatory, five had symptomatic coronary artery disease, and one had previously sustained two myocardial infarctions. Two patients had essential hypertension, one had gout, and the four remaining cases were free of symptoms of major disease when studied. The exercise tracings of these patients were selected only on the basis of showing at least one millimeter of ST segment depression during exercise.

In normal subjects, ECG tracings recorded during two levels of exercise were examined. One level was either 450 or 600 kpm*/per minute carried out on a stationary bicycle ergometer for five minutes. After a five-minute rest, the higher level of exercise 1050, 1200, or 1500 kpm/min was undertaken again for five minutes. The higher exercise level was chosen to be at or near the maximum aerobic capacity for each subject. ECG tracings were taken during the last ten seconds of each minute of exercise. The tracings selected for Fourier analysis were those obtained during the fifth minute of exercise at each level and the rest tracing was obtained before the beginning of the first exercise level.

A somewhat different exercise test was given to the patients. Depending on each patient's clinical status and pre-exercise ECG, exercise was begun at either 150 or 300 kpm/min. The exercise load was then increased by 150 kpm/min, after each two minutes of exercise, according to exercise stress tests developed by one of us (N.C.B.) over several years in the Ergocardiographic Laboratory. Exercise tracings were obtained during the last ten seconds of each minute of exercise. The maximal exercise level reached a range from 300 to 750 kpm/min. Exercise was terminated with the appearance of significant ECG changes (*increase* in ST segment depression of 1 millimeter or more, or the appearance of significant arrhythmia), chest pain or muscular fatigue. In each of these patients, exercise was terminated because of the degree of ST segment depression. In addition, two cases developed anginal pain at the time ST segment depression occurred. In both the normal subjects and patients, a modified lead V_4 or V_6 was mon-

---

*Kilopond meter/min. 1 Kp = force acting on a mass 1 kg at normal acceleration of gravity. 1 kpm/min = 7.238 ftlb/min = .00219 HP = 1.63 watts.

itored during exercise and this lead was the one utilized for Fourier analysis. A description of the electrodes and lead position utilized, has been published previously (4). The data acquisition system employed in this investigation had a measured bandwidth between the half power points which extended from 0.15 cps to 70 cps.

The lowest heart rate present in the records of the twenty-three subjects was 55 beats/min or 0.92 cps. The highest heart rate reached was 198 beats/min or 198 cps at the 60th harmonic. Because of the bandwidth characteristics of the data acquisition system, the amplitudes of the higher harmonics would be attenuated to some degree. This attenuation would affect the results of the normal subjects more than the patients because of the greater energy in the higher harmonics in the normal subjects.

Harmonic analysis was applied to one complex of each cardiogram analyzed, so that each complex was represented by a Fourier series truncated at the 60th harmonic. The particular form of harmonic analysis employed is essentially a computer mechanization of the procedure given in "Sokolnikoff and Redheffer" (5). One complete complex of the cardiogram to be analyzed was manually divided into 120 equal time intervals, after photographic enlargement, which expanded the 1 mm square grid of standard ECG paper to a 10 mm square grid. Values of $y(t)$ were measured at these 120 points. These values of $y(t)$ were used to perform the harmonic analysis for each of the complexes on a GE 605 Computer. Values of A_n and $\emptyset_n$ were thus obtained for 60 harmonics for each complex. The dc term, the constant term $\dfrac{A_o}{2}$, was discarded since the values of $y(t)$ were not measured from the baseline, but instead from an arbitrary and convenient reference line which varied from case to case. The dc term is thus arbitrary. The remaining values of A_n for each series were then normalized by dividing them by the amplitude, A_1, of the fundamental or first harmonic. This normalization procedure was used to eliminate those individual variations in the amplitudes of corresponding harmonics caused by inter-individual differences in heart rate. The number of equidistant values of $y(t)$ chosen is based on Shannon's theorem (6), which states that a continuous function of time is completely determined by ordinates spaced at distances equal to the reciprocal of

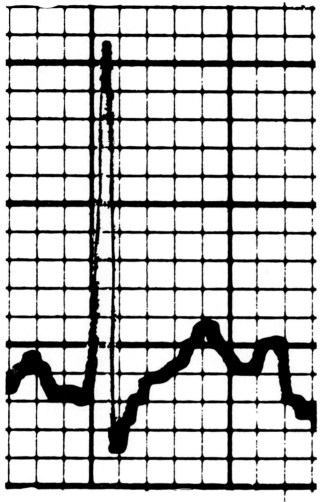

INPUT DATA:

=228	228	228	229	228	233	236	242	246	251	253	256
257	258	263	271	273	273	268	262	258	256	256	251
243	233	226	221	218	219	218	216	216	216	216	216
213	212	211	208	209	208	211	221	239	256	276	322
408	481	558	649	736	816	825	746	568	401	246	138
147	159	166	172	178	187	197	201	203	206	212	222
236	237	241	242	242	243	246	247	251	252	254	256
258	263	266	268	274	277	281	287	291	293	298	304
311	317	322	326	328	328	329	326	324	318	313	306
301	296	291	286	282	278	276	268	266	262	261	261

FIGURE 10-1. Exercise ECG complex from normal subject and amplitude values measured at 120 equidistant points. The ECG recording (modified lead V_6) was obtained during the last ten seconds of a five-minute bicycle ergometer ride at 1050 kpm/min. The amplitude measurements for 120 equidistant points within this complex which are shown in the lower panel were performed on a photographic enlargement ($\times$ 10) of this complex.

BASELINE-ADJUSTED DATA:

228·	228·	227·	228·	227·	232·	234·	240·	244·	249·	250·	253·
254·	254·	259·	267·	269·	268·	263·	257·	252·	250·	250·	245·
236·	226·	219·	214·	210·	211·	210·	207·	207·	207·	207·	206·
203·	202·	200·	197·	198·	197·	199·	209·	227·	244	263·	309·
395·	467·	544·	635·	722·	801·	810·	731·	552·	385·	230·	122·
130·	142·	149·	155·	160·	169·	179·	182·	184·	187·	193·	202·
216·	217·	220·	221·	221·	222·	224·	225·	229·	230·	231·	233·
235·	239·	242·	244·	250·	252·	256·	262·	265·	267·	272·	278·
284·	290·	295·	299·	300·	300·	301·	297·	295·	289·	284·	276·
271·	266·	260·	255·	251·	247·	244·	236·	234·	230·	228·	228·

H#	NORM MAG
1	1.000
2	2.077
3	2.561
4	2.151
5	2.012
6	1.768
7	1.532
8	1.277
9	1.010
10	0.879
11	0.722
12	0.596
13	0.489
14	0.367
15	0.303
16	0.263
17	0.183
18	0.188
19	0.186
20	0.146
21	0.113
22	0.101
23	0.061
24	0.028
25	0.016
26	0.030
27	0.030
28	0.037
29	0.033
30	0.030

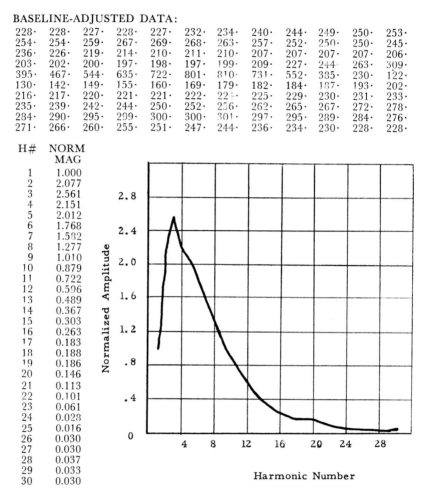

FIGURE 10-2. Baseline adjusted amplitude values, normalized harmonic content, and envelope spectrum plot of single ECG complex. The upper panel shows the 120 amplitude values of Figure 10-1 adjusted for baseline drift. The lower panel shows the computer output for the harmonic analysis based on these 120 inputs and the resulting plot of the spectrum of the ECG complex shown in Figure 10-1.

twice the highest frequency present in the wave. Thus if the highest frequency expected to be present in the cardiogram is sixty times the heart rate, then the complex to be analyzed should be divided into 120 equal time intervals.

RESULTS

Figure 10-1 shows a single ECG complex (modified lead V_6) from a normal subject at the fifth minute of exercise at 1050 kpm/ min. The ordinates for 120 equidistant points in this complex are also shown. Figure 10-2 (*top*) shows these values after correction for baseline drift. The latter values serve as the digital input information for the Fourier analysis computer program. The computer printout of the normalized amplitude values and the plot of the envelope of the amplitude spectrum for the first 30 harmonics are shown at the bottom of the figure. In this subject, at this exercise load, the peak amplitude occurs at the 3rd harmonic (2.8 cps). There is a gradual decrease in amplitude as shown to the 30th harmonic. Data beyond the 30th harmonic was not plotted because the amplitudes decayed very rapidly beyond this point.

Figures 10-3 and 10-4 show the envelopes of the mean values for the Fourier spectra at rest, and at two levels of exercise for the eleven normal subjects and twelve patients, respectively. Table 10-I shows the standard deviation for the individual spectra. In both groups the amplitudes of nearly all harmonics at low exercise levels were larger than at rest. However, the higher exercise load clearly separates the mean spectral ECG responses of the normal and patient groups. In the normal subjects, there was an additional increase in amplitudes at nearly all harmonics with the higher exercise loads. Six of the eleven normal subjects showed this response. The mean amplitude values for the patients, on the other hand, decrease at the higher exercise load to resting levels or below. All twelve patients showed this response.

There are also obvious differences in the locations of the peaks and notches seen in the curves from the two groups of subjects. Tables 10-II and 10-III show the number of normals and patients whose individual spectral envelope showed notching and peaking in the first ten harmonics.

Although the phase angle information is also calculated by this computer program, this information is still under analysis.

DISCUSSION

If the precise functional form of the P, QRS and T waves of the

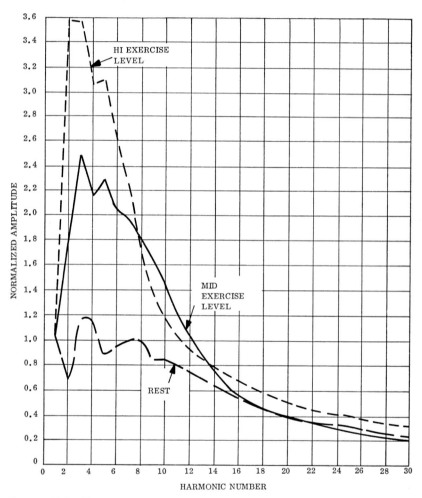

FIGURE 10-3. Fourier spectra envelopes of ECGs at three exercise levels in eleven normal subjects. The amplitude of each harmonic is normalized to the first harmonic for each subject, and the mean values plotted against harmonic number. The dc level has been discarded. Note the increase in amplitude of most harmonics as the exercise load is increased.

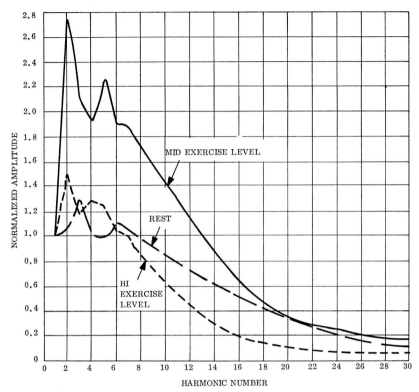

FIGURE 10-4. Fourier spectra enevlopes of ECGs at three exercise levels in twelve patients with ST segment depression. Normalized mean amplitude values are plotted as in Figure 10-3. Note the difference in response at the high exercise level to that of the normal group, Figure 10-3.

ECG were known, it would be theoretically possible to employ equation (1), where the amplitude coefficient A_n is defined by

$$A_n = 2f_o \sqrt{\left[\int_o^{1/f_o} y(t) \sin 2\pi nf_o tdt\right]^2 + \left[\int_o^{1/f_o} y(t) \cos 2\pi nf_o tdt\right]^2}$$

and the phases of the harmonics $\emptyset_n$ are defined by

$$\tan \emptyset_n = \frac{\int_o^{1/f_o} y(t) \sin 2\pi nf_o tdt}{\int_o^{1/f_o} y(t) \cos 2\pi nf_o tdt}$$

together with amplitude and duration measurements for each of the waves to derive the series for any cardiogram. However, the

TABLE 10-I

STANDARD DEVIATIONS OF THE FIRST THIRTY HARMONICS
AT EACH EXERCISE LEVEL

Harmonic Number	11 Normal Subjects			12 Patients		
	Rest	Mid Exercise	High Exercise	Rest	Mid Exercise	High Exercise
2	.823	.857	3.898	.494	2.153	.845
3	.566	1.076	3.784	.623	1.849	.510
4	.521	1.100	2.940	.301	1.393	.432
5	.660	1.288	3.029	.423	1.534	.557
6	.605	1.046	2.450	.468	1.159	.340
7	.538	1.189	1.855	.343	1.298	.367
8	.551	1.082	1.324	.360	1.046	.288
9	.544	1.044	1.071	.360	1.010	.230
10	.507	.941	.993	.320	.876	.192
11	.457	.839	1.036	.331	.804	.142
12	.427	.707	1.059	.316	.669	.118
13	.411	.615	.995	.304	.661	.112
14	.362	.462	.886	.300	.524	.090
15	.334	.343	.835	.280	.482	.083
16	.301	.247	.785	.266	.419	.088
17	.293	.178	.764	.260	.384	.084
18	.264	.144	.729	.247	.345	.082
19	.252	.159	.720	.229	.298	.085
20	.251	.135	.676	.221	.268	.074
21	.246	.163	.618	.213	.238	.068
22	.240	.129	.605	.203	.200	.061
23	.245	.127	.588	.186	.169	.053
24	.254	.104	.561	.176	.151	.038
25	.250	.112	.510	.175	.130	.040
26	.252	.092	.501	.165	.127	.032
27	.249	.103	.479	.151	.112	.033
28	.244	.109	.444	.145	.111	.030
29	.238	.103	.443	.136	.090	.032
30	.233	.108	.431	.125	.083	.037

TABLE 10-II

DISTRIBUTION OF NOTCHES IN AMPLITUDE VS. HARMONIC NUMBER IN PLOTS FOR 11 NORMAL SUBJECTS AND 12 PATIENTS

Harmonic Number:	2	3	4	5	6	7	8	9	10
Exercise Level									
Rest	9*/4**	0/3	1/3	6/5	3/2	0/0	0/0	6/1	0/0
Mid	1/1	2/4	5/5	3/0	1/1	0/0	0/0	0/0	0/0
High	1/2	2/6	5/2	0/1	0/1	0/0	0/0	1/0	2/0

* Number of normal ECGs exhibiting amplitude notch
** Number of patients' ECGs exhibiting amplitude notch

TABLE 10-III

DISTRIBUTION OF PEAKS IN AMPLITUDE VS. HARMONIC NUMBER IN PLOTS FOR 11 NORMAL SUBJECTS AND 12 PATIENTS

Harmonic Number:	2	3	4	5	6	7	8	9	10
Exercise Level									
Rest	1*/2**	4/8	6/1	1/3	4/4	4/4	1/0	1/1	4/3
Mid	0/9	7/1	2/3	2/7	0/0	1/1	1/0	0/0	0/0
High	8/6	2/1	2/8	5/2	0/1	0/1	0/0	0/0	1/0

* Number of normal ECGs exhibiting amplitude peak
** Number of patients' ECGs exhibiting amplitude peak

precise functional form of these waves is not known for any particular situation. The P wave, for example, might be a semicircle, a parabola or the arch of a sine curve. Therefore, in this study, the ECG complexes were described by an approximate Fourier series which consists of a finite sum of terms of the form of equation (1) by the well-known empirical procedure called Harmonic Analysis. Values of $y(t)$ measured at equidistant points in time between the beginning and end of one complex of the cardiogram were used to calculate A_n and $Ø_n$ to yield the spectra of the ECG.

The results of harmonic analysis of the resting ECG tracings in this study are similar to the curves of ECG spectra published by others in that the majority of the energy is found in the first twenty or so harmonics. Obviously, if one includes the data of succeeding higher harmonics, the reconstituted ECG resembles more and more the original signal. Our data indicated, however, that 99 per cent of the energy content can be accounted for within the first twenty-eight harmonics in normal subjects, including the exercise data, and within the first twenty-four harmonics for the patients at rest and exercise.

Of considerable interest is the clear separation of normal subjects and patients in the spectra provided by the higher exercise load. Since the patient EECGs were classified as abnormal by simple inspection, the critical question is whether EECGs from individuals not known to be affected by coronary artery disease and whose tracings appear normal to inspection have a Fourier analysis signature different from that of the normal spectra described here. The wide range of standard deviations in the harmonic content of the normal subjects found does not, in itself, negate the possibility that such a situation may exist. Results of the analysis of phase shift data may provide additional support for this possibility.

Although the difference in response of the EECG to high exercise loads between the normal subjects and the patients cannot be interpreted adequately at this time, it is tempting to speculate on the similarity of this phenomenon to the performance of certain man-made equipment. The response of the patients, for example, might be likened to the decrease in gain of an overdriven amplifier.

Since the cardiograms analyzed in this study were recorded, the half power bandwidth of the data acquisition system has been extended to range from below 0.05 cps to above 200 cps. Data to be used in a study of a much larger sample of subjects is being taken on this newer system.

SUMMARY

Harmonic analysis was performed on ECG complexes recorded from eleven normal subjects aged eighteen to twenty-two years and twelve patients aged forty-four to seventy-two years at rest and at two levels of exercise on a bicycle ergometer. All patients showed ST segment depression of 1 mm or more during exercise. In both groups the amplitudes of nearly all harmonics at lower exercise levels were larger than at rest and in six of eleven normals, further increases in amplitudes occurred at the higher exercise load. In all twelve patients a decrease in harmonic amplitudes occurred at the higher load. Ninety-nine per cent of the energy content of representative tracings could be accounted for within the first twenty-eight harmonics in normal subjects and within the first twenty-four harmonics in the patients including the exercise data. Fourier analysis of exercise ECGs appears to warrant further study.

REFERENCES

1. SCHER, A.M., and YOUNG, A.C.: Frequency analysis of the electrocardiogram. *Circ Res, 8*:344-346, 1960.
2. CADY, L.D., JR.; WOODBURY, M.A.; TICK, L.J., and GERTLER, M.M.: A method for electrocardiogram wave-pattern estimation. Example: left ventricular hypertrophy. *Circ Res, 9*:1078-1082, 1961.
3. THOMPSON, N.P.: Fourier analysis of the electrocardiographic function, *Amer J Med Electronics,* 1962, Vol. I.
4. BARRY, A.J.; DALY, J.W.; PRUETT, E.D.R.; STEINMETZ, J.R.; BIRKHEAD, N.C., and RODAHL, K.: Effects of physical training in patients who have had myocardial infarction. *Amer J Cardiol, 17*:1-8, 1966.
5. SOKOLNIKOFF, I.S., and REDHEFFER, R.M.: *Mathematics of Physics and Modern Engineering.* New York, McGraw, 1958, p. 711, *et seq.*
6. GOLDMAN, S.: *Information Theory.* Englewood Cliffs, Prentice-Hall, 1953, p. 67.

PART THREE

BIOENGINEERING PROBLEMS AND SPECIFICATIONS OF AUTOMATED SYSTEMS OF EXERCISE ELECTROCARDIOGRAPHY

11

Noise Measurement and Quality Control Techniques in Recording and Processing of Exercise Electrocardiograms

DAVID A. WINTER

DURING THE RECORDING of exercise electrocardiograms, or during the subsequent processing of the recorded signal, a quantitative indication is required that the noise content is within some predetermined level. Visual inspection can give a qualitative indication of the quality of the record; however, it is desirable to have a more accurate and more automatic system. Elaborate digital filtering techniques can assist in noise reduction after it has been fed into a digital computer, but these programs cannot be done in real-time, and may be very time consuming. With small special purpose averaging computers the results may not be satisfactory. Rautaharju (1) has reported that about 10 per cent of the exercise records made during submaximal stress produced erroneous results. This was attributed to excessively noisy artifacts perturbing the average as well as causing false triggers, missed triggers and signal distortions such as smoothing error (2).

It is therefore necessary to examine the characteristics of the noise itself. We have defined noise as any additive perturbation, whether random or periodic. A summary of our noise measurement techniques, and the results, have been reported (3) and are summarized in Figure 11-1.

Generally speaking, the higher frequency components such as hum or myoelectric signals can be filtered out by averaging techniques

Note: This work was supported through research grants from the Medical Research Council and the Canadian Heart Foundation.

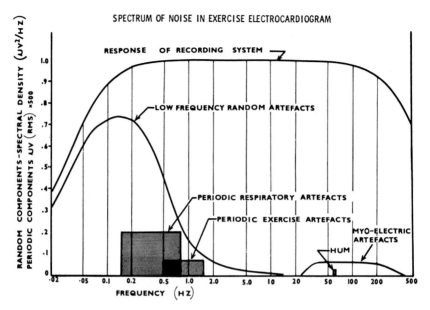

FIGURE 11-1. Summary of spectrum of components of noise present in exercise electrocardiograms. The periodic components are scaled in μv(rms) while the random components are plotted as a density function.

or by a moving average type filter in a digital computer. However, the components that cause problems are the lower frequency random and periodic components plus single large amplitude spikes or step changes. One method recently described (4) works satisfactorily, but is too expensive to realize. A second method (5) recently developed in Halifax is able to assess the total noise content of these latter components within each ECG complex. The circuitry for this analysis is such that at the end of each complex, in the electrically inactive region between T and P waves, a measure of the total noise within that complex is instantaneously known and is recorded. This quality control circuit can be realized fairly cheaply utilizing integrated operational amplifiers now on the market. Components cost about $200.00, a reasonably inexpensive device. A quantitative assessment of the noise is a prerequisite of any system designed to process exercise records automatically or semiautomatically. To operate in real-time, such a system should be able to assess the quality of the record, complex by complex, and be able to reject excessively noisy complexes before

SCHEMATIC DIAGRAM OF REAL - TIME QUALITY CONTROL SYSTEM

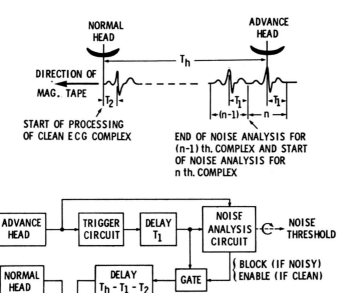

FIGURE 11-2. Schematic diagram of an on-line quality control system designed to reject excessively noisy ECG complexes. For operation of system see text.

they are fed into the computer. An overall schematic diagram of such a system under development in Halifax is shown in Figure 11-2.

The ECG tape is played back from both the normal and advance heads. The signal from the advance head serves two purposes. First it generates through a suitable trigger and delay (T_1) circuit the pulse required to commence noise analysis on the ECG complex about to pass under the advance head. This same pulse also commences the normal interhead delay, T_H-T_1-T_2, required for triggering the ECG signal from the normal head into a computer of average transients. However, if the quality control circuit indicates the presence of an ECG complex noisier than a preset value, a block pulse is generated so as to prevent the generation of this interhead delay just described. Therefore, the noisy ECG complexes will not receive a trigger pulse as they pass under the normal head, while the cleaner signals will be triggered into memory T_2 ms before the R wave of that particular complex.

FREQUENCY CONTENT OF R - WAVE TRIGGER AND RESPONSE OF ACTIVE FILTER

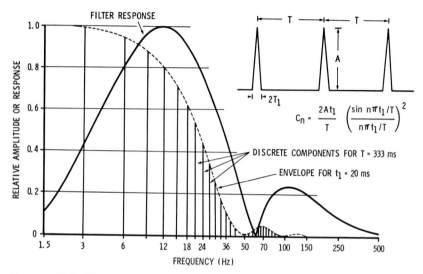

FIGURE 11-3. Frequency response of the active filter section of the trigger circuit compared to the spectrum of typical R waves.

The trigger circuit is described because of its importance to the overall operation of this system. If the trigger produced is false or misses, the noise analysis circuit will be triggered into operation at the wrong time within the ECG complex. The result will be an erroneous analysis of noise over an incomplete ECG complex or over more than one complex. It is therefore essential that a reliable trigger circuit be devised. The active filter section of our trigger circuit has a frequency response as shown in Figure 11-3 compared to the frequency spectrum of typical R waves. The net result of this filter is such that most of the spectrum of the noise is rejected while about 2/3 power in the R wave trigger is passed. The schematic detail of the trigger circuit appears in Figure 11-4, the additional features being designed to further discriminate against all but the R wave. The squaring circuits are nonlinear amplifiers which have a low gain for low amplitude signal and noise components and high gain for the peaks of the R wave. Also available are inputs for two orthogonal components, the X and Z signals. The reason the Y lead was omitted from triggering was because it was found, on the average,

SCHEMATIC OF R - WAVE FILTER AND TRIGGER CIRCUIT

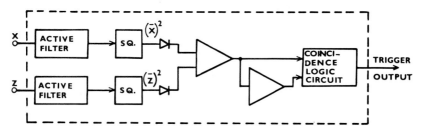

FIGURE 11-4. Schematic diagram of complete trigger circuit.

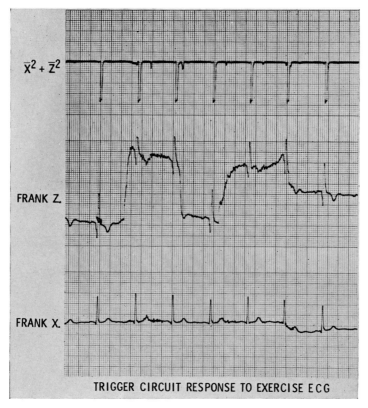

TRIGGER CIRCUIT RESPONSE TO EXERCISE ECG

FIGURE 11-5. Response of active filter section of trigger circuit to a typical excessively noisy input, when dual inputs are used.

to be four times as noisy as either the X or Z lead (3,5) and also had a less prominent R wave required for triggering. A summation of the X^2 and Z^2 signals produced the desirable effect of reinforcing the in-phase R waves and causing partial cancellation of the out-of-phase noise component. This technique is another example of noise reduction by means of spatial averaging (3). As a final discrimination against sharply spiked noise artifacts or sharp baseline jumps, a coincidence logic circuit is incorporated which triggers, on receipt of a filtered R wave of sufficient slope and of duration, not less than 20 ms and not more than 60 ms. Any false triggering from this circuit is the result of an artifact that looks too much like an R wave to be discriminated. Using X and Z signals, in Figure 11-5 are shown some very noisy ECGs with the resultant trigger signal.

One further test was carried out using this trigger circuit on typical noisy records to determine the deviation of the triggering point to see how well it served as a fiducial point in time. These results were compared with similar deviation analyses obtained from triggers derived from unfiltered ECGs. The results of this latter investigation will be presented first in order to indicate the error that can occur. Maximum deviations in the trigger point varied from ± 5 ms in a relatively noise-free exercise record to ± 12 ms in a very noisy record (3). In Figure 11-6, we see the smoothing error due to averaging one of these very noisy recordings (3). It should be noted that the averages shown do not include the residue of noise, but show only the distortion of the QRS signal complex due to variations in the trigger point about the fiducial point. A second important point is the effect of increasing the trigger threshold; the distortion due to smoothing error is actually increased. This is due to the fact that the increased trigger threshold causes more missed triggers when the noise has a negative polarity. Thus a greater percentage of the complexes are averaged when the noise has a positive polarity, and this results in early triggering; thus the extra distortion shown.

By the use of the active filter described the maximum deviation in triggering was found to average 3.5 ms for the X signal itself, 3 ms for the Z lead and 2.5 ms for the combined X and Z signals. The resultant smoothing error from such small deviations would be negligible.

SMOOTHING ERROR DUE TO EXCESSIVE NOISE IN E CG TRIGGER

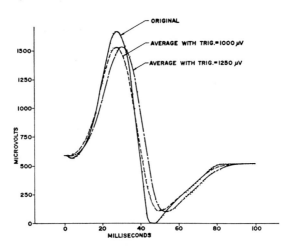

FIGURE 11-6. The mean smoothing error from averaging of a noisy exercise tracing is on the order of 3 msec.

With reliable triggering we can then analyze the quality of the exercise records and process them into a computer. Processing of signals by averaging techniques is a typical method. Here we may have a limited number of ECG complexes available, so there must be some assurance that excessively noisy complexes are eliminated from the averaging process lest they unduly distort the final result. All that is needed is a warning or blocking signal to prevent the averaging of the noisier complexes. Such blocking pulses are shown in Figure 11-7; here they are generated at the instant that the amount of noise present, as indicated by the output of the integrator circuit, exceeds some preset threshold value.

We may do one of two things with these warning pulses. First, we may use them as a visual warning that the recording is getting excessively noisy. Or, we may consider it to be an automatic blocking pulse which can be suitably arranged to prevent the triggering of the noisy ECG complex when it passes under the normal playback lead. Results from the automated system described at the beginning of this paper are given in Figure 11-8. Here we see the average of twelve of the cleanest of a group of signals from about a fifty-second record of an extremely noisy Frank Y lead. It can be seen to have

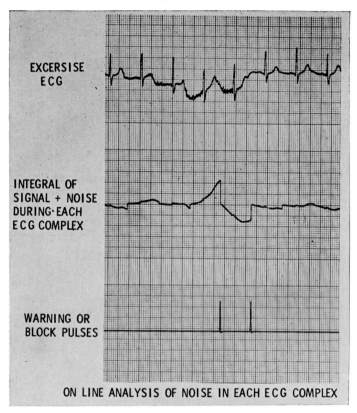

EXCERSISE ECG

INTEGRAL OF SIGNAL + NOISE DURING·EACH ECG COMPLEX

WARNING OR BLOCK PULSES

ON LINE ANALYSIS OF NOISE IN EACH ECG COMPLEX

FIGURE 11-7. Recording of ECG noise analysis system. Measure of noise in each complex is given by the integral of the ECG signal over that complex. Blocking pulses are produced when the integral of the noise and signal at the end of each complex exceeds a threshold value.

distinct Q, R and S peaks, and is a good curve for only twelve complexes. As we permit noisier and noisier complexes to be triggered into memory the average becomes quite distorted, and if we trigger all complexes we see further distortion.

In summary, we can say that it is desirable to have routine processing of exercise ECGs done in real-time, which necessitates some form of instantaneous quality control. The output of the quality control would normally indicate that the noise content had exceeded some predetermined value. It could act as a visual warning when recording the signals, or during subsequent processing; or it could automatically

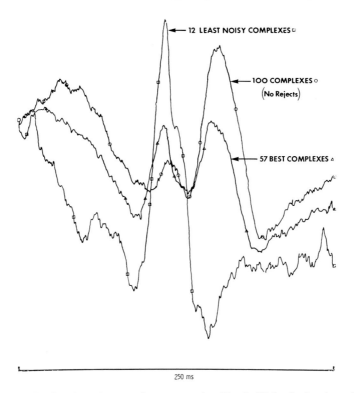

FIGURE 11-8. Results of averaging very noisy Frank Y lead signals utilizing the automatic quality control system in which those complexes above a predetermined threshold were rejected. See text for details.

block the entry of the noisy sections of the record into the computer. The system we have proposed and constructed achieves these goals at a fairly reasonable cost. Associated with this electronic hardware is a reliable trigger circuit which has three desirable characteristics; it minimizes false and missed triggers, and has an acceptable deviation as a fiducial point in time.

REFERENCES

1. RAUTAHARJU, P.M.; WINTER, D.A.; WONG, A.Y.K., and BLACKBURN, H.: Computer analysis of the exercise electrocardiogram. International Symp. on Electrical Activity of the Heart, Univ. of Western Ontario. Springfield, Thomas, 1967 (to be published).

2. RAUTAHARJU, P.M .,and H. BLACKBURN: The exercise electrocardiogram. *Amer. Heart J, 69*:515, 1965.

3. WINTER, D.A.; RAUTAHARJU, P.M., and WOLF, H.K.: Noise content in exercise electrocardiograms. *Amer. Heart J, 74*:324, 1967.
4. WINTER, D.A.: Quality control in recording of exercise electrocardiograms. Digest of 1st Canadian Medical and Biological Conference, Ottawa, Ont., Sept. 8-9, 1966.
5. WINTER, D.A.: Analysis and Reduction of Noise in Exercise Electrocardiograms. Ph. D. thesis, Dalhousie University, Halifax, N.S., 1967.

12

Assessment of Precision and Accuracy of Computer Programs for Analysis of Electrocardiograms

HERMANN WOLF *and* PENTTI M. RAUTAHARJU

INTRODUCTION

AUTOMATED MEASUREMENT and analysis is becoming an increasingly important method in electrocardiography. In many instances, as in analysis of the ECG response to exercise, it is necessary to measure signals less than 50 μv in amplitude in the presence of relatively large amounts of noise, and it would be exceedingly difficult to attempt any quantitative measurements without computer analysis.

Assessment of precision and accuracy of computer measurements has been almost completely neglected throughout the early years of computer-assisted ECG studies. Practically the only method used so far has been comparison of the visual and computer measurements. Computer measurements are regarded as satisfactory if they approximately agree with the visual measurements. A subjective and in many circumstances unreliable and erratic method is used as a standard which prevents improvement of technique beyond the accuracy of visual methods. Procedures have been developed recently to measure the noise and its characteristics from an exercise ECG record (1,2,3,4). Although it is possible to control 60 Hz noise with careful recording techniques, it continues to be the most common problem in routine recordings done in hospitals and field studies. Most of the noise in exercise records is random (2). Once the noise and signal character-

Note: This work was supported through research grants from the Medical Research Council and the Canadian Heart Foundation, and was done during Mr. Wolf's tenure of The Isaac Walton Killam Memorial Scholarship, Dalhousie University.

[169]

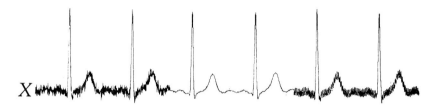

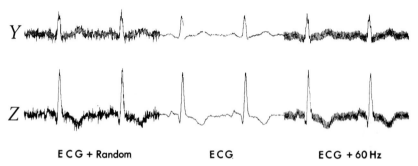

| ECG + Random | ECG | ECG + 60 Hz |

FIGURE 12-1. Examples of records used in noise simulation. The X, Y and Z components of the noise-free control record are in the center. Superimposed on the control record is 60μv rms random noise on the left and 60μv rms 60 Hz noise on the right.

istics are adequately known, it is possible to use simulation techniques for evaluating the precision of computer measurements.

This paper describes one approach for quantitative assessment of the performance of ECG measurement programs in the presence of noise. It also demonstrates the importance of such assessment before any program is accepted for routine use.

The Simulation Principle

Twelve normal Frank lead electrocardiograms were selected for the simulation study. All were high quality resting records digitized at a sampling rate of 500 samples per second per lead. The records were filtered before conversion using a low pass filter with a 3 db point at 150 Hz. Practically no noise could be detected visually from the digitized plots scaled twice the conventional standardization, 1 mv = 20 mm, and it was estimated that the noise level in the original record in the band from 5 to 100 Hz was less than $10\mu v$ rms.

The Mayo IBM program was used for interval and amplitude measurements from the Frank leads (5). The values for amplitudes and intervals measured by the program from noise-free records were accepted as "true" reference values.

Known quantities of random noise and 60 Hz noise were generated by the IBM 1800 computer and superimposed on the digitized records. The noise levels were increased in steps of $10\mu v$ up to a level of $100\mu v$ rms. Interval and amplitude measurements were repeated at all noise levels and the values obtained compared with the reference values of the noise-free records. A total of 46 QRS complexes were measured from the records of twelve subjects at each noise level, a total of 966 QRS complexes. A mathematical description of the characteristics of the noise is given in detail in Appendix B.

Only the precision of QRS interval measurement was evaluated in the present study. A variety of different logic decision rules are used in various ECG programs for defining the onset and offset for QRS. It must be emphasized that all of these are arbitrary and they cannot be related in any simple way to events corresponding to the beginning and end of excitaton of the ventricles. It is very important, however, that the onset and the offset of QRS as defined be located as precisely as possible at all expected noise levels.

Examples of records used in noise simulation are shown in Figure 12-1.

RESULTS

The simulation program makes a list of noise levels where the error in QRS measurement is equal to or larger than 10 msec. This noise level is defined here as the critical level for QRS measurement.

Figure 12-2 shows the distribution of critical noise levels for forty-six QRS complexes measured. In one-half of the records, the critical noise level was about $40\mu v$ for the random noise and $50\mu v$ for the 60 Hz noise. The distribution of critical noise levels for 60 Hz noise is very asymmetric. In eight out of forty-six records (17 per cent)

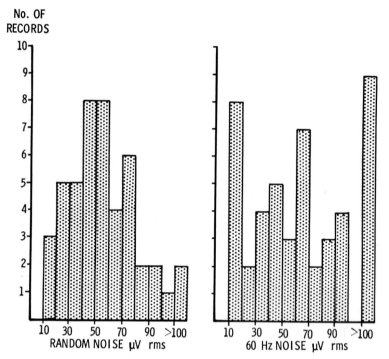

No. OF
RECORDS

FIGURE 12-2. Distribution of critical noise levels for $\geqslant$ 10 msec error in QRS duration measurement with the December 1967 version of the Mayo-IBM program. Critical noise levels for random noise (*left*), and from periodic noise (*right*).

10 msec error occurred already at the noise level of $10\mu v$ rms, whereas in about 20 per cent of records the critical noise level was beyond $100\mu v$ rms. The distribution of critical noise levels for random noise is more symmetric. In three out of forty-six records (6.5 per cent), the critical noise level was $10\mu v$ rms.

It was decided that the performance of the program must be improved to reduce sensitivity particularly to 60 Hz noise. The program was modified by incorporating a digital filter described in Appendix A. The results from measurements with the modified version of the program are summarized in Figure 12-3. The filter considerably improves the performance of the program in the simulation runs with 60 Hz noise. In all but one QRS measurement, the error was less than 10 msec up to noise levels of $100\mu v$ rms. The improvement was

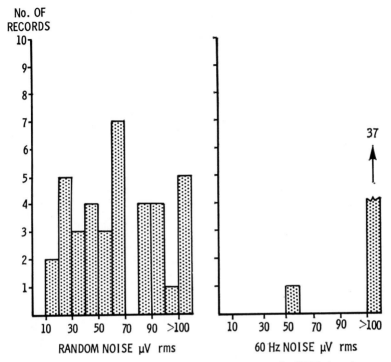

FIGURE 12-3. Critical noise levels for ⩾ 10 msecs error in QRS duration measurement with a modified version of the Mayo-IBM program.

much less pronounced for random noise. The mean value of the critical noise level distribution has shifted only by 10μv, from 40 to 50μv rms. It appears that other forms of filtering are necessary for random noise.

The convenience of the simulation approach in assessing the consistency of the measurements is depicted in Figure 12-4. The onset and offset of the QRS as defined and located by the original and the modified version of the program are shown below the spatial magnitude curve for all noise levels simulated. It is possible to verify with one glance whether modification by a filtering process really improves precision of the measurements. It is also possible to assess separately the reliability of the logic used for defining onset and offset of QRS.

DISCUSSION

Perhaps the most significant result of this investigation is develop-

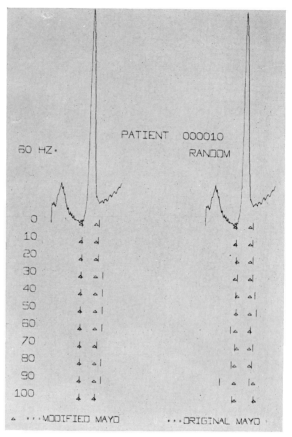

FIGURE 12-4. The QRS onset and offset points at ten simulated noise levels as determined by two different computer programs. The noise levels are given in μv rms. The curve above the onset-offset marks is the spatial vector magnitude computed from the Frank leads.

ment of an automatic technique to evaluate critically and objectively the performance of an ECG measurement program. New programs can be designed and old programs improved and the improvement can be measured quantitatively and documented.

Measurement of the QRS duration was selected as a criterion for performance in this investigation. Measurement of all intervals and amplitudes used for diagnosis must be evaluated in a similar fashion. Determination of the onset and offset of QRS is perhaps the most crucial item in any automated ECG analysis program. These time points are used not only for determination of the QRS duration but also as reference points for most other interval and amplitude measurements. The QRS offset is of particular importance for analysis of exercise electrocardiograms because it defines the QRS-ST junction.

In our opinion, and based on diagnostic needs, the QRS duration should be measured with at least 10 msec precision at all expected noise levels. Frequent errors exceeding 10 msec at noise levels of 10 or $20\mu v$ rms are considered unacceptable.

This investigation indicates that the 60 Hz noise problem can be almost completely eliminated as far as QRS duration measurement is concerned. Elimination of random noise on the other hand, can be considerably more difficult and requires more sophisticated approaches.

The results are based solely on the measurement of QRS duration from reasonably normal types of QRS patterns. Considerably worse performance could be expected from certain abnormal types of QRS patterns.

CONCLUSIONS AND SUMMARY

1. A simulation technique was developed for assessment of the precision of computer programs for ECG measurement. The method is based on evaluation of the effect on interval measurements of known types and quantities of random and periodic noise.

2. The performance of the Mayo-IBM ECG Measurement Program was evaluated. A total of forty-six QRS complexes of twelve subjects was measured at noise levels ranging from 0 to $100\mu v$ rms. The critical noise level was defined for each QRS complex as the noise level where the QRS measurement error was equal to or larger than 10 msec.

3. The critical noise level in one-half of the records was $40\mu v$ rms for random noise and $50\mu v$ rms for 60 Hz noise. In 16 per cent of the QRS complexes measured a 10 msec error in QRS measurement was reached at the level of $10\mu v$ rms of 60 Hz noise.

4. A modified version of the program was tested after incorporating a digital filter into the original Mayo-IBM Program. This version of the program practically eliminated the effect of 60 Hz noise on the QRS duration measurement up to noise levels of $100\mu v$ rms. However, only a slight improvement was achieved in reducing random noise.

5. The simulation technique described demonstrates the feasibility of quantitative assessment of automated ECG measurement problems.

REFERENCES

1. RAUTAHARJU, P.M.: Deterministic type waveform analysis in electro-cardiography. *Ann NY Acad Sci, 128*:939-954, 1966.
2. WINTER, D.A.; RAUTAHARJU, P.M., and WOLF, H.: Measurement and characteristics of overall noise content in exercise electrocardiogram. *Amer Heart J, 74*:324-331, 1967.
3. RAUTAHARJU, P.M.; WOLF, H.; BLACKBURN, H., and WONG, A.: The ac-curacy of computer measurements from the Frank lead exercise electro-cardiograms. VIIIth Internat'l Colloquium on Vectorcardiography. Vienna, 1967.
4. RAUTAHARJU, P.M.; WINTER, D.A., and WONG, A.Y.K.: Computer analysis of the exercise electrocardiogram. Internat'l Symp. on Electrical Activity of the Heart, Univ. of Western Ont., London, Ont., 1967.
5. SMITH, R.E., and HYDE, C.M.: A computer system for electrocardiographic analysis. IBM Engineering Publications, Rochester, Minn., 1966.

APPENDIX A

A Digital 60 Hz - Filter

The filter described here has been designed for rejection of 60 Hz noise from data digitized with sampling intervals of 2 msec.

The filter is a "central" type filter with weighting factors for the samples on both sides of the central point. The formula for the filter is

$$A_i^* = h_o \cdot A_i + \sum_{n=1}^{10} h_n \cdot (A_{i-n} + A_{i+n})$$

where A_i^* is the filtered sample at point I and h_n are the weighting factors. A total of ten sample points on each side and the center point are included in the filter process with weighting factors as given in Table 12-AI.

The transfer function of the filter is given in Figure 12-A1.

TABLE 12-AI

Sample Point	Weighting Factor h
I	0.1966
I—1, I+1	0.1862
I—2, I+2	0.1569
I—3, I+3	0.1143
I—4, I+4	0.0662
I—5, I+5	0.0211
I—6, I+6	—0.0140
I—7, I+7	—0.0350
I—8, I+8	—0.0409
I—9, I+9	—0.0340
I—10, I+10	—0.0191

60 Hz filter weighting factors (h) for the central point I and 10 sample points on each side of the central point.

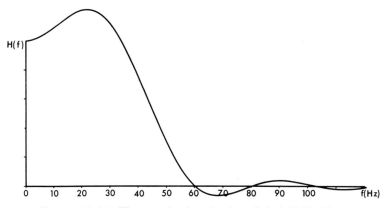

FIGURE 12-A1. The transfer function in a digital 60 Hz filter.

APPENDIX B

Generation of Markhovian Random Noise

The following formula produces random noise with Markhovian characteristics:

$$X^*_i = X_i - c \cdot X^*_{i-1} \qquad (1)$$

where X_i is the ith random sample drawn from a normally distributed population with mean 0 and variance σ^2, X^*_{i-1} is the generated value of the sample point (i-1) and c is a constant; $0 < c < 1$.

The standard deviation σ^* for the X^* population can be calculated from c and the standard deviation σ of the X population using the following expression:

$$\sigma^* = \sigma \cdot \frac{1}{1 - c^2} \qquad (2)$$

Equation (2) can be derived by means of the moment generation function. Rewriting (1) gives

$$X^*_i = X_i - c \cdot X^*_{i-1} = \sum_{n=0}^{i} X_n (-c)^n$$

Hence, X^*_i is a linear combination of n random variables, all of them equally distributed with mean 0 and standard deviation σ. Therefore, the moment generation function is

$$M_{x^*_i}(t) = \prod_{n=0}^{i} M_{x_i}(t) = \exp\left(\frac{\sigma^2 t^2}{2} \cdot \sum_{n=0}^{i} (c^2)^n\right) \qquad (3)$$

For $c^2 < 1$,

$$M_x^*(t) = \exp\left(\frac{\sigma^2 t^2}{2} \frac{1}{1-c^2}\right)$$

$$= \exp\left(\frac{\sigma^2}{1-c^2}\right)t^2/2$$

which is the moment generation function of a normal distribution with standard deviation:

$$\sigma^* = \sigma\frac{1}{1-c^2}$$

The technique of generating random samples from a normal distribution is based on the central limit theorem, which states that the reduced random variable X

$$X = \frac{(Y_n - \mu)}{\sigma/\sqrt{n}} \tag{4}$$

has a normal distribution with mean 0 and standard deviation 1;

$$\overline{Y}_n = \text{sample mean,}$$
$$\mu = \text{population mean,}$$
$$\sigma = \text{population standard deviation and}$$
$$n = \text{number of samples}$$

Assuming a uniform distribution between 0 and 1, the values for μ and σ will be

$$\mu = 0.5, \text{ and}$$

$$\sigma = 1/\sqrt{12}$$

Twelve samples were taken from the uniform distribution and from them, a value X_i was calculated as

$$X_i = (\tfrac{1}{12} \sum_{i=1}^{12} Y_i - 0.5) \cdot \sqrt{\frac{1}{\tfrac{1}{12} \cdot \tfrac{1}{12}}}$$

$$= \sum_{i=1}^{12} Y_i - 6$$

The method used for calculating the samples of the uniform distribution is the "power-residue" method discussed in IBM Manual C20-8011.

Figure 12-B1 shows the amplitude histogram, the power spectrum and the autocorrelation function of the type of random noise used in the present study. A value equal to 0.25 was used for the factor c.

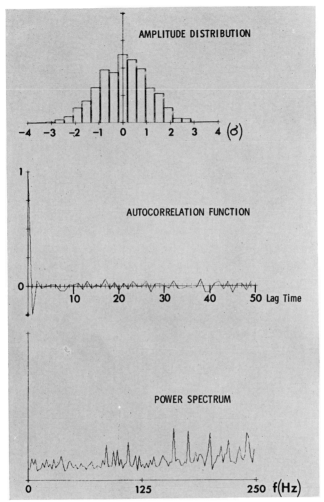

FIGURE 12-B1. An amplitude histogram, autocorrelation function and power spectrum of the random noise used in this simulation study.

ACKNOWLEDGMENT

The authors wish to acknowledge the assistance of Mr. John Sherwood, B. Sc., who wrote the program for the 60 Hz filter.

DISCUSSION

Dr. Blackburn: It is remarkable that after eighty years of electrocardiography and thirty years of exercise electrocardiography nobody knows what really happens to the duration of ventricular depolarization, the QRS duration, during exercise.

Shellong, in the 1930's, used QRS duration as part of the evaluation in a functional test of the circulation. But, it is incorrect to say, as he did, that the QRS is shortened in exercise, on the basis of single lead information. It wasn't nonsense, however, for him to say that normals reacted differently in that one lead than did abnormals. The next look at the total duration of ventricular excitation in exercise was, as far as I know, by Blackburn and Simonson in 1954, using an early orthogonal lead system, the Schmitt SVEC II. Using measurements from ten times magnification of the records we found in ten men exercised an average 3 msec lengthening of QRS duration as a result of moderate "Master" sort of exercise. We didn't have a great deal of confidence in the universality of that finding. This was bolstered, however, by Blomqvist's recent study in which he also found a 3 to 4 msec average lengthening of QRS activation in exercise, using averaged spatial QRS data. Now we see that nobody really knows because as you set definitions and criteria for the onsets and offsets of QRS they are quite affected by the heart rate and by the noise levels. Even at Dalhousie University they still do not know. At least some progress has been made in eliminating the effect of periodic noise and of random noise, and it seems that some day soon we'll know what happens to the duration of ventricular activation under conditions of exercise. We will be able to describe it operationally, computationally and maybe even physiologically.

Now we have a panel of four younger engineers, David Winter, Jerry Meyer, Alan Berson and Hermann Wolf, all with dirty hands from digging in this rich soil. Whether these engineers know it or not they have inherited many genes of ideas from Otto Schmitt. It might be a rather serious confrontation for them to have to sit *across* the table from his presence. I happen to know, however, that it can be a very productive experience to sit *next* to Otto Schmitt, on the same side of the table, for discussion. I would therefore like Dr. Schmitt to come sit with these gentlemen, and contribute or not as he feels moved. Dr. David Winter will chair this panel to discuss general problems in quality control for automated exercise ECG systems.

David, will you take over here?

13

A Panel Discussion on Bioengineering Problems in Measurement of the Exercise ECG Response

DAVID WINTER, *Chairman,* ALAN BERSON, JEROME MEYER, HERMANN WOLF *and* OTTO H. SCHMITT

Dr. Winter: An important aspect of the engineering problem in exercise cardiography is the recording systems themselves—what kind of frequency response they should have, what kind of coupling, what kind of input impedance, etc. I would like Alan Berson to open discussion with comments on this.

Mr. Berson: First I think it is important to understand that even prior to getting concerned with noisy ECGs these ECGs must be faithfully recorded. The low frequency response of the system is important because interpretation of the exercise ECG depends on response at this end. It gets confusing if the recording system is inadequate. We did a study of this problem and came to the conclusion that if you have a poor low-frequency response you indeed would get into diagnostic trouble.

First, there is in almost every application today the use of AC preamplifiers in electrocardiography. I am sure Dr. Schmitt would like to say something about this. Faithful recording requires response down to very low frequencies, something on the order of 0.05 Hertz. Unfortunately, this means the end of using large capacitors and so we are faced with the problem of baseline wandering. To prevent baseline wandering you can sacrifice the low-frequency response which brings the problem of whether the signal you are getting is really the right one, or whether artifacts and distortion are due to your recording system. There is a corrective method—that pointed out by Dr. Schmitt some time ago—whereby you can record with an AC system, even one inadequate in its characteristics, and play this signal back, using another network having characteristics that compensated for the poor response of the initial recording system. The integrity of the data at the low-frequency end is restored. I don't believe this type of system is in routine operation.

I would like to comment upon the belief that to compare a resting ECG with an exercise ECG in the same person it may not matter whether your system happens to be adequate, because the same system is used for recording both events, and all that is desired is to compare those events. This we found to be untrue. The distortion that can occur with inadequate systems varies with different types of wave forms. The QRS duration, the downslope of the R wave, and the heart rate, all may change during exercise, and in changing may cause the system to respond differently, and to distort. Considerable errors are possible and we have estimated these.

Dr. Schmitt: I think we should always do the best job we can in research applications, in contrast to service applications. I think that the records we get are a true response on the surface of the person. Secondly, I don't think we should be compromised by measuring offset potentials.

There are two ways of doing this, one being to bring a very small amplifier to the skin, and the other of bringing the amplified electrode into the amplifier. There are two different objectives. Clinical equipment may require an economical engineering job which deliberately throws out certain features elegance would dictate, making compromises, but knowing that you are doing it. For research sake we all have to make those compromises, and we may find some two or three or four measures that throw out the window most of the careful measurement. On the other side, we should be measuring with increased meaningful accuracy, and know what we are measuring. We are talking about QRS duration. This happy fiction should be defined rather than measured. I think that most of the argument has to do here not with the measurement, but with the definition of what we are allegedly measuring, and of course, once you define it, a thing that is vaguely related to the electrophysiology of the heart, you discover that certain of these mathematical filterings and corrections are essential.

If I may throw in just two remarks with respect to the previous content here, I am sure that the speaker was not intending to say that the baseline and the AC baseline coincide. I think we all realize that this is not true, but somebody might take it seriously. Then if we are going to discuss these various filtering techniques, I wonder that we have so long stayed with quite highly linear techniques, in terms of the frequency domain, rather than dealing in the time domain, which is where we are doing our physiology. Engineering in this linear frequency domain tends to throw out many of the effective techniques that should be incorporated. You understand I am not speaking *against* the frequency domain at all, but speaking *for* time domain analysis in which we conceive of the physiological phenomena and in which consequently we may want to defeat some of the racket and noise of artifacts.

Mr. Meyer: I have investigated the effects, in direct writing instruments, of reducing the high frequency capability, and since most of the literature is in terms of frequency, my approach has been in that direction and my own thinking has been in that direction. However, I would agree. As a matter of fact, when one begins to write about such things, one immediately begins to encounter difficulty in translating from time into frequency, muddying up the whole picture, even in exposition.

I would like to extend Mr. Berson's comments about frequency capabilities to take up the high frequency capabilities of instruments in current use, particularly looking at the capabilities of direct writers, which of course are inherently high-frequency limited. There has been much written about this by many people, a rather popular subject over the years. The shortening of the fast-moving components of the complex is quite well known, and has been commented on extensively. It doesn't end there, however, and on a closer look, again speaking in terms of frequency, it's fairly obvious that in the fast-moving parts of the complex, where one will be high frequency limited, that the frequency content of these sections, that is, between the Q, R and S is different—need not be the same. For instance, the Q R S will be attenuated by an instrument with insufficient high-frequency response, but will not necessarily be attenuated by the same factors, since the S is apt to look quite different from the R, in its time duration certainly. Therefore, when one deals with high-frequency limited instruments, and takes R to S ratios, for instance, as a meaningful parameter, I believe this is quite a dangerous procedure.

I was able to demonstrate in a rather simple-minded run-through using a simulated signal that at about the high-frequency cutoffs of most direct writers you will run into as high as 40 per cent errors on a very ordinary looking S wave, and a good deal less but nevertheless an error on an ordinary looking R.

Dr. Schmitt: Have you not found in many of the available recorders, that the limitation is a slurring limitation, rather than a frequency limitation? I think that many of the recorders are capable, if you will give them a little signal, of responding to fairly high frequencies, and thus pass their proof tests; and yet, when asked to make a quick deflection in a complex wave—you see, this is a case where the sum of a set of sinusoids is not the harmonic sum.

Mr. Meyer: Right.

Dr. Schmitt: The linear slurring rate in the time domain is the limiting factor and may be completely different for the same amplitudes and the same waves, just differently combined into a different composite wave.

Dr. Winter: Associated with the frequency we get into digital conversion, we can cause other problems here—I was wondering if Mr. Wolf would say a few words on digitizing of the analog signal.

Mr. Wolf: To go back to the low-frequency response, I would like to ask Dr. Schmitt, why is everybody specifying the low-frequency cutoff at 0.05 Herz? Why doesn't anybody specify phase distortion at this low cutoff frequency? I found phase distortions are much greater in the low cutoff frequency and commercially available amplifiers show distortions by 180 degrees or even more. Have you looked into this?

Dr. Schmitt: This is one of the very difficult matters with respect to generating standards. The phase data are simply not available. Also a number of manufacturers, by the familiar feedback techniques, have undertaken to sneak in under a specification and still have a good looking response. You know how this can be done, if you throw away some parts of response and still stay at the specified points and specified amplitude sensitivity, letting phase twirl around as it may, you can meet the specifications and get a quiet-looking signal, even if inaccurate. I think it is indeed important, if you are going to specify these in terms of frequency-domain parameters, that we must specify frequency and phase in order to characterize the machine.

Mr. Berson: Dr. Schmitt, in the American Heart Association recommendations did we not attempt to reduce that problem by giving specifications that would prevent the manufacturer from doing things like putting humps in a curve?

Dr. Schmitt: It was a poor attempt at this. We tried, but did not have time to do the arithmetic. We did succeed in putting in some rule-of-thumb limitations to prevent this thing being done vigorously.

Mr. Berson: I want to add something to what you said about the use of buffers. As far as exercise electrocardiography is concerned, this becomes important because as many, including Dr. Schmitt, have pointed out, the shape, the kind of impedance at the electrode-skin interface is one where the impedance goes up drastically as the frequency goes down. You would again expect to find problems in the area where you want to interpret the electrocardiogram in exercise tests. The use of a proper buffer with high input impedance, especially at the low frequencies, is especially important here.

Dr. Schmitt: If I may speak on this for just an instant. We have begun looking into the currently-used small electrodes, especially those used in exercise. We are appalled to see that these things do indeed go up and out, still in this one cycle region, and we have found values in a few individuals but not a negligible number, up to 180,000 to 200,000 ohm impedance level. I think we are not putting this into our thinking. If you are getting nice about measuring the QRS intercept in a tidy fashion, you must discover that this is now a very reactive impedance, and a reactive impedance changes wave forms. I think this has not been considered here, and it is one of the things I'd like to toss at the Dalhousie group, since they've lots of time and money and subjects to do things. I think that it is time to evaluate the relative merits of on-the-patient amplifiers and the simulator on the patient lead amplifier. We have two alternative techniques for making the impedance appear practically infinite. One is to put a little integrated circuit buffer amplifier right in the electrode so the signal never has to go beyond; and the other is to carry the front end of the amplifier up to the electrode so you don't need it, by using now stable methods of negative capacitance and infinite input impedance amplifiers in the amplifier. But we have not seen which of these best handles the problems of noise incidental to exercise, to motion, to displacement currents and fields in a room. Somebody ought to compare the merits of these two—not deciding that you have to use one or the other—but which is the better.

Dr. Winter: Just for the record's sake, all records made in Halifax since 1965 have been with high impedance operational amplifiers as buffers, not on the electrode-skin interface but in the first stage of the recording system. Even impedances of 100 K bother us little.

Dr. Schmitt: How much is the input impedance of your amplifier?

Dr. Winter: I think it was 100 megs. It was just a gain of one buffer amplifier input impedance of about 100 megs, and output impedance of about one ohm.

Dr. Schmitt: You mean then that you didn't use shielded cables out to your patient?

Dr. Winter: No, we didn't and had little trouble there.

Dr. Schmitt: I see. You didn't have some pick-up on the unshielded cables?

Dr. Winter: No.

Dr. Schmitt: Most people do.

Dr. Winter: We were lucky.

Mr. Wolf: I think it is mainly a question of preparing the skin-electrode contact. If you do a good job at this point, you get—

Dr. Schmitt: You have to assume that most technicians are doing it wrong.

Mr. Wolf: Well, maybe it's a question of teaching them.

Dr. Winter: When you go to A to D conversion there's sampling rate involved, and these are, in effect, filters. Could you, Hermann Wolf, make a few comments generally, theoretically, because this affects the analog signal.

Mr. Wolf: As soon as we start digitizing our record, we don't have much trouble. With the low frequency response, we can forget about it. But then we start worrying about the upper frequency, because it's starting to be a question of money and time on the computer.

Dr. Schmitt: Can I ask you a very pointed question about this?

Having settled on a digitizing rate, what is the desirable window compromise with respect to the sample? This is a very important parameter that we've neglected. That is, when you sample, for how long do you sample? You've got, let's say, 1000 μsec in which to sample—how long a window do you open up in that period?

Mr. Wolf: Well, it becomes a question of the machine you use.

Dr. Schmitt: Yes, we can make converters do anything we want. It's up to us to decide. Now what do you decide, and why? I know what we think, but what do you decide?

Mr. Wolf: We use a converter which averages for 40 μsec, and takes this average value and converts it into a digital value.

Dr. Schmitt: All right, I will contend that mathematically you should integrate over the entire intersample period and substitute that for the midpoint. Now why don't you do that. Is this mathematically wrong?

Mr. Wolf: No.

Dr. Schmitt: If it's not wrong, why don't you do it?

Mr. Wolf: It would be mathematically correct, but we don't do it because of a time question. If we don't convert during the time, we can use the computer for something else.

Dr. Schmitt: Yes, but you only need a computer to convert, and then go about doing other things while it's doing this accumulating converting.

Mr. Wolf: Well, another point is, our machine isn't capable of it.

Dr. Schmitt: Oh, *that's* it!

Mr. Wolf: We have to live with those 40 μsec averages.

Dr. Winter: We appear to be getting into semantics on the sampling theorem. I think we'll now have to end the discussion. Thank you all.

14

A Panel Discussion on Functional Engineering Specifications for Automated Systems of Exercise Electrocardiography

Pentti Rautaharju, *Chairman,* C. Gunnar Blomqvist, Cesar
Caceres, Otto H. Schmitt, Ralph Smith, Naip Tuna,
David Winter *and* Hermann N. Wolf

Dr. Rautaharju: The terms of reference for our panel this morning are drawn from a resolution of a recent workshop in Halifax on minimal performance requirements of ECG measurement programs. We solicit opinions from the panel members and the audience about the following issues:

1. Is it sensible at the present time to suggest minimum performance requirements for automated ECG measurement programs, and particularly for programs designed to measure ECG response to exercise?

2. If so, which features of the ECG should be identified as the minimum of accepted reference points for amplitude and interval measurements?

3. How accurately and precisely should the desired items, amplitudes and intervals be measured?

4. How much noise, and what kind of noise, should the measurement system be able to tolerate and still provide measurements with defined precision?

MEASUREMENT AND STANDARDIZATION PROBLEMS

May I invite Dr. Lepeschkin to open discussion with a statement about engineering specifications for ECG instrumentation and problems in ECG measurement.

Dr. Lepeschkin: It is an honor to be here. I am one of this group interested in instrumentation who has been concerned also with the basic electrophysiology as well as clinical application of the electrocardiogram. I also am on the electrocardiographic standardization committee of the American Heart Association, and it is unfortunate that not all of us can participate in the meetings of that committee.

The reason why the new American Heart Association specifications for ECG instrumentation were higher than most manufacturers or even people who have to work with computers would like was that the existing specifications and criteria were developed throughout this century largely by clinicians using inferior equipment. Because of engineering progress, we are able now to shoot high for quality and fidelity in electrocardiography. We must make a conscious effort to discern how much is compromise and how much is true representation of the electrocardiogram. Otto Schmitt quite aptly said yesterday that the engineers of these machines often introduce artifacts into the electrocardiogram or suppress features which may not be of diagnostic interest now but may be in the future. Small variations in the QRS complex, such as the notches, may not have practical significance now, but the beginning and the end of the QRS complex certainly contains high frequency components of potential interest. The action potential of the single heart cell has frequency components up to 1000 cps, and the plateau in the repolarization process goes way down to D.C., to zero. Anything less than fidelity throughout this range is compromise. What we should not do is to filter out the so-called artifacts, but rather try to prevent and to recognize them. The human can recognize them but the computer cannot, so we neutralize them by various feedback mechanisms. For instance, we have heard here about a notch filter to reduce 60 cycle hum, but it will certainly reduce that component of the QRS complex. For instance, the QRS may begin with a 60 cycle component, then during exercise, because of the increased speed of conduction, it becomes 65 or 70 cycles; instead of the true beginning we will have a smooth line because the filter will filter out that particular part. We get a false change in the direction or duration of QRS.

The same applies to the computer averaging processes described at this Conference. We know there are respiratory changes in the form of the complexes. For instance, if the ECG begins in inspiration, it may begin with a Q wave; in expiration, it may begin with an R wave. If we average blindly, even for a few beats, these differences may average out to zero and even the QRS duration may appear shorter than in reality. What we should do is to average beats at the same phase of the respiratory cycle, and for that purpose it would seem to me that the respiratory cycle must be recorded to influence the program. The more we tamper with the electrocardiogram the more we are likely to introduce distortion. It seems to me that it would be absolutely necessary, in addition to what we feed into the computer or an analogous network, to have available, stored, an undistorted curve containing all the artifacts. Maybe a few days, or years, from now someone will come out with a new study on the high frequency components, or on the very low frequency components. Then we may want to go back into our results and analyze them with these in mind.

It is very well to have rejection circuits for large artifacts; but when we apply stress to a person, the time when we want to see the electrocardiographic changes may be at the same time where the artifacts are greatest, so we cannot make the computer blindly reject this artifact.

Now what are artifacts? Artifacts are electrical events not produced by the depolarization and repolarization of the ventricle. Because of their importance in sustaining circulation it is the ventricular electrocardiogram in which we are most interested. The repolarization wave of the atrium is, so to speak, an artifact as far as the ventricular complex is concerned. The U wave is part of the ventricular complex, but I believe that it may be an electrical-mechanical artifact caused by mechanical events. Because something appears rhythmically with the heartbeat does not mean that it is not artifact, because just the mechanical activity of the blood vessels and of the heart may produce an artifact. For instance, sometimes arm electrodes are put over the radial artery causing an arrhythmic mechanical artifact. The same is certainly true whenever precordial leads are taken because the movement of the chest wall created by the heart itself may cause artifacts. This is why I believe that any recognition circuit should be able to distinguish between an atrial wave and a false displacement of the baseline. When the heart rate is fast, the U wave prevents us from recognizing the true baseline.

PRECISION AND ACCURACY OF ECG MEASUREMENTS

Dr. Rautaharju: The paper presented by Mr. Wolf demonstrated that it is possible to assess quantitatively the *precision* of computer measurements. The reliability of defined amplitude and interval measurements can be evaluated in the presence of noise of such type and in such quantities as can be expected in an exercise ECG.

In a sense, the simulation technique described also provides a method of measuring the *accuracy* of a computer program against a standard which in this case was the set of measurements made by the program from the noise-free records.

The Halifax resolution, published in these proceedings as the Report of a Technical Group, calls for a precision of 10 msec for interval measurements and a precision of 20uv or 10 per cent of the signal amplitude, whichever is larger, for the amplitude measurements. This does not dictate what kind of logic an investigator should use, for instance, for detecting the onset of QRS, but expects that a reasonable effort is put into defining the onset so that measurements of crucial QRS durations are not perturbed unduly by small amounts of noise. Furthermore, it is important that measurements provided by various programs agree with each other within reasonable limits. If this is the case, then it matters not what kind of logic was used for the detection.

Dr. Schmitt: What do you mean by accurate? I am pointing out the difference between precise and accurate.

Dr. Rautaharju: Yes, go ahead, please.

Dr. Schmitt: It may be very precise to define a point most meaninglessly, but if you go to millisecond precision, then you must have something that is definable and meaningful to millisecond precision. You must convince yourself that the events you are looking at are repetitive in the feature that you are looking at in this detail. This is all.

Dr. Rautaharju: Correct. This is exactly why we have tried to be so careful with our statements about ECG measurement accuracy and precision. Before we proceed it may be important for somebody to tell us what we mean by precision and accuracy. Who would volunteer? What about our medical engineer, Dr. Winter?

Dr. Winter: May I put a diagram on the board?

Dr. Rautaharju: Yes, please.

Dr. Winter: [blackboard presentation] Here we have a meter measuring something—it could be time intervals, or amplitudes, or anything. If the pointer is a great big thick blob, like that, it may be the most accurate meter in the world, but it is impossible to read it with any degree of precision. Take the reverse situation, a meter with a very fine pointer with a mirror on the dial. This meter gives you a very precise reading, allowing use of the full accuracy of that instrument. Suppose now that either the dial or the pointer is displaced, or bent. The instrument now gives very precise readings, all very inaccurate.

Dr. Rautaharju: Thank you, Dr. Winter. Is this engineering definition of precision and accuracy acceptable?

Dr. Schmitt: This is a fine definition of precision and accuracy, but what about the electrocardiographic case?

Dr. Rautaharju: The question is, is it possible by any means to know the true values of the items we are trying to measure? Do we know the truth so that we can find out how accurate our measurements are?

Dr. Schmitt: Would you be willing to define accurately the truth that you are seeking? What are the things we would like to detect? I mention this because I think we should bring into this the notion of dispersion of index.

THE FIDUCIAL POINT AS A REFERENCE POINT

Dr. Rautaharju: Let us elaborate a bit on this notion. In some instances, investigators cannot agree which items to measure from the ECG and even less agree how to define them. Everybody seems to agree, however, that it is important to identify the existence of every ventricular excitation event, i.e., the QRS complex. For certain noise reduction purposes, such as averaging in its elementary form of time-coherent amplitude summation, it is important to have accurate reference points from each QRS complex.

I remember an incident back in 1961 in Dr. Schmitt's office when we discussed design of a filter needed for a trigger circuit for averaging ECGs. The problem came up because we did not know what to call the electronically derived reference point for averaging. Dr. Schmitt started talking about "the fiducial point." This is what we have called it ever since, but not until yesterday did I really know what it meant. Yesterday I looked it up in a dictionary of legal terms. But maybe Dr. Schmitt could tell us what "fiducial" is.

Dr. Schmitt: It means a faithful point, a point that you can trust, that you can refer to.

Dr. Rautaharju: All right, so it's a true, prudent, faithful, reproducible point, a reference point. Now, is it always necessary to recognize a fiducial point for ECG analysis, and if so, how accurately should one attempt to locate it?

Dr. Schmitt: I would suggest that we be careful not to identify this more accurately than we can define it.

Dr. Rautaharju: Could you elaborate on that point, please?

Dr. Schmitt: Yes, I mean that we can, as we have done so often with computer programs, purify out all the things we don't like and define a particular place and detect it very accurately and think we have done something marvelous, when in fact what we have has no relationship to a particular phase, or feature, of excitation. I think we are really trying to identify some particular phase in the excitatory cycle, and we must not overdefine this fiducial mark—beyond the meaning of it. For example, if excitation is a distributed thing, if the pattern of excitation changes from beat to beat, we mustn't define that fiducial mark to the point where we think it defines something unique, when that uniqueness disappears in the definition of it.

Dr. Rautaharju: Fine. Perhaps you could now elaborate also on the meaning of *the notion of dispersion of index* which you just brought up a while ago.

Dr. Schmitt: I think you want to suppress the idea that one beat is different from another beat, and want to detect something that is stable and firm and identical about each beat to tie the rest of it onto. Now, I think we should recognize that this is not exactly true, and verbalize what it is we would like to determine and find an index that has the narrowest dispersion, that is to say, the least variance of the measures of it in the several cyclic measures. Do you remember when we were working on this some time ago, we noted that by picking a point early in the QRS for the fiducial mark, by taking the clustering of high frequency components and using a fiducial mark in the middle of them, the time dispersion became less important on the two sides? It is this kind of index that I think we should be seeking. But we should be recognizing that it is a spatial entity producing it and define the fiducial mark in terms of a feature of that three dimensional entity.

Dr. Blomqvist: May I first suggest that the transmembrane action potential should be the starting point in our attempts to define the onset and offset of waves. Ideally, you would like to define the onset of QRS in statistical terms, e.g., as the point where 1 per cent of the cells in the ventricles have depolarized.

Dr. Schmitt: That wave form, the transmembrane potential, is I think what you're plotting. This could be given as a histogram, could it not, for the entire myocardium?

Dr. Blomqvist: Yes, that is what I am getting at.

Dr. Schmitt: Well, the rapid onset is a good fiducial mark in itself. The question is, what portion of the histogram do you want to detect? That is, you might be setting off an explosion; there is a faltering term which we all think of as the phase of excitation, which is now spread through the tissue, and then there are a few lagging cells. Now is it the earliest ignition phase that you want to detect? Is it the explosive phase; is it the mid-point of it? Which feature gives us the best advantage and why? This, I think, is what we're trying to settle.

Dr. Blomqvist: But I think I'm just trying to say that you probably have to think of it in statistical terms.

Dr. Schmitt: Yes, that is what a histogram is, and where in that histogram should we be choosing our fiducial mark.

Dr. Rautaharju: We all realize that all these definitions we are using now are quite arbitrary. There is no way out; they are bound to be arbitrary. The important thing is to reach an agreement for a common language, to define our measurements so that we can at least document how closely the measurements provided by different programs agree with each other.

Dr. Schmitt: You mean it doesn't make any difference if we're wrong, just so long as we say the same thing?

Dr. Rautaharju: Of course it makes a difference but as long as there is no way of knowing who is right, it is better to be consistently wrong than to have an unnecessary array of different inconsistent definitions.

Dr. Caceres: I agree with you that we have to have some sort of a standardization. If we don't come to some agreement on terms, we certainly will not be able to discuss the same things. You were talking for example, of truth in the electrocardiogram. What is the truth? Well, the ECG is a nonrepetitive pulse, and if each complex is a wave train of nonrepetitive pulses, every pulse is truth. It is a unique thing, it exists, that's it. I think one of the problems in electrocardiography is that we fail to accept that these things are nonrepetitive, and this has brought in great diffculties in the use of machinery and terminology. I think that we have to go back and start at this very basic level, starting from the point of view that the electrocardiogram is nonrepetitive. Once you've done that you've clarified a great many things about whether or not you can average, and what you do if you do average. You end up, for example, with an interesting item, which, if it is not necessarily true, might be useful in some fashion, but with a misconception about what you are doing when you are averaging. I would like to stress that we do have to standardize the very basic terminology and standardize it on the machinery, and finally on the output terms we are going to use.

Dr. Rautaharju: I have to make a further simplifying assumption to proceed here. Let us say that half a dozen of us in different medical centers have agreed to use a certain definition for the onset and another definition for the offset of QRS. There is no question in my mind that this can be done consistently, in such a way that we have a common language. These time points are then used as reference points for a set of interval and amplitude measurements. The question is, how accurately in time and how accurately in amplitude should we try to do our measurements from an exercise electrocardiogram?

Dr. Caceres: This depends on the instrumentation you are using. If you've recorded your data digitally to start with, you are going to have a very high degree of accuracy; this is the first point.

Dr. Rautaharju: You are asking for trouble unless you clarify your point.

Dr. Caceres: If you have said, "This is the first point," and you have recorded it digitally on some machine, there is no other choice because the machine selected that point for you. If you record your data on an analog tape, and play that analog tape back through an analog-digital converter, your accuracy is going to be very different; I think it might depend on the instrument you use.

Dr. Rautaharju: Now we are getting into controversy. Dr. Schmitt.

Dr. Schmitt: Quickly let us point out that a digital record merely gives precision—it gives the same answer, repeatedly, so it is not necessarily accurate.

Dr. Caceres: I agree with you. Now if you are going to use an analog record, and obtain repeatability, we may be able to do that with an extremely sensitive instrument. I don't know of anyone around here who has that type of instrument. If you are now going to refer to biologic variability, for instance, if you are going to refer to a measurement that has something to do with biological systems, it's very difficult to say ever that you were anywhere near accurate or precise, because you do not know where you are in the scale of distribution of values.

Dr. Rautaharju: Would you agree that at the present time the limiting factor is not the precision of measuring instruments? There are other factors that are much more serious, such as noise in the records and weaknesses in the measurement logic of computer programs. Mr. Wolf, would you say that it makes any difference, regarding the noise level, how we record, digitally or otherwise?

Mr. Wolf: I do not think that the type of recording, analog or digital, makes much difference. However, even if the instrumentation is the limiting factor, I think we should never adjust our requirements to the precision available in commercial instruments. If we need higher precision, we can get it by investing more money. Our aim here is to agree on necessary precision of data analysis and this means we can assume raw data of any degree of precision. The problem we face is the precision of our pattern recognition.

Dr. Rautaharju: Let us assume that we agree to use instrumentation which meets at least the specifications proposed by the American Heart Association ECG Instrumentation Committee, hoping that the instrumentation used is not the limiting factor for measurement precision and accuracy.

I would suggest that we should not attempt to force every medical center and every computer program to use an identical definition for, say, QRS onset. In my opinion, it would not really matter what logic is used provided that various programs provide measurements which agree with each other within reasonable limits. This then means that we should not tell exactly which logic the programmer should use but we have to tell him what measurements we want, the precision required and we also have to give him enough information about the noise and the signal expected. Does somebody disagree?

Dr. Schmitt: Yes, I disagree. If you're going to say that you are now going to train your programmers to be good biophysicists so that they can use the judgment you are not going to contribute, of course, fine; but if he is merely a programmer who competently programs what you tell him to program, I think you are going to get into severe difficulty unless you convey to him the physiological feature that you are trying to discriminate.

Dr. Rautaharju: If you give specifications for a measuring instrument to a design engineer, you don't tell him how he has to design it. You give the specifications, and the performance requirements, but you don't care how he does it. For an average consumer, it is a black box. Automated ECG measurement programs are beginning to be more and more complicated and sophisticated and very few persons can follow in detail the logic used. Fortunately, this is not necessary as long as the performance is satisfactory.

Dr. Caceres: I would agree with you.

Dr. Schmitt: I don't believe you're willing to accept a program without knowing something about it even if it works.

Dr. Caceres: No, I think it depends on the specific individual. You may be very fortunate and have a programmer that understands the physiological reality of things. You are totally dependent on the individual. Ordinarily you would not be able to turn over a problem to the conventional, though good, programmer available to us. It would have to be a very special person that you could give this type of problem to.

Dr. Rautaharju: It seems to me we are still avoiding the issue. Dr. Sheffield, tell us, is it possible to define the offset of QRS so that we can all understand what we mean, and secondly, can you suggest to us now, with what accuracy should we attempt to measure the timing and the amplitude at that particular reference point?

Dr. Sheffield: I'd like to start by saying that we can either make arbitrary definitions or attempt to do with a computer program what we think we have been doing clinically by eye. [blackboard demonstration] I think it is possible to define a point like this without knowing for certain whether this is the end of the QRS complex. But we do know that it is the thing that we have been measuring for fifty years or so. We can suggest a definition for QRS offset which is derived from the time point of the maximum deceleration, or slope change, that occurs within a window following a specified recognition point in the QRS, and which is followed by an electrically relatively quiet interval.

Now just to suggest something that the rest of you can criticize (I notice everyone has been particularly reticent to suggest figures), I'll be brash and suggest figures; I suggest that we might accept a tolerance of plus or minus 3 msec for locating QRS offset and onset, just as a figure to talk about.

Dr. Rautaharju: As Dr. Caceres said, there is a true event that we call QRS with every heartbeat, and it has a certain duration in time from onset to offset. We can define the offset and the onset. Now, if we have to measure it with a precision of plus or minus three msec, what does it imply? If we repeat the same measurement one hundred times, perhaps with a variable amount of noise in the signal, we get a certain average value and a certain standard error of measurement. How do you suggest we define the precision, as a 95 per cent guaranteed precision, or do you insist that not a single measurement be off more than 3 msec?

The latter alternative is a very strict requirement. If the tolerance is defined as a standard error, we would occasionally tolerate in some very difficult situations a few measurements to fall beyond these limits. Would this be acceptable?

Dr. Schmitt: I think that a fundamental feature enters into it; that is your sampling band theory enters into what you mean by this measurement. When you make a measurement, the way in which you measure it is subject to a statistical fluctuation. Consequently, it becomes a matter of special definition as to what you mean by measurement accuracy within so many microvolts and so much time.

Dr. Rautaharju: I would like to ask Dr. Ralph Smith how precise measurement he obtains with his program, from relatively noise-free resting records.

Dr. Smith: We think that we do reasonably well with standard waveforms within the noise that we have. We measure peak-to-peak noise instead of rms values and we try to keep our system noise below 25 μv when referred back to the patient. This is in resting ECGs and is achievable in our system; the reproducibility with normal R complexes I think is within 4 to 8 msec.

Dr. Rautaharju: Eight msec? Would you say that 95 per cent of your measurements from the resting QRS are within 8 msec?

Dr. Smith: Yes. Now, I'm talking about fairly normal wave forms. When we go to abnormal forms, they are within 16 msec.

Dr. Rautaharju: All right, now we are talking about reasonably noise-free *resting* records and a rather good measurement program. Dr. Caceres, what is your impression, what kind of precision can we hope for in present-day programs for the resting QRS interval?

Dr. Caceres: Our program was intentionally made to simulate measurements that a physician makes eighteen inches away from an electrocardiographic record. This is what we reproduce; this is what we intended. In other words, we were quite arbitrary; whatever we were measuring initially was changed to come up with values that are like those obtained by the physician. Some rounding is made in our program. This actually means we are not going to have this type of repeatability. I am not sure that you can have this high a repeatability, for example, if you were to play back the analog tapes.

Dr. Rautaharju: Is it better than 8 msec? In 95 per cent of the cases?

Dr. Caceres: I would say that we come within about 5 per cent.

Dr. Rautaharju: Of QRS duration?

Dr. Caceres: Of all measurements. We can repeat these within about 5 per cent.

Dr. Rautaharju: This means an error range of 10 msec for a QRS duration of 100 msec?

Dr. Caceres: I think your error factor within your total system has to also be considered when you come up with these values. What I'm saying is that it depends on the total system, that an individual component in the system has very little to do with it. The 5 per cent error refers to the total system error.

Dr. Rautaharju: Notice that we are now talking about reasonably stable noise-free resting records. What about the precision standards for exercise electrocardiograms. Dr. Tuna has made some exercise ECG analysis. Would you care to comment?

Dr. Tuna: Just a comment on the repeatability of measuring the beginning and end of a QRS complex. In normal patients my guess is we get probably between 5 and 10 msec, but I cannot give exact figures. I would say that in pathological material our wave recognition program is not this repeatable, but in clean, normal records this may be within the limits mentioned.

Dr. Rautaharju: My feeling is that even with the best available programs it is tough to get a precision of QRS interval measurement from exercise ECGs better than 5 msec standard error. Results from a pilot study conducted by Mr. Wolf indicate that in one half of the records the measurement error in QRS duration exceeds 10 msec at a noise level of 40 to 50 μv rms. Dr. Bruce has used averaging to reduce noise from exercise ECGs, and of course it is possible that by averaging and filtering, one can get more consistent measurements. I wonder if Dr. Bruce would care to say something about what kind of accuracy and precision we can expect from exercise electrocardiograms using averaging techniques?

Dr. Bruce: I think we are in the same boat in terms of what we are trying to get and actually achieving. "What are the minimal measurement requirements?" We also have to ask the question, "What are the effects of the measurement?" This is a question you haven't touched on at all. You should put the question in this framework.

From biophysical considerations, I would like to add one thing about averaging which has been mentioned so many times; that is, the sample size and the variance of measurements. By computing the variance we get additional information from every point. It was amazing to discover that there was useful information here that we'd overlooked. In the consideration of Dr. Rautaharju and Dr. Blackburn, sixteen samples is enough to average, and one hundred beats which we were doing was burning a lot of time unnecessarily. Here was a new point. It turns out that when we look at the mean of sixteen and the mean of one hundred samples, they're almost exactly the same, but the variances are quite different. There is greater variance with a small sample.

Dr. Rautaharju: Thank you, Dr. Bruce. That is a valuable point. Any further comments on precision requirements in ECG measurement?

Dr. Schmitt: Well, I think you can say that you can probably afford the luxury of slightly overinstrumenting and overrecording and then discard data liberally. We know that for most of the instrumentation we are using, about a nine or ten bit sample precision exceeds any reasonable interpretive accuracy. As a start, supposing one were to suggest that you maintain approximately ten bit precision of integrals between sample point measurements. This is saying something concrete, isn't it? This is a class measurement that is achievable, that is slightly more than realistically precise, and is fairly easy to do with computer programs. Is that a place to start?

Dr. Rautaharju: How would it sound if we specify as 95 per cent tolerance limits for amplitude measurement precision 20 μv or 10 per cent of the signal amplitude, whichever is larger? Is it adequate for research and clinical purposes at the present time?

Dr. Schmitt: That is accuracy for full scale?

Dr. Rautaharju: Yes.

Dr. Schmitt: I don't know of any system I have investigated that was holding one per cent system accuracy, and that is what you imply.

Dr. Rautaharju: 20 μv?

Dr. Schmitt: Yes, do you have a system with that precision?

Dr. Rautaharju: Yes, we do. With a gain of 1,000, 20 μv is equal to 20 mv on tape. The signal to noise ratio of 42 or 48 db is required depending on whether you need a span of 2.5 or 5 v. Also, for ECG measurements we are never using an instantaneous measurement at any one time point. It is always a question of utilizing measurements from several points, filtering and other statistical procedures. The noise in the raw data is not necessarily the limiting factor. As an extreme case, a precision better than 10 μv has been reported by Bruce from exercise ECGs with averaging techniques, despite rather noisy records. Dr. Blackburn, you have measured thousands of electrocardiograms with your eyes. What kind of precision do you expect from the ST amplitude measurement?

Dr. Blackburn: The precision you are talking about, as Dr. Schmitt pointed out, is quite beyond any diagnostic precision that we now think we need. Diagnostic criteria for ST depression require identification of 0.05 mv changes.

Dr. Rautaharju: This requires a resolution better than 50 μv with routine ECG recording techniques and visual measurement. For computer measurements, from records made with a decent tape system, 20 μv precision would seem a realistic and necessary requirement.

Dr. Schmitt: There should be different requirements for different parts of the measurement, don't you think?

Dr. Rautaharju: Yes, this is exactly what I specified, 20 μv *or* 10 per cent of the signal amplitude, whichever is larger. Ten per cent is not too tough; you get it even if the overall system precision is 5 per cent. At the ST segment, QRS-ST junction, etc., we hope to have better than 50 μv precision. If we aim at 20 we may get it.

Dr. Schmitt: You have been saying amplitudes. This implies that you have defined amplitudes.

Dr. Rautaharju: Yes, it is not a question of measuring the amplitudes of the analog signal but items like QRS-ST junction amplitude which is a difference of two defined items, the baseline and the so-called J point.

Dr. Schmitt: Then you chop the definition all to pieces.

Dr. Rautaharju: On the contrary, we must define the precision of measurement for items which are actually used for ECG analysis. The precision of sampling, analog-to-digital conversion, etc., in itself is of secondary importance and is not the limiting factor.

Dr. Bruce: I think we are struggling with a very difficult problem and I would like to suggest a brief analogy. Suppose we have the engineering problem of trying to find out what happens when we go from here to the airport on a particular highway in vehicles, and we have a sensing device that determines the number of vehicles that went by per unit time and measure the speed of conduction. Now you come out with the number 39.3567 and so forth miles per hour average speed. That's one set of information that's useful, but that doesn't tell about every vehicle, and you know and I know that there is a wide variation. Some go fast, some go slowly. Maybe the same thing happens here sometimes. You can also with the same sensing device measure the length of each vehicle, with precision, the width of each vehicle, the pathway of the conduit, and get a mean, a standard deviation of how it varies on this channel for a certain period of time. You'll be getting samples from certain times when there's no traffic and other times when there is very congested traffic and you won't get the same number, and every so often someone deviates from the pathway and goes off the road. The same thing happens in real life in this situation, where you get a different type of conduction, and then you've got the problem in repolarization, and in this analogy, can you use the same sensing device, and the same characteristics to ascertain the amount of air turbulence and circulation of the air, the air pollution from this vehicle going by at frequent intervals, and come out with useful information? There are many different questions here, and are all built into the same problem we're talking about with the electrocardiogram.

Dr. Rautaharju: Perhaps we could ask Dr. Schmitt to make a few final remarks on the basic philosophy of this measurement problem we have discussed here today.

Dr. Schmitt: I think that our chatter here today has precipitated a couple of important considerations. Let me get one of them off first. We have talked about what accuracy or what precision we demand of a measurement. Let me put on an engineering hat for a moment and say that every measurement of the accuracy of anything involves the comparison of a particular experimental procedure with some idealized or perfect reference standard. The fact that nobody here has defined the accuracy in this way implies that we are not talking about real qualifications of absolute accuracy at all. We're trying to convince each other that our procedures are satisfactory, and whistling in the dark. I would suggest that we behave like good engineers and say, "This is the standard we are trying to meet and, experimentally or theoretically, this is the deviation that we must or will expect." We have two separate standardization jobs to do here, and I think we should meet them separately. We must specify what it is that we would like to characterize from beat to beat, or for an individual heart cycle, and say that the electrical embodiment of this is best exemplified by the following measurements, and then go about specifying those measurements. We should try not to tell each other how he shall write his computer program, but rather say what the epitome is that he is trying to determine in this exemplification of the physiological principles he wants to measure.

Dr. Blackburn: Thank you all. We have considered the functional engineering problems and seen the difficulties in arriving at specifications. We are very grateful to Dr. Rautaharju for considering these problems, the definitions, the type and range of noise to be dealt with and the precision we need in these programs. Those who are actively involved in this will together in a back room knock out the specific criteria required. Else, by free enterprise, we will follow some standard based on logic or perhaps on popularity. The results of deliberations of a technical group will be published in the proceedings as guidelines, or, more modestly, as provocations to guidelines.

15

Report of a Technical Group on Performance Specifications for Automated Exercise ECG Analysis Programs

Tentative Requirements for Noise Tolerance and Precision

P.M. Rautaharju, *Chairman*, H. Blackburn, C.G. Blomqvist,
A. Freiman, L. Jackson, P. Rochmis, L.T. Sheffield,
D. Winter *and* H. Wolf

Tнe purpose of these arbitrary specifications for exercise ECG analysis programs is to provide guidelines for program design. It is recognized that we are now in the early phase of program development and that any guidelines are likely to be inadequate and bound to change along the way. An attempt is made here to provide *minimal* performance criteria in the light of present knowledge about diagnostic contribution and about characteristics of the signal and the noise in exercise ECG records.

1. Specifications for the Recording System

The recording and data acquisition systems should conform to the standards specified by the American Heart Association Committee on Electrocardiography (*Circulation, 35*:583-602, 1967).

2. Exercise Conditions

Dynamic analysis is desired throughout the exercise period regardless

---
Note: The meetings of this group were supported in part by the Heart Disease and Stroke Control Program, U.S. Public Health Service.

of the type or load of work. Analysis is required of the resting electrocardiogram which precedes the exercise record. Measurements from
each phase of the exercise are compared both with the resting and
previous exercise values to cover a wide range of possible values. Heart
rate range from 40 to 220 beats per minute is to be accommodated.

3. Expected Noise Levels

Even with the best present-day techniques, a considerable amount
of hum, periodic and random noise and sudden baseline transients,
can be expected, especially during maximal exercise, and the program
should accommodate the following commonly encountered conditions:

    a. Hum. Up to 100 μv rms.

    b. Periodic low frequency baseline shifts with a slope up to 1 mv/
       sec.

    c. Random noise. 100 μv rms, in the bandwidth of 0.1 to 100 Hz.

    d. Recognition and rejection of portions of the signal affected by
       "spikes" of short duration, sudden bursts of white noise and
       other sudden transients detrimental to the measurement ac-
       curacy despite noise reduction methods.

4. Precision of Amplitude Measurements at Defined Points

In the presence of noise an initial guideline is proposed that the
guaranteed precision of amplitude measurements shall be $20\mu v$ or
10 per cent of the signal amplitude, whichever is greater. The guaranteed precision of $20\mu v$ implies that in a series of repeated measurements
from digitized records containing $100\mu v$ rms simulated noise, 95 per
cent of the measurements will not deviate more than $20\mu v$ from
the value as measured from the control record with no added noise.
Separate tolerance tests are required for random and 60 Hz noise.
The noise simulation procedure is described elsewhere in this monograph (H. Wolf and P. Rautaharju).

5. Precision of Interval Measurements

A guaranteed precision of 5 msec is proposed for QRS interval and
20 msec for other measured intervals. Guaranteed precision is defined
and determined as described in part 4 above.

6. Storage of Measured Items

For exchange of results from exercise ECG tests, it is proposed that the measured amplitudes be stored from 5 msec intervals in the QRS and 20 msec intervals from other parts of the complex, with identification of onsets and offsets of P, QRS and T.

Measurements reported from any program should be accompanied by a statement describing the confidence of the measurements. If the quality of the record does not meet acceptable limits, the program should recognize and warn of this situation.

The program should recognize and warn of the onset of certain arrhythmias, defined limits of rate, ST depression and other ECG responses considered a potential hazard to the subject. Criteria for these conditions will be the subject of future discussion.

PART FOUR

CONCEPTUAL AND PROCEDURAL PROBLEMS IN STANDARDIZED MEASUREMENT OF THE EXERCISE ELECTROCARDIOGRAM

16

Conceptual Problems in Stress Electrocardiography

PAUL G. ROCHMIS

INTRODUCTION

THE EARLY HISTORY of stress electrocardiology has been reviewed elsewhere (1, 2, 3). The key points are its fortuitous origins (4,5), the early clinical applications (6,7), and the somewhat later adaptation of a "standard" exercise regimen by Master (8). Since that time, stress, or in this case, exercise electrocardiography has achieved a certain fame and notoriety. The fame stems from its proven clinical usefulness, the notoriety from uncertainties of interpretation inherent in any process generated by empiricism.

Presently, we are involved in a healthy upheaval which is characterized by a reappraisal of the entire procedure. This procedure can be thought of as a sequence of events starting with the type of stress and its application (usually physical exercise) and ending with techniques of ECG waveform analysis and interpretation. The use of stress testing has broadened to encompass many areas of cardiovascular research, e.g., work physiology, drug testing and epidemiologic investigations, in addition to the clinical uses of diagnosis and function testing.

PRESENT PROBLEMS

There seem to be four major groupings of problems in the development of stress electrocardiography:

1. Inadequate statement of the objectives of stress testing.
2. Harboring of outdated and inappropriate concepts.
3. Technical problems.
4. Insufficient use and inappropriate interpretation of testing result.

A brief review of the first three of these follows.

THE OBJECTIVES OF STRESS TESTING

The development of exercise electrocardiography has focused on the means of the process and not its ends. The *uses* of a procedure must be defined before it can be intelligently designed.

When the use is for a problem in diagnosis of coronary heart disease (CHD) in an individual, *specificity* and *sensitivity* of the test are of concern whereas economy of cost, speed of performance and, to some extent, relative safety may be partly sacrificed. The needs here are for careful pre-exercise evaluation, near-maximal stress loading, multiple ECG leads, continuous in-test and post-test ECG analysis, and carefully validated diagnostic criteria.

By contrast, if the use is for screening large populations for CHD then some specificity and sensitivity may be sacrificed to economy of cost, speed and convenience of performance, a high level of safety, etc. Other dimensions of use include study in various special populations (e.g., women, high-risk, youth) and in various degrees of disease state (the apparently healthy, latent disease, etc.). Exercise electrocardiography is a tool which can be applied to perform several tasks and its development should be with regard for the *task*.

HARBORING OUTDATED CONCEPTS

Inevitably, each era carries over concepts of the previous one with more or less detriment to progress. An example is in terminology, such as the "horseless" carriage, the "wireless" telegraph. In exercise electrocardiography the "graphy" indicates a classical mode of data display, a result of a visually oriented culture, which limits our ability to extract full information.

Consider the terminology, "ST segment." Is this terminology and its underlying concept still relevant in view of new techniques of ECG signal analysis? Einthoven's descriptive sequential labeling of the ECG waveforms was unrelated even to knowledge of that time about underlying myocardial events. Is it reasonable now to require a computer program to locate the "ST onset" in order to perform certain amplitude measurements? Couching this decision-making process in terms of waveform slope changes, relative to fiducial points, is an empiric transmutation of "eyeball" logic into magic numbers through the pseudosophistication of a computer program.

The dynamic process of ischemia (usually due to CHD) affects various electrical events of the cardiac cycle, notably ventricular repolarization. The signal generated by repolarization is available at the body surface, and under certain circumstances including exercise, in certain patients, has special informational value. But the processes of ventricular depolarization and repolarization overlap in time and space. May not *visual* description of "ST onset" simply distract us from a physiologically open-minded, instrumentation-oriented analysis of the signal? The changes we see in the ST-segment the computer can measure, and with greater accuracy.

Consider the alternative of basing data collection from a point determined by capabilities inherent in the computer such as relating the intersection of the R wave downslope with a constant voltage line (this could be the baseline-adjusted iso-electric line).

Additional information from terminal QRS vectors in the exercise response is suggested by the work of Blomqvist (9), and Kahn and Simonson (9a).

Dedication to a fictional "baseline" from which to measure waveform amplitudes is another outdated concept. One technique reproduces the "eyeball" iso-electric line by connecting computer-determined points such as QRS onsets. In the absence of absolute direct current electrocardiographic amplification the reference "line" might better be determined by comparison of a *series* of points on each complex with similar points on neighboring complexes and subsequent derivation of an "average," ultra-low frequency waveform by "best-fit" methods.

Other examples of the persistence of outdated or inappropriate concepts surely occur to you. At best they make terminology archaic while at worst they sabotage progress.

TECHNICAL PROBLEMS

Quantitation

Quantitation is a freeing process. The end product of work described in this symposium will be in part a new and more efficient language. Elimination of "fuzzy" thought is inherent in an enumerative process. It should free us from some ambiguities in present concepts, much in the way that the introduction of a number system fostered trade and later mercantile societies. Primitive man's communications were limited in efficiency and extent by lack of adequate numerical concepts (10).

We should be better able to communicate with our data and with the machines which generate them, and the machines will be better able to communicate with each other.

Standardization

A major practical problem now is *standardization*, a term which implies regimentation. Standardization of techniques, systems, criteria, validation measures, etc., is desirable to facilitate communication, to enhance the ongoing process of validation in exercise electrocardiography and to increase contributions to common knowledge. Finally, as history reveals (i.e., "Master" test), the medical community is attracted to "standardized" procedures which bear the seal of authority and are practical and useful.

A specific problem in standardization of exercise electrocardiography is the type of stress. Exercise predominates, but considered in the past and perhaps worthy of reconsideration are the following: (a) hypoxia tests (11, 12, 13); (b) drug responses (a wide variety), and (c) combinations of exercise, hypoxia and drugs.

Various modes of exercise have been used, including arm work (cranking) (14, 15) and leg work, and arm and leg work combined. Arm work is interesting from two points of view. First, for a given oxygen uptake there seems to be a greater heart rate response than with leg work, and quite possibly this may be better provocation of the ischemic response (16). Also, arm work may be useful in testing people unable to use their legs.

Most of the pros and cons of leg work have been listed elsewhere and are well-known. Narrowing of this field should be possible once criteria for equipment cost, size, ease of use, quality and quantity of data desired, and other factors are decided upon.

Techniques of imposing the work load will not be considered here except to note that the time-course of the changing ST segment morphology throughout exercise and recovery should be continuously related to the time-course of heart rate change. The latter is determined in large part by the technique of exercise used. Little thought has been given to determining *dynamic* criteria for waveform interpretation *during* the actual exercise.

Regardless of the technique of imposing exercise, a higher yield of "ischemic responders" will be obtained by near-maximal or maximal stress in contrast to a submaximal procedure. We would like to know whether this additional yield represents identification of (a) an increased incidence of "false positives;" (b) a population with the same disease process but at an earlier stage; (c) a population with a somewhat different disease process, or (d) some combination of these.

Regardless of the exercise technique used, certain broad attempts at standardization can be accomplished. First, in terms of the *external work load,* this standard favors certain apparatus and is favored by some work physiologists. The relation of external work to ischemic response, however, is indirect and it seems to me useful only in the following areas:

1. Testing the efficacy of so-called "coronary" drugs.
2. Demonstrating a patient's work capacity in relation to ECG responses.
3. Research in work physiology.

Standardization is also attempted in terms of *cardiac work.* This necessitates some measure of cardiac pump function, the ability of the organ to impart an acceleration or velocity to a mass of blood, or the resultant pressures. We turn to indirect methods by necessity and this leads us into the somewhat bewildering area of sensor/transducer systems, including the ballistocardiograph, displacement devices (e.g., Wayne-Kerr), the body impedence plethysmograph and various ultrasound instruments. All of these must be validated with direct measurements.

Finally, standardization of stress can be attempted in terms of the *determinants* of the ischemic response. To learn more about these requires more understanding of the mechanisms by which alterations in cellular metabolism influence cell membrane potential, and in turn how these events manifest themselves as alterations in the ECG waveform at the body surface. However, heart rate is a major determinant of the ischemic exercise ECG response and is increasingly used for standardization purposes.

Systems Design

The concept of systems design is not new but its application to clinical and experimental medicine has lagged in many areas. Its rationale has been outlined by Caceres (18).

Up to the present the various instruments and procedures of exercise electrocardiography have been treated in a compartmentalized manner. Systems design takes some cognizance of the new "medium" inherent in the generation, transmission, analysis and feedback of information also inherent in exercise electrocardiography. Systems design tends to blur the boundaries between the compartments of treadmill, electrodes, amplifiers, transmission network, A/D converter, computer, etc., by mating components so that their functions blend and support each other. A historical analog of this is the implosion of cultures brought together by air travel, communications satellites and other technological advances.

Systems design also forces a comprehensive view. For example, choice of a lead system for exercise electrocardiography entails the following:

1. The adhesive, electrical and mechanical properties of available electrodes.
2. Ease of skin preparation in areas chosen.
3. Relative "noise" of electrode positions.
4. "Best" signal; (a) giving the greatest absolute or relative ST depression, or (b) the greatest ability to detect "positive" ST responses in a population (20, 21).

Systems design also means mating of component specifications, such as those for electrodes (22), amplifiers (23, 24), (i.e., coupling, input impedance, frequency response), data transmission systems, and for the "accuracy" of computer programs.

Data Handling

The final technical problem is that of data handling. Not only does the new medium change the *content* of the data (attested to by those who have rooms overflowing with punch cards), but it also changes the *form* of the processes from which it springs. Methods of display should be reexamined. Indeed, we may question the need for waveform display at all. Eyeball-oriented techniques and criteria have been failing us, and our own failure to realize their limitations has hindered progress. An example is the masking of our lack of knowledge about physiological and biochemical processes of repolarization by "looking at" these phemonema through the "window" of the ST segment.

Display should be data-oriented, i.e., it should be the servant of our classification techniques (normal vs. abnormal, Group A vs. Group B, or whatever) (25). Pipberger *et al.* (26, 27) have published valuable information and approaches in this area.

Display can also mean *array*. The numbers generated by our efforts must not be hidden by awkward tabulation; rather their full value must be exploited by intelligent array into forms such as, for example, covariance matrices.

Future analysis of the data from the exercise ECG response will involve in all likelihood a variety of techniques such as multivariate probability-density functions with multi-dimensional mathematical models, error-correcting training procedures (9), discriminant function analysis, adaptive computer programs (i.e., a perceptron), factor analysis and multiple regression.

FUTURE USE OF EXERCISE ELECTROCARDIOGRAPHY

Preventive or prophylactic medicine becomes increasingly important. I think that among the tools of multiphasic screening one will find stress electrocardiography important in *early* diagnosis of coronary heart disease, the detection of latent or subclinical coronary heart disease. Epidemiologic applications will increase understanding of coronary heart disease as it exists in the general population and will provide identification of susceptibles for the effective application of preventive measures.

In the future, use of exercise electrocardiography will be what I should like to call *data-oriented/clinically-validated*. This means that having achieved a certain measure of standardization, we can turn our attention to handling the mass of data generated by our activities. Clinical validation will be possible by longitudinal study techniques. The pioneering work of Mattingly (28), and Robb and Marks (29) has been gaining widespread acceptance by the general body of physicians. There is much to be gained in application of electrocardiographic techniques to large groups of people. The final product I suspect will be an individual *process* of data gathering and analysis developed on-line by computer techniques. It will judiciously select and apply diagnostic techniques, one being stress electrocardiography, to help the physician answer the question which has existed since before Hippocrates: "How can I best minister to the health needs of my patient?"

REFERENCES

1. KAHN, R.M.: Das Elektrokardiogramm. *Ergebn Physiol, 14*:1, 1914.
2. SCHERF, D., and SCHAFFER, A.I.: The electrocardiographic exercise test. *Amer Heart J, 43*:927, 1952.
3. LARSEN, K.H.: *Om Forandringer i Elektrokardiogrammet hos Sunde og Syge under experimental Iltmangel.* Copenhagen, Ejnar Munksgaard, 1938.
4. EINTHOVEN, W.: Weiteres über das Elektrokardiogramm. *Arch Ges Physiol, 122*:517, 1908.
5. FEIL, H., and SIEGEL, M.L.: Electrocardiographic changes during attacks of angina pectoris. *Amer J Med Sci, 175*:256, 1928.
6. WOOD, F.C.; WOLFERTH, C.C., and LIVEZEY, M.M.: Angina pectoris. *Arch Intern Med, 47*:339, 1931.
7. GOLDHAMMER, S., and SCHERF, D.: Elektrokardiographische Untersuchungen bei Kranken mit Angina Pectoris ("ambulatorischer Typus"). *Z Klin Med, 122*:134, 1932.
8. MASTER, A.M.; FRIEDMAN, R., and DACK, S.: The electrocardiogram after standard exercise as functional test of heart. *Amer Heart J, 24*:777, 1942.
9. BLOMQVIST, G.: The Frank lead exercise electrocardiogram. A quantitative study based on averaging technic and digital computer analysis. *Acta Med Scand, 178* (suppl.):440, 1965.
9a. KAHN, K.A., and SIMONSON, E.: Changes of mean spatial QRS and T vectors and of conventional electrocardiographic items in hard anoerobic work. *Circ Res, 5*:629, 1957.
10. DANTZIG, TOBIAS: *Number, The Language of Science.* Garden City, Doubleday, 1954.
11. ROTHSCHILD, M.A., and KISSIN, M.: Induced general anoxemia causing S-T deviation in the electrocardiogram, *Amer Heart J, 8*:745, 1933.
12. LEVY, R.L.; BARACH, A.L., and BRUENN, H.G.: Effects of induced oxygen want in patients with cardiac pain. *Amer Heart J,15*:187, 1938.
13. BIORCK, G.: Anoxemia and exercise tests in the diagnosis of coronary disease, *Amer Heart J, 32*:689, 1946.
14. KNIPPING, H.W., and VALENTIN, H.: "Vita-maxima" problems in the management of cardiac patients. *Postgrad Med, 35*:68, 1964.

15. SALTIN, B.: Aerobic work capacity and circulation of exercise in man. *Acta Physiol Scand, 62*(suppl.):230, 1964.

16. HASKELL, W., personal communication.

17. BRUCE, R.A.; ROWELL, L.B.; BLACKMON, J.R., and DOAN, A.: Cardiovascular function tests. *Heart Bull, 14*:9, 1965.

18. CACERES, C.A.: Computers in Biomedicine. Presentation at N.I.H. Conference on Future Goals for Engineering in Biology and Medicine, Sept. 8-9, 1967.

19. McLUHAN, M.: *Understanding Media: The Extensions of Man.* New York, New Am. Lib., 1964.

20. BLACKBURN, H.; TAYLOR, H.L.; VASQUEZ, C.L., and PUCHNER, T.C.: The electrocardiogram during exercise. *Circulation, 34*:1034, 1966.

21. BLACKBURN, H.: The electrocardiogram in cardiovascular epidemiology: problems in standardized application, *Ann NY Acad Sci, 126*:882, 1965.

22. WINTER, D.A.; RAUTAHARJU, P.M., and WOLF, H.K.: Measurement and characteristics of over-all noise content in exercise electrocardiograms. *Amer Heart J, 74*:324, 1967.

23. BERSON, A.S., and PIPBERGER, H.V.: The low-frequency response of electrocardiographs, a frequent source of recording errors. *Amer Heart J, 71*: 779, 1966.

24. MEYER, J.L.: Some instrument-induced errors in the electrocardiogram. *JAMA, 201*:351, 1967.

25. ABRAHAM, S.; CALATAYUD, J.B.; GORMAN, P.A., and CACERES, C.A.: Application of statistical techniques in analysis of electrocardiography. *Ann NY Acad Sci, 134*:573, 1966.

26. PIPBERGER, H.V., and CARTER, T.N.: Analysis of the normal and abnormal vectorcardiogram in its own reference frame. *Circulation, 25*:827, 1962.

27. BATCHLOR, C.D.; BERSON, A.S.; NAVAL, I.A., and PIPBERGER, H.V.: Computer search for electrocardiographic lead directions to optimize diagnostic differentiation. *Circulation, 36*:320, 1967.

28. MATTINGLY, T.W.: The post exercise electrocardiogram. Its value in the diagnosis and prognosis of coronary arterial disease. *Amer J Cardiol, 9*:395, 1962.

29. ROBB, G.P. and MARKS, H.H., Post-exercise electrocardiogram in arteriosclerotic heart disease. *JAMA, 200*:918, 1967.

17

The Exercise Electrocardiogram
Technological, Procedural and
Conceptual Developments

HENRY BLACKBURN

RAPID CHANGES taking place in exercise stress testing with electrocardiography are related to several conceptual developments and to technological and procedural improvements. It is inevitable that some methods which have served well for many years will be replaced by new methods and standards. Meanwhile, there is a state of chaos in which different techniques and approaches are applied, the results of which are not comparable. Unfortunately this has happened at a time when many physicians have become interested in the practical uses of exercise stress testing in cardiac diagnosis, in functional evaluation, and in prediction of future risk of a coronary event. The absence of an acceptable standard procedure based on newer physiological concepts and technology may be considered an indication of active research in a field of considerable theoretical and practical importance.

Many of the concerns about measurement in exercise electrocardiography exposed in this conference are not immediately or universally applicable to the practitioner's needs. This report attempts to consider some of his interests and to fill in certain of the uses and developments not treated in other presentations of this monograph.

USES OF EXERCISE ELECTROCARDIOGRAPHY

Historically the development of exercise electrocardiography has

Note: This report is based on studies sponsored by USPHS Grant Nos. HE-04697, HE-04967, HE-03088 and HE-06314 and by the Heart Disease and Stroke Control Program, USPHS Contract PH 86-68-170 for a Technical Group on Exercise Electrocardiography, by the American Heart Association, Minnesota Heart Association and Graduate School Awards of the University of Minnesota.

been an amalgamation of the older European tradition of circulatory function testing with the newer diagnostic observations of "ischemic" change in the electrocardiogram (ECG) (15, 19). Some conceptual impediments to more effective exploitation of information available from the exercise ECG have to do with confusion over its uses. The ECG response to exercise is used in the following manner:

In Diagnosis

1. To confirm a clinical impression of angina pectoris.

A clearly "ischemic" exercise ST depression, or even a "borderline" ST-T change or arrhythmia, increases the probability that a chest pain is of coronary origin when other obvious etiology is excluded, such as valvular disease.

2. In the differential diagnosis of chest pain, as in *1*.

3. To detect latent coronary artery disease.

In the absence of other obvious etiological forms of heart disease, a clearly "ischemic" ST depression in an exercise ECG, without such finding at rest, is usually due to a perfusion defect, in turn probably due to coronary atherosclerosis. The degree of probability that the finding represents an early manifestation of coronary insufficiency is greater: the more "ischemic" and the greater is the amount of the ST-T depression and the longer it lasts in recovery; the more are the ECG leads in which is appears (40, 41), and very likely, the less is the amount of stress required to induce the finding.

In Risk Prediction

4. To predict future risk of coronary attack, as in *3*.

High risk of heart disease is a preventive medical concept with the same portent generally as diagnosis of a latent or early disease condition. It means in this case that of individuals otherwise equal (in age, weight, etc.), those who have an "ischemic" ECG response to exercise are at greater risk, over the short and the long term, of a coronary event and death than are those with no such response. As in diagnosis, the risk is greater the more "ischemic" is the character, and the more severe and prolonged the change; and, very likely, the more easily induced with respect to work load.

In Function Testing

5. To test function of the heart and circulation.

The ECG and heart rate response to a peak work effort are a part of an overall evaluation of myocardial function and circulatory capacity.

6. To assess work capacity.

The ECG and heart rate response during and after a given work load provide an estimate of the capacity and safety of performing peak work. They have been extrapolated empirically to the capacity for endurance work at energy levels lower than those of the test.

In Population Research

7. To investigate effects of therapy, as in clinical trials.

Change in the ECG response to a standard exercise test provides, in the living subject, an assessment of the efficacy of therapy, including direct surgical interventions on the myocardium or cardiac valves or coronary circulation, or indirect effects on the heart of drugs, physical conditioning, diet, etc.

8. To make population comparisons.

Objective comparisons of populations are attempted on the basis of ECG responses to standard procedures and physiological stress (9).

Not all these applications are met effectively by the common clinical method which is a single-stage, short-term step test, followed by paper recording of conventional ECG lead data as sequential traces and finally by impressionistic interpretation. Possibly *no* standard exercise test procedure could be devised to meet requirements of all these uses, though this, along with measurement, would be highly desirable.

CONCEPTUAL IMPEDIMENTS TO EFFECTIVE APPLICATION OF EXERCISE ELECTROCARDIOGRAPHY

Exercise ECG tests are performed in a ratio of 1 for 250 resting ECGs in University of Minnesota teaching hospitals. At the Mayo Clinic fewer than 10 per cent of patients suspected to have coronary disease are subjected to exercise stress testing (12). Though this is inadequate exploitation of the method it is true that the contribution of stress testing to diagnosis in such referral centers is limited. The patient population in these centers, where most physicians are trained, is an extreme segment of the diseased population and a very small segment indeed of the general population. Most referred patients in middle age and beyond are so involved by vascular disease that little information of a purely diagnostic nature is added by stress testing. Other patients may present such a diagnostic and therapeutic quandary that direct coronary artery visualization with catheter studies is entertained. Often overlooked in these centers are the value of (a) personal observation by the physician of the patient's symptoms, often evoked in life-like reproduction but under controlled conditions of work, and (b) the quantitative information provided about the degree of disability or impairment of function.

In the "real world" of out-patient centers, the physician's office, annual preventive examination programs and insurance risk appraisals, the proportion of subjects diseased is much smaller and their identification more difficult. In these real-life situations one needs all the help available to diagnose latent coronary artery disease. Here, a carefully monitored exercise electrocardiogram should be among the first methods to follow the traditional medical history-taking and physical examination. More expensive, traumatic or hazardous procedures which require hospitalization are reserved for later stages of the clinical investigation.

There are other comprehensible but unfortunate impediments to effective training for and use of the exercise ECG test and other assessments of circulatory function. A whole generation rejects most muscular activity as unpleasant, unintelligent or "lower class" activity. Many physicians are of this generation or are still influenced by it. Fortunately this attitude is disappearing. Many physicians hold the concepts of preventive and rehabilitative medicine as outside the main line of physician training and interest and outside their responsibility. This, too, is changing, though slowly. Stress tests require supervision of the hospital physician who finds it inconvenient to schedule and monitor such tests in the ECG department during his busy days. In the office situation it is much easier to supervise the test and monitoring devices with oscilloscopes are available for beat-to-beat displays, so that this impediment is disappearing.

There has been confusion of the diagnostic with the functional testing applications of exercise electrocardiography. Now it is appreciated that functional evaluation of work capacity is abetted by the test and that with proper precautions it is safe to stress cardiac patients. Another confusion has been the dictum that an exercise ECG test is never performed in the presence of an abnormal rest ECG. In a stable clinical situation assessment of function and prognosis is improved, though knowledge is still meager about the significance, in these terms, of an exercise-induced change in an *already abnormal* rest ECG. This question begs investigation among subject groups large enough, and followed long enough, to develop the answers.

FACTORS INFLUENCING THE ECG RESPONSE TO EXERCISE

The results of an exercise ECG test have been regarded simplistically as "positive or negative" based on the postexercise response to a particular work prescription of Master (28). Actually many factors influence the ECG response to exercise. Some of these are listed here:

TABLE 17-I

PREVALENCE RATES OF "ISCHEMIC-TYPE" ST-T DEPRESSION (MINN. CODES 11.1, 2, 3) IN THE POSTEXERCISE ECG (NONE AT REST) BY AGE AND AREA
(Rates per 1000 men)

Area	Total N	Ages 40-49	Total N	Ages 50-59
U. S. Rail Clerks	349	59.5	498	120.1
Italian farmers (M)	369	52.5	347	65.3
Yugoslavian farmers (S)	284	28.9	415	43.2

Age

Table 17-I indicates that the frequency of classifiable ST-T findings ings in the immediate postexercise record increases with age in many populations, irrespective of the apparent burden of coronary or other heart diseases in the population (9).

Sex

A few studies show that, at a given age, women have more frequent "ischemic" ST-T depressions than men (1, 25, 32). This important observation needs elucidation.

Physical Characteristics

Figure 17-1 illustrates the association between marked "ischemic" postexercise ECG responses (Minnesota Code 11.1) and physical characteristics of skinfold thickness (obesity), blood pressure and serum cholesterol, discussed in detail in the section on the prognostic power of the exercise ECG (p. 000) (9, 22).

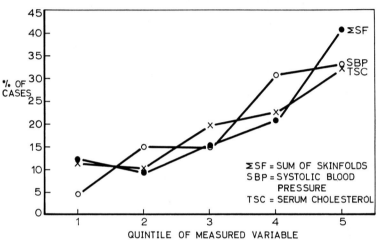

≥ 1.0 MM POST-EXERCISE ISCHEMIC S-T DEPRESSION (XI.1) VERSUS PHYSICAL CHARACTERISTICS

FIGURE 17-1. The proportion of cases is plotted with distinctly positive (≥ 1.0 mm flat or downward sloping) "ischemic" postexercise findings in the conventional ECG after a three-minute step test, according to physical characteristic. If there were no relationship between the positive test and the characteristic 20 per cent of the positive cases should fall in each 20 per cent class of the measured variable, Σ SF sum of skinfolds, SBP systolic blood pressure and TSC total serum cholesterol. In fact there is a significant positive relationship of the ECG response to each physical characteristic. The problem is that these characteristics are themselves interrelated (9).

Habits

There is an inverse frequency of "positive" exercise ECG responses to a standard single-stage test according to increasing habitual physical activity of occupation; and no apparent association with cigarette smoking habits (9, 22). The confounding variables in these associations are examined elsewhere (9, 22).

ECG Instrumentation

The fidelity of the recording system, especially at the lower range of ECG frequencies, has a great influence on the display and measurement of the exercise ECG and on the frequency of errors and distortion (4, 23).

ECG Lead Systems

The performance, strength and orientation, and number of ECG leads affect the contour, amount and interpretation of ST-T exercise responses, as pointed out later in this presentation and elsewhere (8).

Technical Quality of the Record

The "noise" level and general technical quality of the record and its mounting affect measurement and interpretation (36, 39).

Recording Conditions

Posture, ambient temperature, meals, tobacco smoking, hyperventilation, emotional state and drug therapy (especially digitalis) affect the ECG response to an exercise stress probably by resetting the relationship between work load, heart rate response and myocardial oxygen requirement.

Work Load

The type of work, amount of work, work posture, rate of work, program of work, and monitoring intervals during and after work affect the exercise ECG response (4).

Measurement and Criteria

Measurement or its lack, and the criteria used for classification, affect the reliability and validity of exercise ECG interpretation (36, 39).

Many of these influences can be eliminated by improved technology, reduced by measurement and definition, or accounted for by standardizing or randomizing the test conditions. A simplified approach to interpretation of the ECG response to stress which ignores these influences results in confusion, at best, and error at worst.

Let us now consider some of the technological and procedural problems in exercise electrocardiography and certain developments leading toward their solution.

THE SKIN-ELECTRODE CONTACT

Means of improving the skin-electrode contact, and awareness of its importance, are as significant as any factors affecting the use of electrocardiography in dynamic states. Improvement of the recording quality at the "source" allows improvement all along the line of instrumentation, procedure and analysis. After years of admonitions from a few (31, 45), the need for good skin preparation is now more generally realized. The crucial factor in a good preparation is elimination of the horny layer of epidermis. This is often inconsistently attained by superficial cleansing and daubing of electrolytic paste on the skin. However, it may be accomplished uniformly by dermal abrasion with a sterile needle or dental burr lightly and momentarily applied to the electrode site after cleansing the skin with a fat solvent. The procedure is painless and no blood is drawn. With the dental burr a shiny shallow pit about 2 mm in diameter is obtained which heals promptly.

The family of lightweight, liquid-contact relatively nonpolarizing silver-silver chloride electrodes with plastic housing and small flexible cables have provided a major contribution to exercise ECG technology. The electrodes in effect go into solution with tissue fluids when the horny layer of skin is removed and liquid junction established. Sources of motion artifact which derive from change in contact resistance between skin and electrode are thereby avoided, and the electrode-electrolyte interface is very stable. Somewhat larger electrode surface areas would be desirable as would a reduction in the price of these electrodes. An input impedance in excess of 3 megohms or buffer amplifiers (18) are required to avoid loss of signal amplitude.

INSTRUMENTATION

Frequency Response

The wider recognition of the importance of faithful recording at the lower end of the ECG frequency range is a significant development in instrumentation for electrocardiography in dynamic states. Earlier

American Heart Association instrument specifications were below those required to reproduce always accurately the slower components of the ECG, including the gradual wave forms of the ST region and T wave. The distortion effect of short amplifier time constants, equivalent to filters which exclude slow wave components, has been known for many years but recently was restudied by Berson and Pipberger (3) and is discussed in this volume by Mr. Berson (p. 000). They estimate a 3 per cent frequency of ST segment displacement errors amounting to 1 mm or more ($\geqslant$0.1 mv) from instruments built to the A.H.A specifications which existed until 1967. They illustrate how heart rate and QRS configuration determine different frequencies of error and types of ST-T distortion.

Discussion continues whether differences in phase angle of the slower ST-T components are entirely accounted for by the new 1967 A.H.A. specifications for ECG instrumentation (37, 38), but the possibility for distortion is vastly reduced. The new specifications require errors of less than 0.5 mm (0.05 mv) in the early part of ST-T (0.05 Hz cutoff with a 6 db per octave rolloff).

Buffer Amplifiers

Schmitt has proposed that amplifiers having high input impedance relative to the source, with low output impedance, be placed close to or within the electrode (44). Signal transmission to the later stage amplifiers should be accompanied by less noise from the contact source and pickup of induced hum. Use of such amplifiers appears to have been helpful in studies reported in this volume (see van der Groeben, p. 000) but no systematic comparative experience is available. They happen to have come into use simultaneously with great improvements in the skin-electrode contact, patient cables, amplifiers and grounding procedures.

Many technical aspects of ECG recording during muscular activity are clearly interdependent. Improvement at one stage has resulted in improvement in and attention to developments all along the system. For example, poor frequency-response characteristics are found in many ECG apparatus in current use, including portable tape monitoring devices and FM radio-telemetry systems. These were engineered to provide a "pretty" record, actually to be insensitive to baseline shifts from changing electrode contact and respiration. It happens that these artifacts occur at the low end of the frequency range just where diagnostic ST-T information exists. As motion artifact has been reduced by improved skin-electrode contact and lightweight cable arrangements it follows that the fidelity of the recorder may be improved, still producing technically acceptable records. As impedance at the skin-electrode source is reduced by better skin preparation, electrodes or buffer amplifiers, so are the problems of hum, distortion and attenuation in the record. Internal amplifier hum which occurs when excessively high input impedance is required by high source impedance can be avoided. And so it goes, throughout the recording system. Systems for noise reduction and quality control are described in this monograph (see Winter, p. 000), and elsewhere (36).

Magnetic Tape Recording

Little has been said in this conference about special problems in the use of tape recorders. No summary will be attempted. It may suffice to indicate that magnetic tape recording is integrated into most of the systems of ECG measurement considered here. The available tape apparatus are generally more than adequate for faithful ECG recording. Many of the problems of the recent past in systems design, of "noise" contributed by the tape recorder itself, of control units including calibration and coding, etc. have been met successfully.

Computer Programs and Technology

Automated programs for quality control, wave recognition and machine measurement or "diagnosis" in exercise electrocardiography make up the substance of other presentations in this monograph.

ECG LEAD SYSTEMS

Three general classes of ECG lead system are used in exercise ECG tests:

> Conventional limb and Wilson precordial leads
> Simple bipolar chest leads
> Orthogonal "vector" X, Y, Z lead systems

The use of one or another system depends upon the sensitivity desired, the engineering support available and exigencies of time and cost. Each type of lead system has practical advantages and disadvantages, different degrees of sensitivity, specificity and effectiveness of ST-T display, and different performance during muscular activity. Use of a system other than conventional leads requires careful documentation. Standards do not exist for using other leads, procedures or interpretive criteria.

It is important that clinical studies with the exercise ECG be comparable to others using conventional lead standards. New studies such as in population research and therapeutic trials, are less constrained. In the collaborative project between the Laboratory of Physiological Hygiene and Dr. Rautaharju at Dalhousie University, six simultaneous channels of data are recorded on magnetic tape. Potential differences are recorded between a reference electrode and each exploring electrode located at the Frank lead sites (modified by Blomqvist [11]). Any desired lead data can then be synthesized in a computer program which provides the particular lead weighting factors at the processing stage rather than at the time of recording.

Simple bipolar chest leads are considered here in recognition of their extensive use and in an attempt to provide some information on the meaning of responses occurring in them. This should not be construed as a recommendation for their use.

Conventional Leads

Conventional leads I, II, III, aVR, aVL, aVF, V_1 through V_6 have the advantage of wide use and familiar criteria and the disadvantages of redundancy, distortion and relative insensitivity to ST display. Virtually all the information from the ST-T response in conventional postexercise records is found in six of the twelve leads, II, aVF, V_3, V_4, V_5, V_6, and most of it (89 per cent) in lead V_5 alone (5). However, practical problems arise in attempting to reduce for exercise tests the number of conventional-type ECG leads. Overall, V_5 or a simple bipolar chest lead give the best ST-T display in the most people (8). This is not sufficient for evaluation of the individual problem case though it is useful in screening or comparisons among large populations.

The relative frequency of "ischemic" findings in more vertically oriented leads versus right-left oriented chest leads has been examined in this laboratory in both conventional and Frank lead records. The conventional-type ECG was obtained from one hundred middle-aged U.S. men having "ischemic type" ST-T depression ($\geqslant$ 0.5 mm. horizontal or downward sloping segment depression) in one or more of the twelve leads following a three-minute standard step test. Codable ST-T depression was found in one or the other "vertical lead" (II, III, aVF) in thirty men. Of the thirty men with "positive" S-T findings in the vertically oriented leads, twenty had associated "positive" findings in one or another of the "left lateral leads" (I, aVL, V_4 through V_6). In this series of middle-aged men the ratio is 10 to 1 of left lateral lead location to vertical lead display of "ischemic" ST-T. The "ischemic" finding was confined to lead III in 1 per cent, to lead aVF in 3 per cent and to both III and aVF in another 3 per cent.

Scalar records of the Frank lead ECG were obtained in another group of middle-aged men (N = 84) having at least 0.5 mm horizontal or downward-sloping ST-T segment in one or more of the three leads. Sixty-five per cent of cases displayed the "ischemic" finding only in the horizontal lead X, 25 per cent in both the horizontal and vertical leads X and Y (25 per cent), and 10 per cent uniquely

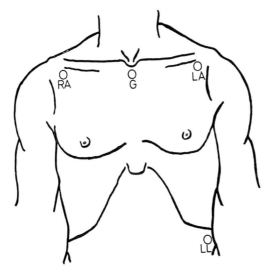

FIGURE 17-2. Limb electrodes for right arm (RA), left arm (LA), left leg (LL) and ground (G) are fixed to the torso to reduce motion artifact during the exercise tests. See Mason and Likar (27).

in the vertical Y lead, a similar distribution to that found in comparable conventional ECG leads in a quite different but randomly chosen group of men.

Motion artifact resulting from the usual placement of the conventional limb electrodes is greatly reduced by their attachment on the trunk at sites illustrated in Figure 17-2. This does not appear to affect significantly the amplitudes obtained, though precise and systematic comparisons have not been made (27). Conventional leads may not be as sensitive to ST display as certain distorted bi-polar leads or specially synthesized lead configurations (8).

Bi-polar Leads

Simple bi-polar leads in various configurations across the chest, or from head to chest, are used in many monitoring situations and in exercise testing. Practical advantages of a two or three electrode system include the little time required to prepare the subject, the great reduction of the amount of ECG data, less chance of motion artifact than in multiple central terminal leads and optimal distortion for display of ST responses (8). But little information is available about the diagnostic power of findings in these leads. Theoretically, a portion of "positive" ST displays will be missed in *any* single lead approach. Information is available, however, on the relative lead strength, orientation and discriminative power of several simple bi-polar chest leads (8).

The "mean maximum ischemic ST vector" is found 180° away from the mean maximum QRS vector (8, 11). Most but not all of the lead difference in amplitude of ST segment depression is explained by different amplitude of the R wave in a given lead as shown in Figure 17-3. Diagnostic discrimination may be sharpened by correcting or normalizing ST segment amplitude for R wave amplitude but this has not been studied adequately.

Several simple transthoracic bi-polar lead configurations have been examined because of their demonstrated superiority in earlier studies, or their use by centers reporting at this conference. The exploring electrode was common to all five systems, at C_5 (V_5) chest position (left anterior axillary line at the horizontal level of C_4). The position of the reference electrode for each lead is illustrated in Figure 17-4.

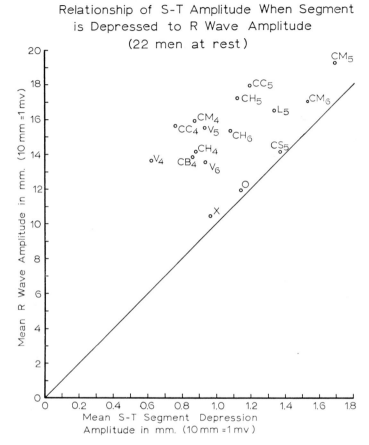

Figure 17-3. ST amplitudes are plotted according to R wave amplitude for numerous individual ECG leads. All men had measurable ST depression. All leads were recorded from each man. There is a crude relationship, but the 45° line is not a regression line.

The ground electrode is placed at any convenient chest position, usually symmetrically opposite on the chest to the reference electrode.

Amplitude comparisons were made from records taken simultaneously in the same middle-aged men, mixed normal subjects and cardiac patients, and in a subsample, twenty-five men were exercised to maximal work capacity with all leads recorded simultaneously. The noise level and frequency of baseline shifts were visually measured and averaged.

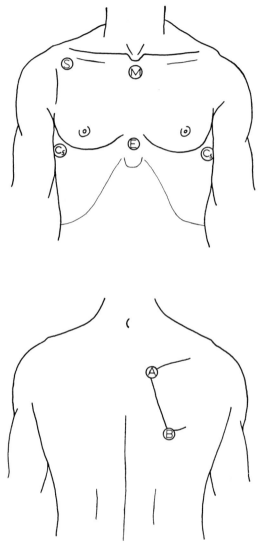

FIGURE 17-4. Simple bi-polar transthoracic leads found to give strong QRS and ST display as well as good performance during muscular activity. The bipolar systems compared utilize the same positive exploring electrode at standard C_5 (V_5) position in the left chest and different negative reference electrodes, below the right clavicle (CS), on the manubrium of the sternum (CM), at C_5 on the right chest (CC) and over the right scapula CA and CB.

TABLE 17-II

FOUR SIMULTANEOUSLY RECORDED BIPOLAR MONITORING
ECG LEADS IMMEDIATELY POSTEXERCISE AMONG A MIXED
GROUP OF NORMAL SUBJECTS AND PATIENTS*

		CB N=25	CA N=25	CS N=25	CM N=25
Q wave amplitude	M	0.5	0.8	0.9	1.4
	SD	0.7	1.0	0.9	2.0
R wave amplitude	M	16.0	19.0	17.9	19.9
	SD	7.3	9.1	9.2	9.8
S wave amplitude	M	4.5	5.8	4.8	3.4
	SD	2.5	3.7	2.2	2.6
T wave amplitude	M	2.3	2.7	2.7	2.5
	SD	2.1	1.9	2.0	2.2
ST junction	M	—2.5	—2.6	—2.3	—2.4
Maximum amplitude	SD	1.6	1.8	1.9	1.9
ST midpoint amplitude	M	1.8	1.8	1.8	1.9
	SD	0.4	0.3	0.3	0.4
ST segment maximum amplitude when depressed	M	—3.8	—6.0	—5.0	—4.9
% *Total Depressed*		48	36	36	44

		Reference Electrode	*Exploring Electrode*
	CB	inferior scapular angle, right	Common to all in
	CA	medial scapular ridge, right	position C_5
	CS	subclavicle, right lateral	
	CM	manubrium sternum	

*Amplitude in mm (10 mm = 1 mv) Means (M) and Standard Deviations (SD).

The comparison in Table 17-II and others indicate that generally during exercise similar QRST contours and amplitudes are obtainable from several simple, obliquely oriented bipolar chest leads. These leads, with the exploring electrode at position C_5, resemble the contour of conventional left precordial Wilson leads, especially V_5. Small and usually insignificant amplitude and orientation differences exist between some of these bipolar leads and, in turn, between these and Wilson chest leads. While the mean differences are rarely significant there are lead differences in the frequency of "positive" responses by a given criterion so that study results using different electrode placement are not interchangeable.

Bipolar chest leads which combine highest R wave amplitudes and greatest display of ST depression are CM_5 (manubrium -C_5) and CS_5 (right clavicle - C_5). There is little to recommend one of these leads over the other. CM_5 is slightly more likely than CS_5 to have "false positive" negative T waves at rest standing (4 per cent vs. 3 per cent). CM_5 is more likely than CS_5 to be sensitive for any

TABLE 17-III

DIAGNOSTIC POWER OF ST-T CRITERIA IN THE RESTING ECG
ACCORDING TO LEAD SYSTEM EMPLOYED AMONG A
POPULATION SAMPLE OF MEN AGED 45-64

| | | *Sensitivity*[†] | |
Specificity[*]	*12 Leads*	*Bipolar*	*XYZ*
85%	59%	58%	38%

[*]The proportion of "normals" correctly identified
[†]The proportion of "cardiac cases" correctly identified

ST depression (28 per cent vs. 18 per cent of older men). CM_5 may perform slightly better than CS_5 in regard to noise and baseline shifts (4.3 versus 4.8 average baseline shifts greater than a 5 per cent slope).

The real sensitivity-specificity relationships with respect to an independent assessment of coronary heart disease are not known for any of the special bi-polar leads. The crude first approach in Table 17-III suggests they may be more sensitive than other leads, and indeed perhaps "too sensitive." Their use can be justified, mainly for cost-expediency reasons, in long-term patient monitoring, or for screening and larger collaborative studies where internal comparisons are possible.

XYZ Orthogonal Leads

There are several special considerations in the application of orthogonal leads to electrocardiography in dynamic states, in addition to those general questions of the dipole model which are widely investigated and reviewed elsewhere.

Data reduction and redundancy are central concerns in processing the many beats obtained in prolonged testing or monitoring. Three XYZ leads represent an appreciable data reduction compared to twelve conventional leads.

Recognition of the onset and offset of waves is crucial to any system of automated ECG measurement and analysis. A particular problem of identification exists in exercise cardiography when these points are buried in the "noise" of muscular activity. Determination of these points based on time-coherent spatial magnitudes is more precise and reproducible than is extraction of the ECG signal from the "noise" found in numerous single and sequentially recorded leads (36).

Reduction of data variability is particularly relevant to problems of the exercise ECG in which the stress situation introduces new sources of measurement and biological variability. Data from corrected orthogonal leads may show less individual variations and smaller group limits for important ECG-VCG items (33) though this has been challenged (11a). If true, the implications are clear for enhancing the diagnostic and prognostic power of the method.

But Frank leads (16), the most widely used of the theory-based orthogonal systems, have certain limiting features for exercise application. The lead strength of the vertical component Y leaves something to be desired, since this is an important coordinate for "ischemic" ST-T display. The interdependence of X, Y and Z leads with common electrodes and networks means that "noise" or errors originating in one electrode or lead affects data from more than one lead. None of the vector lead systems was designed with performance during activity as a consideration.

The Frank Y lead is particularly susceptible to "noise" during many types of exercise, even when electrodes are moved to relatively "quiet" regions on the trunk (36). Partial cancellation of "noise" having random properties has been achieved with a technique of multiple electrodes (30). A better system may be to record potential differences between a reference electrode and each of the Frank electrode positions as raw data for subsequent manipulations by computer programming (46).

Diagnosis According to Lead System

Attempts have been made to compare sensitivity-specificity relationships of ECG lead systems, exercise tests, and various analytical programs using the independent reference of clinical heart disease diagnosis (10).

In Table 17-III is a first approach to study of the relative power of conventional lead data, simple bipolar leads, and Frank leads to discriminate between heart disease patients and normals, assessed independently from the electrocardiogram. With this particular set of measurements and clinical classification criteria little difference was found between conventional and bipolar leads, but the XYZ leads were less sensitive. Remarkable shifts of the rank order of cases and controls resulted from small changes in criteria in this analysis. In addition, these data are based on ST-T findings only and not on all the information obtainable from the ECG-VCG, so that the results are very tentative.

Hornsten and Bruce report (21) that, using the same kind of ST-T amplitude information, diagnostic power is similar between Frank leads and a simple bipolar lead, but a reference independent of the ECG was not employed.

IMPROVED CHARACTERIZATION OF THE ST RESPONSE

The cardiologist looking at an exercise ECG is concerned mainly with the amount and contour of ST segment depression. He describes the ST-T contour as upward sloping, flat or sagging and measures the ST amplitude in millimeters or fractions of a millimeter displacement from a "baseline," an imaginary tangent to the P-R segment or a horizontally projected line from the onset of QRS.

The ECG measurement programs described at this conference are primarily occupied with producing measurements of ST amplitude and slope comparable to visual ones. Most programs measure amplitudes at some defined J point, and other amplitudes later in the S-T segment and at the peak of the T wave. Some programs tie the ST-T sampling point to one or another fixed interval following a time marker in the rapid part of QRS. Others divide the ST-T region into several equal parts, so that any ST segment amplitudes measured are corrected, or "normalized," for differences in heart rate.

Rautaharju and I have attempted to combine several characteristics of the ST-T region into manipulable values representing average ST amplitude and slope, and characteristics of convexity, concavity and higher order terms of waveform analysis. The curve-fitting procedure is described elsewhere (7, 35, 36). Values of the coefficients describing the ST-T form are used in a simple ranking program. The system is then tested for its ability to discriminate between independently classified "cardiacs" and normal subjects and this performance is compared, for example, to the power of analysis with individual ST segment amplitudes and slopes. The results of these analyses are not given here because small changes in classification of groups compared produce inordinate changes in the discriminatory power of the rest and exercise ECG, probably from the wide chance fluctuations of games with small numbers. (These sorts of occurrences led us necessarily to attitudes about the "uncertainty" principal expressed in the introduction to this monograph.)

Improved characterization of the ST-T segment of this or another approach may improve discrimination (36). Meanwhile we must deal with descriptive contours and amplitudes.

Using the simple approach of individual ST segment amplitudes to discriminate between normal and abnormal groups, Rautaharju and I find that the third and fourth of eight ST-T amplitude samples taken from the spatial magnitude curve between J point and T peak, are more powerful discriminants than J or T peak or any intermediate ST-T value. Blomqvist finds ST sample 3 of eight between J and the end of T to be more consistently discriminatory (11). Punsar utilizes the amplitude of the ST segment at onset of T as a discriminatory criterion (34). The QX/QT criterion of Lepeschkin has long been used in which ST-T depression beyond the halfway "vector" between onset of QRS and the end of T is discriminating. Clearly these independently arrived at discriminatory points are similar. A simple amplitude in this midregion may prove useful until the characteristics of the ischemic configuration or other characteristics not yet obvious are found to improve discrimination.

Figure 17-5 attempts to illustrate the problem which arises in the use of ST-T slope values in computer programs for ECG diagnosis, and is related to the differences in spatial orientation of the J point vector and later ST segment vectors. The two middle illustrations might represent, depending on lead location, a "normal" J point depression on the left and an "ischemic" sagging segment depression on the right. The slope values, diametrically opposite, would discriminate well between the cases. In different leads both findings with opposite slopes might be "normal." In the lower figures the slopes are also opposite but the contours are "abnormal," "near ischemic" and "ischemic," and have similar, or nearly similar, clinical importance. Takahashi, Iwatsuka *et al.* (50) regard the pattern on the lower left, called "near-ischemic" by Robb and Mattingly (40), as a combination of heart acceleration-induced, physiologic J point depression plus a degree of early depolarization from ischemia. J de-

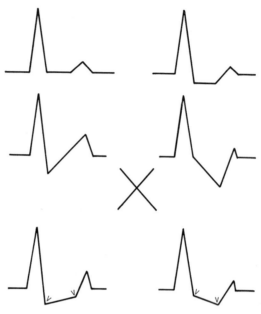

FIGURE 17-5. Diagrammatic representation of ST-T contours, and the fact that slopes opposite in sense may have opposite or similar clinical significance. This explains in part why values for ST-T slope contribute little over values for amplitudes in diagnostic computer analyses.

pression often develops first in the forward evolution of an ischemic ST response. They consider the "near-ischemic" contour a combination of influences because J point depression does not reappear as the ischemic response disappears.

A simple but objective method of characterizing this "intermediate ischemic" manifestation would be useful and the mid-ST vector amplitude described may prove to be it.

The Atrial T Wave

Another important problem of ST segment characterization is the influence of the atrial repolarization wave on ST amplitude and contour. This is especially important at higher heart rates and in vertical leads (11). Dr. Lepeschkin has admirably covered the problem, if not the solution, in this volume (p. ——).

OBSERVER VARIATION IN INTERPRETATION OF THE EXERCISE ECG

One of the great gains anticipated from the computer programs discussed in this conference is reduction in ECG measurement-classification error. The Technical Group on Exercise ECG has made a simple demonstration of the seriousness of the problem of human observer variation (39). Classification of exercise ECG responses was made as "normal, borderline or abnormal" without defined criteria. The frequency of "positive" diagnoses in a set of exercise ECG records varied, between fourteen experts, from about 5 to 55 per cent. The conclusions are that useful comparisons cannot be made of the frequency of "positive" exercise ECG tests reported in the literature and that collaborative studies cannot be undertaken on the basis of impressionistic ECG interpretation. The variation is also great within a given center, and by a single reader at different times. Random error is important and systematic variations between readers or in one reader over time weaken seriously any study based on exercise electrocardiograms. This is aside from any consideration of physiological, instrumental or other procedural sources of variability. The chief sources of the observer differences are as follows: (a) interpretation of J point ST depression, or "combined" J point and ischemic configurations variously labeled as "near-ischemic"; (b) "noise" and technically poor records, and (c) the absence of stated criteria or measurements.

Substantial reduction of disagreements is possible, even for visual inspection, in paper records of the exercise ECG response. Classification of the ST response into relatively unambiguous categories based on simple measurements reduces observer variation (39).

Technical personnel are more consistent than cardiologists, and as accurate, in classifying ST-T "abnormalities" according to Minnesota Code criteria (4, 42). At the Laboratory of Physiological Hygiene and at the London School of Hygiene many university student part-time employees, clerical, statistical and technical personnel have been trained over the past five years to code disease-related ECG findings (42). Table 17-IV shows a recent comparative reading of 1879 mixed records from a national collaborative study. Four classes of ST-J or segment depression were coded with overall agreement on

TABLE 17-IV

Clerical Observer Variation in ST-T Coding

Of Hospital Outpatient Records

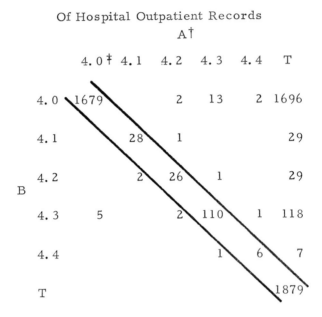

B	A†					
	4.0‡	4.1	4.2	4.3	4.4	T
4.0	1679		2	13	2	1696
4.1		28	1			29
4.2		2	26	1		29
4.3	5		2	110	1	118
4.4				1	6	7
T						1879

† A and B are different observers who read
blinded the same set of 1879 ECGs.
‡ 4.0 indicates "no codable ST finding"
while 4.1-4.4 inclusive are Minnesota
Code Classes of ST depression (42).

the presence of some ST code in *178* records out of the 200 called
"positive" by one or the other of the reader pairs. *Complete* agreement
on detailed subclass of ST depression was obtained in 170. For the
clearly ischemic class, i.e., $\geqslant$ 1.0 mm ST segment depression (code
4.1), there was *no* disagreement on its presence or absence, and disagreement of only one subclass in three out of thirty-one cases so
classified. For the more borderline class of downward sloping ST
segment with no J depression (code 4.3), there was disagreement on
its presence or absence in only eighteen out of 132 cases coded by one
or the other observer.

These results of student technician coding represent something close to an irreducible minimum of observer variation based on visual inspection and simple measurement. They are probably "acceptable" levels of agreement for most large scale comparisons. More detailed measurement, amounting to manual analog-to-digital conversion, has been successful in smaller clinical investigations but is impractical for larger studies. A few tangents and perpendiculars superimposed on the records, along with simple magnification, further reduce the measurement error and variability of classification (26, 39, 47).

There is no satisfactory way for the clinician or investigator to weight quantitatively the effect of inevitable misclassifications, either those from classification error to those arising from "biological" variability, i.e., actual changes in the individual myocardial response to stress at different times. But it is desirable to measure the contribution of observer error as a starting point. From these data, in a highly controlled situation, 10 per cent variability in classification must be exceeded before one can even begin to consider significant any group difference in the frequency of codable exercise ST responses. Practically, the confidence level for a given observation of an exercise ECG response in an individual diagnostic problem is greater the better the record technically and the greater the ST displacement.

In summary, impressionistic interpretation of the ECG exercise response is inadequate for the comparisons and assessments now needed. Classification of the ECG by specially trained technical personnel in a central processing facility allows useful comparisons of data. An irreducible minimum of observer variability is obtained with experienced ECG coders utilizing simple measurements on the tracing and employing magnifying devices. The concern then becomes the validity and standardization of criteria for classification of the ST response.

RECORDING PROCEDURES AND TEST CONDITIONS

It is feasible to conduct an exercise test which incorporates most of the standard conditions of past years while adding new conditions imposed by developments in concept, instrumentation and procedure. However, it is cumbersome and the question is whether it is worthwhile to maintain comparability of the old and new. Certainly clinically oriented studies should make this effort which would include making records in the supine position, with conventional-type leads both before and after exercise. The new conditions dictate adding a control resting record made in the upright posture and recording before, *during* and immediately after upright physical work, before reassuming the supine position for the conventional series of postexercise records.

Centers represented at this conference, and others engaged in population research, can now process information from large numbers of men, utilizing theory-based lead systems recording during and after upright work administered in a progressive multistaged stress test. Validating criteria are available from clinical-pathological and population studies by a number of centers using improved technology, with ECG measurement and diagnostic computer programs. It would seem unnecessary for these new, larger, adequately engineered studies to be burdened with less efficient procedures for the sake of obsolete standards. These studies will, in fact, develop the next standards.

Standardization of the conditions for conducting an exercise test includes minimizing the acute effects of meals and glucose administration, smoking, temperature-humidity extremes, physical exertion, hyperventilation and orthostasis. Use of any of these factors in attempts to *increase* the sensitivity of the exercise test are on occasion fruitful in individual diagnosis (12) but little can be generalized about the diagnostic or prognostic meaning of responses occurring under these influences. No qualitative difference is discernible between significant ST responses related to these influences and those related to disease. No prognostic data are available to segregate further these influences. There are impressions, including the observations made by Dr. Lepeschkin in this monograph, that responses to hyperventilation or orthostasis are benign, as are those occurring in vertically oriented lead configurations, in younger subjects with vertical electrical heart positions.

The best approach available is to reduce the effect of these influences by appropriate scheduling of the exercise ECG test. The test should follow by at least an hour any meal or smoking or unusual activity. Anxiety and hyperventilation are allayed by increasing the subject's familiarity through repeat encounters with the test procedure. Orthostatic changes are reduced by avoiding prolonged standing in the rest and recovery records. They may, of course, be demonstrated and identified by recording an "orthostatic test," eight minutes of quiet standing. Systematic validating experience is not available but the sitting position probably provides comparable data to standing position without the same tendency in the subject to pooling, lowered cardiac output and syncope.

Where a given condition cannot be standardized, such as the meal effect in populations appearing for outpatient or field examination, randomization of the effect should be sought in the study design.

THE WORK LOAD

The amount and program of the work load are predominant influences on the ECG response to exercise. The topic is discussed by experts in this monograph (Taylor *et al.*, p. 000). Chief reasons for current interest about the work load in exercise electrocardiography, and for its brief consideration in this review of developments, are the possibilities that greater stress administered in multiple levels of exercise can give a larger yield of diagnostic and predictive information and improved standardization.

Increased Yield of Information

It has been known for years that an increase in work load may induce angina pectoris and ECG changes inapparent at lower levels of work. This information has recently been exploited and quantified (14, 26, 27). The frequency of "ischemic" ST-T depressions among middle-aged men is several times greater following work near maximal capacity than after the double Master two-step test (14, 26, 47). This presupposes that the criteria are the same for the different tests. However, this does not mean that the significance of the "ischemic" finding is the same in terms of the degree of myocardial perfusion defect present or of subsequent mortality risk. In other words, it may become necessary to adjust the diagnostic criteria, and it is quite likely that an individual who develops "ischemic" findings at low level work is at greater risk than one who develops them only after work at near capacity. The answers are not yet available.

We cannot yet accept the "ischemic" finding after maximal effort as diagnostic in itself. The efficiency of various work levels to identify the population at risk is the practical question and must be answered before the possible risks and distinct inconvenience of general testing at high work loads can be accepted.

Equivalent Work Loads

Perhaps the greatest source of variability in exercise testing, between individuals or groups, and over time, is the lack of a standard stress. The stress we seek to standardize is the circulatory stress, stress of the aerobic metabolism. The load should provide testing at an equivalent myocardial oxygen consumption. This would elicit differences in capacity of the coronary circulation or degrees of perfusion defect.

The ECG "ischemic" response is not an all-or-none phenomenon; neither is it linearly related to the external work applied or to the proportion of maximal work capacity at which subjects are tested (11). A standard external work load results in selective penalization of smaller individuals who perform more work, relative to the capacity of their oxygen transport system, than larger persons. For example, a young male mouse would perform the Master two-step test at a much greater fraction of his cardiovascular capacity than an elderly female mammoth, according to the prescription of the Master two-step table, despite similarity of the absolute amounts of oxygen consumed.

The attempts described in this monograph and elsewhere to test at equivalent physiologic work loads are handicapped by our inability to measure, conveniently and indirectly, the blood pressure against which the heart works and the rate at which myocardial tension develops. This leaves only heart rate as a readily measurable major determinant of cardiac work. Fortunately, heart rate is the single greatest determinant of myocardial oxygen consumption and coronary flow. Efforts to predict work capacity and oxygen consumption from heart rate provide the current, if inadequate, basis for practical standardization of the work load.

Until measurement is possible of the other variables in cardiac work, two approaches to work load standardization available are the following: (a) work to a predetermined heart rate based on a predicted fraction of maximal work capacity, for age and sex; (b) work to an end-point at or very close to maximal oxygen consumption.

Though valuable information has been obtained for years using less standardized stress, quantitative comparisons and evaluation are now needed.

DURING EXERCISE VERSUS THE POSTEXERCISE ECG RESPONSE

A controversy has developed about the relative diagnostic contribution of the ECG response *during* versus that postexercise. It might be worthwhile to outline the approach used in the collaborative study with Rautaharju and to see whether a reasonable tentative conclusion is now possible (7, 36).

TABLE 17-V

DIAGNOSTIC POWER OF MAJOR "ISCHEMIC" ST-T FINDINGS IN THE CONVENTIONAL ECG IN SEPARATION OF CARDIAC CASES AND NORMALS IN A SAMPLED POPULATION OF MEN AGED 45-64 YEARS

	Resting ECG Alone	*Resting plus Postexercise ECG*
Sensitivity (for "true cases")	34.0%	42.6%
Specificity (for "normals")	94.4%	91.5%

We studied a sample of men aged forty-five to sixty-four in Finland, a group under long-term observation in the International Program of Ancel Keys (22). A conventional 12-lead scalar ECG was registered supine, at rest and following a step test on a 30 cm step at twenty steps per minute for three minutes. At least a half hour later in the examination schedule, a Frank lead ECG was recorded in a subsample of one in four men, in seated position on a bicycle ergometer, before, during and after a four-minute test at an external work load of 600 kilopond meters per minute.

Unambiguously defined major and minor criteria for ECG abnormality, from the Minnesota Code, were used to classify the conventional ECGs read blinded, from resting and immediate postexercise records. The efficacy was determined of major, minor, or combined ECG criteria to discriminate between men with definite heart disease or none, according to a clinical judgment made independently of the ECG. This contrived use of the ECG provided a basis for evaluating diagnostic power of more sophisticated ECG systems as well as a gross estimate of the sensitivity of the ECG when used as a screening tool.

Table 17-V gives the sensitivity of criteria for major ischemic ST-T abnormality in the conventional 12-lead ECG in identification of manifest heart disease in a general population. In this study it is 34 per cent from the resting ECG and 43 per cent from the resting and postexercise record combined. Adding the postexercise ECG response lowers specificity, "false positives" increase from 5.6 to 8.5 per cent. Sensitivity is increased at the cost of specificity; the problem is to find the "best" discriminative combination for the application desired.

Frank lead records were analyzed in the same men. After averaging and smoothing by computer, the ST-T region of the spatial magnitude curve was characterized by curve-fitting. A score was obtained from the values of the coefficients which represent the aspects of amplitude and contour of the ST-T. Scores for the men with heart disease were ranked alongside scores of men without heart disease, independently for rest records, for exercise, and for recovery records. Sensitivity in this isolated fashion utilizing only the ST-T region of the ECG was assessed for each phase of the test while holding specificity constant at the arbitrary and not especially desirable level of 80 per cent, i.e., a 20 per cent "false positive" rate. The postexercise response alone was the single most highly discriminating record, followed by the resting ECG, and by the record made during exercise. Independent or additive information was obtained from the ECG at rest, as well as that during and after exercise, justifying analysis of each.

THE DIAGNOSTIC POWER OF EXERCISE ELECTROCARDIOGRAPHY

This conference is concerned primarily with measurement of the exercise ECG response. Measurement must be accomplished before an effective reconsideration is possible of the diagnostic and prognostic meaning of the test. However, remarkable diagnostic claims have been made for the Master two-step regimen often and from many platforms, and as frequently refuted. The issue has attained the stature of a major scientific polemic. I believe this unnecessary situation could be resolved, without reflection on the protagonists or antagonists, by acceptance of a few simple facts.

Diagnostic effectiveness of a medical method is often tested first by comparisons of independently classified contrasting polar groups of "normals" and cases, as they exist at one cross section in time. Consider the claim of Master that his test procedure and criteria result in identification of 93 per cent of well-defined, extreme, typical coronary cases while separating out 98 per cent of the normal controls (28). This claim is based, among other things, on the occurrence of coronary disease over a considerable period of observation (therefore combining diagnostic with predictive information). It is inappropriate to extrapolate from the test situation used by Master to the quite different one confronting the physician: a patient with an atypical clinical manifestation or with no complaints whatever, who may or may not have heart disease of a determinable etiology other than coronary. The physician would like to make a diagnostic appraisal now rather than waiting for several years. In this realistic application there is, I believe, no medical diagnostic method, in any medical field, which operates at such a high level of discrimination, i.e., 93 per cent sensitivity for diagnosing "true" cases, at a level of 98 per cent specificity, or a 2 per cent "false positive" rate.

Any real-life diagnostic situation must account for the range of severity of disease and an inevitable overlap of values between those involved and those apparently uninvolved by the disease. This is particularly so in chronic degenerative diseases of gradual development and multifactorial origin. Sensitivity and specificity of a diagnostic method exists on a continual scale and may be altered by resetting the value of the diagnostic criterion. This has been shown with the exercise ECG as a particular example, with varying "severity" of criteria for a "positive" exercise test (7, 17).

Any claim that a "negative" response to a two-step test excludes coronary artery disease, and its corollary, that a "positive" test indicates the sure presence of coronary artery disease, fails to recognize these facts: (a) etiologic causes of heart disease, other than coronary, must first be excluded; (b) the severity of coronary artery disease is on a continuum; (c) any myocardial perfusion defect is also on a continuum, and (d) the ECG response to a perfusion defect at the cell level is on still another continuum. This many-variable system, operating on the basis of a many-variable methodology, negates any simplistic all-or-none concept of the diagnostic meaning of an electro-cardiographic exercise response.

THE PROGNOSTIC POWER OF THE EXERCISE ECG TEST

A distinctly abnormal and "ischemic" ECG response to exercise, in the absence of heart disease of other clear etiology, is generally regarded as an indicator of inadequate myocardial perfusion or due to coronary artery atherosclerosis. It may be considered an indication of increased future risk of manifest coronary event or death. These different and related concepts indicate only a different medical background or philosophy. It is quite appropriate to hold either of these views consistent with concern over individual diagnosis and with the broader public health.

Robb, Marks and Mattingly demonstrated that people with "positive" ECG responses to a Master two-step test have significantly greater mortality and coronary attack rates than "negative" responders (40, 41). This largely unqualified conclusion is responsible for much interest and investigation of the exercise ECG test as a method to identify high risk individuals among the apparently healthy. But in any medical test found to predict future risk, it must be established how much of the excess risk is related to the phenomenon measured and how much is related to common factors of risk. In other words, how much added and independent information about risk does the exercise ECG response provide above that of the subject's age, weight, blood pressure, or other known factors of cardiovascular risk?

None of the studies which have related the exercise test response to future risk has given sufficient consideration to confounding risk variables. In Figure 17-1 we summarized experience from 185 "ischemic" postexercise responders among 9,757 men, aged forty to fifty-nine years, submitted to the three-minute, constant rate step test described; a frequency of 1.9 per cent "positive" tests. The proportion of "positive" cases is given according to quintile cuts in the distribution for each physical characteristic, from lowest to the highest 20 per cent of values. If no relationship exists between the "ischemic" ECG response ($\geqslant 1.0$ mm. ST-T depression) and obesity (Σ skinfolds), blood pressure or serum cholesterol, 20 per cent of ischemic cases, or a horizontal line relation, should occur in each quintile class of the physical variable.

A highly significant concentration of "positive" ST-T responses is found in the more obese (by skinfold thickness). A linear, highly significant increased frequency of ST-T depression is found according to increasing blood pressure, as well as a statistically significant relationship to serum cholesterol level.

In addition to demonstrated relationships of the exercise ST-T response to age and sex, there are strong associations with obesity, blood pressure and serum cholesterol as well as with physical activity habits (9, 22). This affects the interpretation of the prognostic power of a "positive" test. How much *independent* information is obtained from the exercise test over that from simple measures of other "risk factors?" The problem is that build, blood pressure, blood lipids and activity habits are strongly intercorrelated. Detailed and quantitative definition of the power of the exercise ECG response requires vast numbers of cases to make the appropriate comparisons of ST-T depression and coronary risk according to the many possible combinations of age and risk variable. No study has yet produced adequate numbers.

However, it is likely that a "positive" exercise ECG response represents an additional risk above that contingent upon any level of blood pressure or obesity. It is also likely that, having screened out of a group those with other elevated coronary risk factors, a "positive" ECG response among the residual would provide important risk information. Confirmation of this estimate, and measurement of the risk, requires the pooling of information from large collaborative studies, longer term follow-up in existing studies, or a reanalysis of the extensive insurance data by Robb and Marks to account for characteristics confounding the risk picture.

SAFETY

Practitioner and investigator alike are concerned about the actual risk of a stress test. Master two-step tests are widely administered to asymptomatic subjects having normal, or nearly so, resting electrocardiograms with no special safety precaution other than the presence nearby of the physician.

For suspected or definite cardiac patients and for higher level stresses, constant monitoring of the ECG during work and recovery should be carried out, with oscilloscopic or continuous paper display. Bruce has stated that most accidents from syncope, and the rare serious or fatal arrhythmias and infarction, occur following, rather than during the exertion. It is not yet possible to predict such reactions from findings at rest or during the work stages, so that beat-by-beat cardiac monitoring is recommended.

Bruce has summarized in a committee report the safety procedures for testing at higher work levels (13). Briefly, the test is interrupted as as follows:

1. When the patient signals he has had enough or when he complains of discomfort.
2. When an ataxic gait appears.
3. When runs of three or more ventricular premature beats or other arrhythmia develops.

Seated recovery, with legs elevated, avoids most syncopal problems. Training and equipment for resuscitation must be first-class. A recent unpublished summary of these safety considerations is available from Drs. Hornsten and Bruce, University of Washington, Seattle.

CRITERIA FOR INTERPRETATION

It is emphasized that no single reasonable criterion or set of criteria can be given for diagnoses of "positive or negative" exercise ECG responses. This is due to the great number of interrelated influences on the response and to the continuous rather than dichotomous characteristic of both the response and the disease process. Furthermore, it is not yet clear whether "criteria" devised for the postexercise response following moderate work are relevant to records recorded at high heart rates during heavy work.

But it seems that investigators might come to agree upon general defined classes of ST-T response, since there is unanimity about the characteristics of the response which interest us. Use of agreed classes might allow data comparability if other conditions were standard. If testing conditions were not similar, there would result at least a better comprehension of each others reported findings.

Astrand and her committee (2) have discussed a practical approach to visual classification of the ST segment which considers, as does the Minnesota Code on which it is based, the amplitude of the ST junction (J) and slope of the segment. Importance is given to the amount and configuration of ST displacement having a zero or negative slope, i.e., a flat or sagging contour. This is provided for in the first ST classes of the Minnesota Code (4.1, 2, 3) (6, 42). Junctional depression with an upward-sloping segment is accounted for though possibly as a "physiological" manifestation. But the principal problem in ST coding lies with responses having an important degree of J depression and a flat though positive slope, described by Astrand's committee as "ST segment straight and slowly ascending." Most would concur that this is a phenomenon of diagnostic and prognostic interest and many attempts have been made to dissect, explain, describe, measure and classify this phenomenon. As mentioned earlier, the group at Nagoya University consider the pattern a mixture of "physiological" J depression and "ischemic" response (50). Robb, Marks and Mattingly classified the finding qualitatively as "near ischemic." Various measurements in the midregion of the ST, discussed on pages 000, are means of describing this characteristic.

The Scandinavian approach is a useful one until such time that adequate characterization of the segment is obtained, based on firm measurement and reassessment in well-designed studies of diagnostic and predictive power. But for reasons cited in the Scandinavian Committee report it may be wise to classify the intermediate contour separately from the "accepted" flat or downward "ischemic" contour. The mortality and infarction cases on which their pooling is based are not yet sufficiently numerous to indicate clearly that these contours have the same level of clinical significance (34). Moreover, very high reproducibility is attainable in coding distinct $\geqslant$ 1 mm "ischemic" ST depression (Minnesota Code 4.1) as seen in the figure for technician readers in this laboratory. Experience with reproducibility of the "near ischemic" contour suggests that its classification is less reliable (39).

ST-T Classification

Characteristics of ST-T requiring classification include the following:

1. Several classes of magnitude for distinct "ischemic" flat or sagging ST-T segments.
2. One or two classes of "physiological" type J point depression with a convex and upward sloped ST-T segment.

3. A type of response intermediate between 1 and 2, if it can be adequately defined.

The classes should include absolute values of ST depression and elevation as well as *change* relative to the resting ECG classification.

The classification should provide for findings and changes in T waves and conduction and rhythm characteristics.

The classification should be in mutually exclusive subclasses or in some rank order of presumed "severity."

The classification should be tested for the reasonableness of the distribution obtained, for the reproducibility of detailed subclasses and for discriminatory and predictive power.

ACKNOWLEDGMENTS

John Mazzarella, M.D., of the University of Washington, Seattle and Noboru Okamoto, M.D., of Nagoya University, Nagoya, Japan collaborated in the detailed comparison of bi-polar chest leads.

The opinions and experience reported are the responsibility of the author, but many contributions to the development of concepts, procedure and technology in this field are acknowledged to come primarily from members of a technical group on exercise electrocardiography, as follows:

Members: Gunnar Blomqvist, M.D.
Robert A. Bruce, M.D.
Alvin Freiman, M.D.
Robert E. Mason, M.D.
Pentti Rautaharju, M.D.
Paul Rochmis, M.D.
L. T. Sheffield, M.D.
Larry Jackson, M.D.
Consultants: Joseph T. Doyle, M.D.
Richard S. Gubner, M.D.
Herman K. Hellerstein, M.D.
T. J. Reeves, M.D.

REFERENCES

1. ASTRAND, I.: Exercise electrocardiograms recorded twice with an 8-year interval in a group of 204 women and men 48-63 years old. *Acta Med Scand, 178*:27, 1965.

2. ASTRAND, I., Chairman, The Scandinavian Committee on ECG Classification: The "Minnesota code" for ECG classification. Adaptation to CR leads and modification of the code for ECG's recorded during and after exercise. *Acta Med Scand,* 1967, suppl. 481.

3. BERSON, A.S., and PIPBERGER, H.V.: The low-frequency response of electrocardiographs, a frequent source of recording errors. *Amer Heart J, 71*: 779, 1966.

4. BLACKBURN, H.: The electrocardiogram in cardiovascular epidemiology. Problems in standardized application. *Ann N Y Acad Sci, 126*:882, 1965.

5. BLACKBURN, H., and KATIGBAK, R.: What electrocardiographic leads to take after exercise? *Amer Heart J, 67*:184, 1964.

6. BLACKBURN, H.; KEYS, A.; SIMONSON, E.; RAUTAHARJU, P.M., and PUNSAR, S.: The electrocardiogram in population studies. A classification system. *Circulation, 21*:1160, 1960.

7. BLACKBURN, H.; RAUTAUHARJU, P.M.; WONG, A.; BARRY, A.; KARVONEN, M.; ORMA, E., and KEYS, A.: The discriminatory power of the electrocardiogram in population studies. Proceedings of the VII International VCG Colloquium, Smolinice, Czechoslovakia, September 1966.

8. BLACKBURN, H.; TAYLOR, H.L.; OKAMOTO, H.; MITCHELL, P.L.; RAUTAHARJU, P.M., and KERKHOF, A.C.: The exercise electrocardiogram. A systematic comparison of chest lead configurations employed for monitoring during exercise. In *Physical Activity and the Heart.* Karvonen, M.J., and Barry, A. (Eds.), Springfield, Thomas, 1966, chapt. 9.

9. BLACKBURN, H.; TAYLOR, H.L.; KEYS, A., and collaborators: The postexercise electrocardiogram. The frequency of abnormal responses and their relationship with other coronary risk factors among 10,000 men aged 40-59. (In preparation)

10. BLACKBURN, H.; RAUTAHARJU, P.M.; KARVONEN, M., and KEYS, A.: Diagnostic sensitivity and specificity of the electrocardiogram in a random sample of a total population. *Circulation (Abstract), 34*(III): 57, 1966.

11. BLOMQVIST, G.: The Frank lead exercise electrocardiogram. A quantitative study based on averaging technique and digital computer analysis. *Acta Med Scand, 178*(suppl):440, 1965.

11a. BORUN, E.R.: Variability of electrocardiographic data recorded with orthogonal leads. *Amer Heart J, 76*:62, 1968.

12. BURCHELL, H.B.: The value of exercise tests in the diagnosis of coronary disease. Symposium on coronary heart disease. Supplement to *Circulation,* January 1961.

13. BRUCE, R.A.; KATTUS, A.A., and MAZZARELLA, J.A.: Report of the committee on safety procedure. In *Physical Activity and the Heart.* Karvonen, M.J., and Barry, A. (Eds.), Springfield, Thomas, 1966.

14. DOAN, A.E.; PETERSON, D.R.; BLACKMON, J.R., and BRUCE, R.A.: Myo-

cardial ischemia after maximal exercise in healthy men. *Amer J Cardiol, 17*:9, 1966.

15. FEIL, H., and SIEGEL, M.L.: Electrocardiographic changes during attacks of angina pectoris. *Amer J Med Sci, 175*:256, 1928.

16. FRANK, E.: An accurate, clinically practical system for spatial vectorcardiography. *Circulation, 13*:737, 1956.

17. FREIDBERG, C.K.; JAFFE, H.L.; PORDY, L., and CHESKY, K.: The two-step exercise electrocardiogram. A double-blind evaluation of its use in the diagnosis of angina pectoris. *Circulation, 26*:1254, 1962.

18. GEDDES, L.A.; BAKER, L.E., and MOORE, A.G.: The use of liquid-junction electrodes in recording the human electrocardiogram. *J Electrocardiol, 1*:51, 1968.

19. GOLDHAMMER, S., and SCHERF, D.: Elektrokardiographische Untersuchungen bei Kranken mit Angina Pectoris. *Z Klin Med, 122*:134, 1932.

20. HELLERSTEIN, H.K.; PROZAN, G.B.; LIEBOW, I.M.; DOAN, A.E., and HENDERSON, J.A.: The two-step exercise test as a test of cardiac function in chronic rheumatic heart disease and in arteriosclerotic heart disease with old myocardial infarction. *Amer J Cardiol, 7*:234, 1961.

21. HORNSTEN, T.R., and BRUCE, R.A.: Comparison of ischemic ST responses in Frank X, Y, Z, leads with those in a simple bipolar chest lead. (in press)

22. KEYS, A., and collaborators: Epidemiological studies related to coronary heart disease. Characteristics of men aged 40-59 in seven countries. *Acta Med Scand, 180*(suppl.):460, 1967.

23. LEPESCHKIN, E.: Electrocardiographic instrumentation. *Prog Cardiovasc Dis, 5*:498, 1963.

24. LEPESCHKIN, E.: Exercise tests in the diagnosis of coronary heart disease. *Circulation, 22*:986, 1960.

25. LEPESCHKIN, E., and SURAWICZ, B.: Characteristics of true-positive and false-positive results of electrocardiographic Master two-step exercise tests. *New Eng J Med, 258*:511, 1958.

26. LESTER, F.M.; SHEFFIELD, L.T., and REEVES, T.J.: Electrocardiographic changes in clinically normal older men following near maximal and maximal exercise. *Circulation, 36*:5, 1967.

27. MASON, R.E., and LIKAR, I.: A new system of multiple lead exercise electrocardiography. *Amer Heart J, 71*:196, 1966.

28. MASTER, A.M., and ROSENFELD, I.: Monitored and post-exercise two-step test. *JAMA, 190*:494, 1964.

29. MASTER, A.M.; FRIEDMAN, R., and DACK, S.: The electrocardiogram after standard exercise as a functional test of the heart. *Amer Heart J, 24*:777, 1942.

30. MURAYAMA, M.; MURAO, S.; HARUMI, K.; SATO, C., and UEDA, H.: Studies on the lead system for telemetering the exercise electrocardiogram. *Jap Heart J, 5*:312, 1964.

31. OKAJIMA, M.; SCHMITT, O.H., and BLAUG, M.: Factors influencing meas-

ured electro-augmentation ratios. *Digest of the 1961 International Conference on Medical Electronics.* p. 235.

32. Ostrander, L.D., Jr.; Brandt, R.L.; Kjelsberg, M.O., and Epstein, F.H.: Electrocardiographic findings among the adult population of a total natural community, Tecumseh, Michigan. *Circulation, 31*:888, 1965.

33. Pipberger, H.: Advantages of three lead cardiographic recordings. *Ann NY Acad Sci, 128*:873, 1965.

34. Punsar, S.; Pyorala, K., and Siltanen, P.: Classification of electrocardiographic ST segment changes in epidemiological studies of coronary heart disease. *Scand J Clin Lab Invest (Abstract), 19*(Suppl. 95): 112, 1967.

35. Rautaharju, P.M.: Deterministic type waveform analysis. *Ann NY Acad Sci, 128*:939, 1966.

36. Rautauharju, P.M.; Winter, D.A.; Wong, A., and Blackburn, H.: Computer analysis of the exercise electrocardiogram. In *Electrical Activity of the Heart.* Manning and Smith (Eds.), U. of W. Ontario, 1967.

37. Report of Committee on Electrocardiography, American Heart Association: Recommendations for standardization of leads and of specifications for instruments in electrocardiography and vectorcardiography. *Circulation, 35*:583, 1967.

38. Report of Subcommittee on Instrumentation, Committee on Electrocardiography, American Heart Association: Recommendations for standardization of instruments in electrocardiography and vectorcardiography. *IEEE Trans Bio Med Engin, 14*:60, 1967.

39. Report of a Technical Group on the Exercise Electrocardiogram: Differences in interpretation. *Amer J Cardiol, 21*:871, 1968.

40. Robb, G.P.; Marks, H.H., and Mattingly, T.W.: The value of the double standard two-step exercise test in the detection of coronary heart disease. A clinical and statistical follow-up study of military and insurance applicants. *Trans Assoc Life Insur Med Dir Amer, 40*:52, 1956.

41. Robb, G.P., and Marks, H.H.: Post-exercise electrocardiogram in arteriosclerotic heart disease. *JAMA, 200*:918, 1967.

42. Rose, G.A., and Blackburn, H.: *Cardiovascular survey methods. WHO,* Monograph Series #56, Geneva, Switzerland, 1968.

43. Rowell, L.B.; Taylor, H.L.; Simonson, E., and Carlson, W.S.: The physiologic fallacy of adjusting for body weight in performance of the Master two-step test. *Amer Heart J, 70*:461, 1965.

44. Schmitt, O.H.: Averaging techniques employing several simultaneous physiological variables. *Ann NY Acad Sci, 115*:952, 1964.

45. Schmitt, O.H.; Okajima, M., and Blaug, M.: Skin preparation in electrocardiographic impedance. *Digest of the 1961 International conference on Medical Electronics.* p. 236.

46. Sheffield, L.T.; Lester, F.M., and Reeves, T.J.: Investigation of elec-

trocardiographic manifestations of angina pectoris by multichannel recording. *Circulation* (Abstract), *34* (suppl.) III:215, 1966.

47. SHEFFIELD, L.T., and REEVES, T.J.: Graded exercise in the diagnosis of angina pectoris. *Mod Conc Cardiovasc Dis, 34*:1, 1965.

48. SIMONSON, E.: *Differentiation Between Normal and Abnormal in Electrocardiography.* St. Louis, Mosby, 1961.

49. SOLVAY, H., and DENOLIN, H.: L'electrocardiograme d'effort. Technique et interpretation. Hopital Universitaire St. Pierre, Brussels, 1967.

50. TAKAHASHI, H.; IWATSUKA, T.; OHASHI, I., and HOTTA, S.: Some observations of the ST depression in the exercise electrocardiogram. *Jap Heart J, 4*:105, 1963.

18

Exercise Tests: A Summary of Procedures and Concepts of Stress Testing for Cardiovascular Diagnosis and Function Evaluation

HENRY L. TAYLOR, WILLIAM HASKELL, SAMUEL M. FOX, III
and HENRY BLACKBURN

INTRODUCTION

A TECHNICAL GROUP composed of those listed* met in conjunction with this conference to consider the status of procedures and concepts of stress testing and where possible to unify methods and thinking. This report summarizes and expands the discussion. The authors take responsibility for any direction taken or recommendations contained. The report considers a number of aspects of stress testing, including current use in clinical and field applications, details of the modes and loads of work imposed, end-point manifestations and criteria for tests including heart rate and electrocardiographic responses.

The clinician or investigator who begins to look into the literature on exercise tests for the measurement of work capacity or the evaluation of the exertional electrocardiogram is usually appalled by the multiplicity of work test protocols, many of which are beset by obvious

Technical group members: Irma Astrand, M.D., Stockholm, Sweden, Henry Blackburn, M.D., Minneapolis, C. Gunnar Blomqvist, M.D., Dallas, Robert Bruce, M.D., Seattle, Samuel M. Fox, III, M.D., Heart Disease and Stroke Control Program, U.S.P.H.S., Burt B. Hamrell, M.D., Minneapolis, William Haskell, Ph.D., Heart Disease and Stroke Control Program, U.S.P.H.S., T. Joseph Reeves, M.D., Birmingham, Loring Rowell, Ph.D., Seattle, Thomas Sheffield, M.D., Birmingham, and Henry L. Taylor, Ph.D., Minneapolis.

Discussions of this Technical Group were supported in part by grant No. CD-00118 from the U.S.P.H.S.

pitfalls or designed for highly specialized applications. This chapter is an effort to present and evaluate the protocols based on different theories of how to measure the cardiovascular capacity for work including electrocardiographic evaluation of myocardial perfusion.

Since the level of work which patients can tolerate without significant symptoms is of considerable interest to the cardiologist, work capacity measurements are discussed in detail. However for those who wish to concern themselves primarily with examining the electrocardiographic responses to work the material in Part II will be of more interest.

Part I

USES OF EXERCISE TESTS

Consideration of the questions to be answered by the use of an exercise test is the first step in selecting the procedure. Any of several purposes may be of concern:

1. To detect electrocardiographic responses related to inadequate myocardial perfusion in individual subjects, cardiac patients or among population groups.
2. To determine the intensity of work at which a cardiac patient develops symptoms.
3. To study details of respiratory, circulatory, metabolic or other functions under the stress of defined work loads in normals or patients.
4. To study limiting physiological factors to work performance in "normals" (bedrest, extremes of ambient temperature, starvation, physical conditioning) and in patients with well-defined disease.
5. To estimate the relative aerobic capacity of individuals and groups for comparative studies including controlled trials.
6. To determine maximal oxygen intake both to characterize individuals and groups and to provide the basis for comparisons of individuals with divergent capacities for work at submaximal work loads and at comparable proportions of their maximal cardiovascular performance.

Other factors which determine the choice of an exercise test procedure include age, sex, general state of health, aerobic capacity, subject motivation, the frequency of tests to be administered per day, the size of the test sample, the staff available, and the location, whether in the laboratory, the clinic or in the field. Finally, because of the degree of stress, potential risks, and medico-legal considerations, the experience and training of those who conduct the procedure is a determinant of the test used.

CHARACTERISTICS OF EXERCISE TESTS

Characteristics of an exercise stress test include the type of exercise, the work load and the pattern and rate of applying the work load.

Figure 18-1 illustrates different types of exercise and mode of imposing the work load. Four types of frequently used tests are characterized on the ordinate: step or bench climbing, walking or

EXERCISE TEST METHODS

ERGOMETER	SINGLE LOAD TEST	MULTIPLE LOAD TESTS		
		INTERMITTENT	CONTINUOUS	
		VARIABLE WORK INCREMENT	SMALL WORK INCREMENT	LARGE WORK INCREMENT
STEPS	Master (42) Simonson (56)	Sheffield (54) Wyndham (66)	Shephard (55)	
TREADMILL	Cureton (19) Robinson (48) Simonson (56)	Astrand,I. (5) Mitchell (45) Taylor (59) Wyndham (66)	Balke (9) Kattus (35) Naughton (47)	Bruce (15,16,24) Wyndham (66)
UPRIGHT BICYCLE	Tornvall (63)	Allard (1) Astrand,P-O (8) Hellerstein (31) Wyndham (66)	Binkhorst (10)	Astrand,I. (4) Denolin (21) Sjöstrand (57)
SUPINE BICYCLE	Frick (26)	Holmgren (33)		Westura (65)
MODE OF APPLICATION →				

FIGURE 18-1.

running on a motor-driven treadmill, sitting on a bicycle ergometer or supine pedaling of a bicycle ergometer (used frequently in the cardiac catheterization laboratory). On the abscissa are modes of application of the work load.

SINGLE-STAGE TEST PROCEDURES

In Figure 18-1 the best known test among physicians is the Master Two-Step Test (42). Other single-stage tests widely-used are a treadmill test with a work load of 3 mph and 5 per cent grade used by Simonson (56), a single-stage bicycle test and a step test of 30 cm height with a constant stepping rate employed by Keys and associates in comparative studies of the epidemiology of coronary heart disease (38).

Single load procedures are based on the principle that measurement of some variable related to cardiovascular performance, such as pulse rate or blood pressure, provides a measure of the ability of the individual's cardiovascular system to adapt to a given work load. The procedures are simple, of little duration and safe in eliciting diagnostic or prognostic ECG responses. The disadvantages, discussed below, include lack of standardization based on myocardial oxygen consumption and in most cases a relatively low yield of "diagnostic" ECG findings.

MULTISTAGE TEST PROCEDURES

The second, third and fourth columns describe multistage procedures which impose work loads considerably higher than those usually employed in single-stage tests. Some of these tests are designed specifically to determine maximal oxygen intake and all of them require safety considerations. For example, all these tests are considered to be without important risk in children and in young men certified by a physician as free of cardiovascular disease. But in testing men over the age of thirty-five years and women forty-five years detailed requirements of personnel, instrumentation and procedure should be decided on in advance to provide protection for both investigators and patients or subjects (15, 16, 34).

Intermittent Tests

The second column of Figure 18-1 gives references and the mode of application for multistage procedures in which increasing work loads are interrupted by rest periods. Examples of this test are Hellerstein's version of the work capacity test (P. W. C. 150) (31), the widely-used Swedish bicycle regimen (6, 57) and the treadmill test employed by Taylor *et al.* (59) or its modification by Mitchell *et al.* (45). These intermittent procedures give the subject a chance to recover between bouts of work. They allow work at higher levels in individuals whose capacity is not symptom-limited (11). Performance is not as vulnerable to local muscle fatigue as it is in continuous testing.

The recovery time allowed between loads varies widely. Taylor *et al.* (59) allowed twenty-four hours or more between bouts of work. Åstrand, Åstrand and Rohdal (7) preferred to limit the subject to two work periods in any one day. Mitchell *et al.* (45) allowed ten minutes between tests and generally were able to elicit a maximal oxygen intake in one visit to the laboratory.

Continuous Tests

In the third column are examples of multistage tests with no rest periods between increasing work loads. The duration of work load at each level is usually one minute so that a physiological steady state does not occur. The Balke-Ware treadmill test at 3.4 mph with 1 per cent increase of grade per minute is an example of this procedure (9). The principal disadvantage of either multistaged procedure is the time consumed.

The far righthand column of Figure 18-1 gives examples of a progressive and continuous multistaged procedure in which work periods are sufficiently prolonged to approach a steady state at each load. Examples are the Bruce procedure (15, 16) which employs three-minute work increments and the P. W. C. 170 bicycle test popularized by Sjostrand which requires intermittent six-minute work and six-minute rest periods (6, 57).

STANDARDIZATION OF SINGLE-STAGE SUBMAXIMAL TESTS

The Bicycle

Table 18-I presents some of the physiological consequences, assump-

TABLE 18-I

COLUMN ONE PRESENTS CERTAIN PHYSIOLOGICAL CONDITIONS AND OBJECTIVES REGARDING WORK TESTS. COLUMNS 2 THROUGH 5 PRESENT THE ERGOMETERS WHICH CAN BE USED TO ACHIEVE THESE CONDITIONS UNDER EACH OF THE SEVERAL PROTOCOLS, ALONG WITH COMMENTS ON THE OBJECTIVES

Physiological Conditions and Objectives	*Single Load Tests*	*Multiple Load Tests*		
		Intermittent	*Continuous*	
		Variable Work Increment	Small Work Increment	Large Work Increment
Constant external workload	Master's Two-step Upright or supine bicycle	Bicycle Treadmill (interpolated)	Bicycle Treadmill (interpolated)	Bicycle Treadmill (interpolated)
Workload proportional to body weight	Treadmill constant load step test	Treadmill Bicycle (interpolated) Step test	Treadmill Bicycle (interpolated)	Treadmill Bicycle (interpolated)
Steady state	Treadmill Bicycle Step (time dependent)	Treadmill Bicycle Step (time dependent)	No	6 min work load period— approximate
Work to a predetermined pulse rate	No	Work level for given pulse rate may be interpolated	Small work increments make estimate precise	Intermediate work increments will require some interpolation
Estimation of max VO_2	Pulse rate response can be used to estimate extra- polation	Work to VO_2 plateau determines motivation independent end-point	Self-determined end-point motivation dependent	Self-determined end-point motivation dependent

tions and objective characteristics of the several types of test protocols and ergometric equipment. Submaximal single load tests are treated in column one. In a bicycle test with the brake fixed at a single load, all subjects are presented with a single external work load which is independent of the weight of the subject. Differences in oxygen intake between individuals are related to individual differences in mechanical efficiency. When one uses a fixed load on the brake of the bicycle to examine the ECG response to work, one asks whether the individual can perform the work load specified by the test without abnormal ECG findings. One assumes it is not important that the small man will be working at a larger fraction of his maximal oxygen intake (a good measure of cardiovascular stress) than the large man. In the absence of S-T depressions the cardiologist can certify that both men will be able to perform the given work intensity without evidence of myocardial ischemia. This system makes sense in the case of an industrial physician who is examining men for specific jobs in which the peak work loads are known, although assumptions regarding stress other than the physical work load are involved.

Oxygen consumptions which are proportional to the body weight can be obtained with single-stage bicycle tests but with a variable work load based on a calibration designed to produce a constant oxygen consumption per kilogram of body weight (64). A single-stage bicycle test can be used to predict the maximal oxygen intake from a nomogram developed by Åstrand and Rhyming and modified for the adult age range by I. Åstrand (5). The prediction has a standard error of estimate of ± 10 per cent.

In practice, this means that for a man with a maximal oxygen intake of 3.0 liters per minute, the 95 per cent confidence limits are 3.6 and 2.4 liters/min. The nomogram can be used as a rough guide to the aerobic capacity of an individual. It also provides an opportunity to characterize groups of individuals (49). The characterization of groups must be qualified by the recognition that in the untrained individuals the maximal oxygen intake is understated compared to men who are in good condition (50). In addition, care must be taken to be sure that the ambient temperature is not above 80° F with a relative humidity of 60 per cent or less.

The Treadmill

In contrast to the bicycle with a fixed brake load, walking on the treadmill results in a load and an oxygen consumption proportional to the body weight. It has been proposed (56) that since the weight of the heart is proportional to body weight, the treadmill provides a more uniform stress with which to evaluate the perfusion of the myocardium with the ECG. Consideration of the determinants of myocardial oxygen consumption has invalidated this position (see Part II), but the measurement of pulse rate during work is related to the fitness of the cardiovascular system to withstand the stress of the physical work involved. For example, the work pulse rate of young men walking on a 10 per cent grade at 3.5 mph is markedly elevated by bed rest, and physical conditioning with grade walking or running reduces the work pulse rate from 170 to the control level (60). The responses to other forms of stress have been discussed elsewhere (29). For studies of cardiovascular fitness for physical work in which single level submaximal work loads are to be used, the treadmill is the instrument of choice since the men are working against their body weight.

Treadmill Tests: Speed of the Belt Travel

Speed of belt travel is an important consideration which is dependent on the age and activity status of the group to be studied. For example, Taylor *et al.* (59) found that groups of young men from college populations or from the army always contained individuals who could not comfortably keep up with 8 or 9 miles per hour. It was necessary to standardize the test conditions at 7 miles per hour. Mitchell *et al.* (45) attempted to use this test format with middle-aged men and concluded that 6 miles per hour was more appropriate for their age group.

Bruce *et al.* (15, 16) found that the 3.4 miles per hour used by Balke and Ware was too fast for many patients who had restricted their activity. These authors begin their continuous multistage test at 1.7 mph. Naughton, Balke and Nagle (47) have recommended starting patients with low aerobic capacity at 2 mph on a zero per cent grade. Speed is held constant and the grade is increased 3.5

per cent every three minutes. In dealing with patients with angina, Kattus (35) used a 10 per cent grade with the speed selected for the case in question. The lowest beginning speed was 1.0 mph and the work increments were achieved by increasing speed one-half mile per hour every three minutes up to and including 4 mph.

Step Tests

A step test which employs a constant rate of stepping results in oxygen consumptions which are related to body weight. Accordingly, a well-conducted step test will produce pulse rates which are related to cardiovascular conditioning. Investigators should be aware, however, that while intelligent, coordinated men perform well on step tests, there are some individuals in large groups who need coaching and close attention if the proper pace is to be maintained. Some of these individuals may never produce reliable data.

Standardization of Oxygen Consumption

The effects of the several devices for standardizing the work load are illustrated by data recently published by Blackburn *et al.* (11). The data are presented in Table 18-II which shows the oxygen consumption and pulse rates of ten men who performed five different single-stage test protocols. The sequence of tests was assigned by randomization. The conventional graded Master's test required the largest oxygen consumption per unit time of the five tests, and the treadmill the smallest. The coefficient of variation allows comparisons with regard to variability between tests regardless of the absolute oxygen consumption. Since the bicycle ergometer provides a constant external work load and a mechanical efficiency with a small variability, the lowest coefficient of variation is found when the oxygen consumption is expressed as liters per minute. However, since the work load on the bicycle ergometer is independent of body weight, a marked increase of inter-individual variability is found when the oxygen consumption is expressed as ml/kg/min. The treadmill imposes a work load which is weight dependent and shows a decrease in variability when the results are expressed as oxygen per ml/kg/min. In the Master test, the coefficients of variability for both liters/min. and

TABLE 18-II

OXYGEN CONSUMPTION AND PULSE RATE IN TEN MEN PERFORMING FIVE COMMONLY USED, SINGLE-STAGE STEP TESTS

3-minute work periods, 5-minute recovery periods and random test assignment

(from Blackburn, 11)

Item	Conventional Master	Constant Rate Step Test Single Step	Two Step	Bicycle 600 kpm	Treadmill 3 mph, 5% grade
O₂ Cons. liter/min					
$\overline{X}$	1.63	1.51	1.45	1.34	1.21
S.D.	0.16	0.19	0.13	0.09	0.18
S.D. in % of $\overline{X}$*	9.81	12.6	9.0	6.7	14.9
O₂ Cons. ml/kg					
$\overline{X}$	23.04	21.30	20.42	18.94	16.94
S.D.	3.11	2.38	2.05	2.50	1.57
S.D. in % of $\overline{X}$	13.5	11.2	10.04	13.1	9.3
Pulse r/m					
$\overline{X}$	121.9	117.3	114.2	116.9	104.6
S.D.	14.3	12.1	13.6	13.9	12.2
S.D. in % of $\overline{X}$	11.7	10.3	11.9	11.9	11.7
Reference to test procedure	Master (42)	Keys (38)	Rowell (51)	Astrand (5)	Simonson (56)

*Coefficient of variation.

ml/kg/min. are larger than those for the bicycle ergometer. The difference between these values are similar for the step and the bicycle test. The constant rate step tests (Master two-step and single-step) show little or no difference in the coefficient of variation between total oxygen consumption and that corrected for body weight. This does not conform to theory as well as one would wish.

When oxygen consumption is not measured it can be predicted from the bicycle work load and on the treadmill from the body weight using a previously determined rate in ml/kg/minute. The bicycle has a small advantage over the treadmill in predicting oxygen consumption due to its slightly lower coefficient of variation.

In this series illustrating the principles of standardization of single-stage tests, the body weights of the subjects ranged from 133 to 190 pounds. A wider range of body weights illustrates more effectively the differences in energy cost and variability between the graded Master test routine, by age, sex and weight, and a test involving a constant rate of stepping (51).

In these single-stage submaximal tests, the standard deviations of the pulse rates are of the same order of magnitude. All these tests probably represent non-steady-state situations since the time of the work period is three minutes. Some improvement in reliability and capacity to predict maximal oxygen consumption has been noted by extending the duration of work periods. However, it appears that the improvement is small compared to the cost of the additional time in the field or clinic situation. In laboratory investigations with small numbers of subjects, the added precision obtained from steady-state data of six to ten minute time periods appears to be worth the effort.

STANDARDIZATION OF SUBMAXIMAL MULTIPLE-LOAD TESTS

Heart Rate Criteria

Multiple load tests are used to achieve a predetermined heart rate for the purpose of recording the electrocardiogram at a given constant heart rate. Reasons for this will be discussed later. They are also needed to obtain a measure of work capacity, when the rate of work necessary to elicit a predetermined pulse rate becomes the measured variable. The advantage is that the reliability of the work pulse rate increases as the work becomes more intense and the pulse rate increases (20).

The increments of work and time periods at each work level must be considered. One has the option of small frequent increments which shorten the test or large infrequent increments which allow steady-state recording of ECGs, pulse and/or oxygen consumption.

In the Balke-Ware type of test (Column 3, Table 18-I) the small increments of work load make it easy to identify accurately the work load at which the desired pulse rate criterion is reached. In contrast a pulse criterion may be missed using the procedures described in Columns 2 and 4 in which increments between work loads are moderately large and the time at each load relatively long. However, it is possible to improve the precision for tests in these columns by interpolating between work loads and to determine the work load or oxygen consumption equivalent to the target pulse rate. If oxygen consumption is not to be measured, the work load can be described as kpm with the bicycle ergometer, or as grade walked (at a constant speed) with the treadmill. The assumption here is that oxygen consumption can be calculated with precision from these values, which holds a little better with the bicycle than with the treadmill (see standardization of single load tests). Treadmill tests which use standard speeds and vary the work load by increasing the grade by increments of 1, 2.5 or 5 per cent provide the best opportunity to make precise interpolations. When speed is changed as well as grade, as in the procedure used by Doan *et al.* (24) and Lester and his associates (39), interpolation becomes less precise, particularly as the subject begins to run since the variability between individuals in the ml/kg/minute of oxygen is markedly increased (23). For most purposes the calculation is satisfactory however.

In the above scheme, the rate of increase in pulse rate during recording of the ECG is not considered by some investigators to be excessive. However, if steady-state pulse rate recording is considered to be important, small alterations in grade (if the treadmill is used) or brake (if the bicycle is being employed) can be employed to produce a relatively stable pulse rate for one to two minutes at the target level. This device has been used by Sheffield (54) in administering the graded pulse rate test and by investigators using the 300/kpm/min step between levels employed by the Swedish investigators.

ATTITUDE AND FAMILIARITY OF THE SUBJECT WITH THE TEST

Pulse rates in standard submaximal tests decrease in a variable proportion of a study group with increasing exposure to the test procedure. At least two factors enter into this decline in work pulse rate: (a) learning to walk or run skillfully on the treadmill, or ride the bicycle, or mount the step, and (b) emotional involvement with the test procedure and its outcome. Examples from this laboratory's experience have been provided elsewhere along with evidence that apprehension can produce substantial changes in submaximal work pulse rates (60).

Isolated examples of excessive pulse rate response which occur in special laboratory situations are not impressive unless documented by field or clinic experience. The initial visit to a survey site provides an environment in which (a) the subjects have usually had no previous experience with the personnel of the survey team or on the ergometric equipment to be used, and (b) the subjects have come for a cardiovascular examination. In a railroad survey of coronary heart disease described in detail elsewhere (38), ninety-four men were asked to walk on a motor driven treadmill for three minutes at 3 mph on a 5 per cent grade on three occasions separated by at least a year. The mean work pulse rate at the first exposure was 124.5, at the second 112.4 and on the third 111.5. Distributions of the pulse rate differences between the first and second and the second and third exposures reveal that the change in the mean was due to substantial changes in pulse rate in roughly one-fourth of the population. The work pulse rate changes from the first to the second exposure in 4 per cent of the men were −41 to −52 beats per minute, in eight per cent −24 to −40 and in 13 per cent −20 to −28. Since 95 per cent of the changes between the second and third exposures lay between +11 and −13, it can be concluded that these changes were a good deal larger than those found in the situation where men were accustomed to the equipment and the purpose of the test. Increase in skill of walking seldom produces changes in oxygen consumption of more than 5 per cent. A decrease in oxygen consumption of this magnitude at 3 mph and 5 per cent grade will not account for more than 4 to 6 beats a minute in the observed decreases in pulse rate. It follows then that excitement or apprehension associated with the initial contact was an important factor in producing the elevated work pulse rates in many of the men who sustained large decreases in pulse rate. It is reasonable to speculate that catecholamine activity was very high in some of these men. Since changes in the catecholamines in the cellular environment of myocardial fibers can greatly modify the myocardial oxygen consumption, ECG abnormalities at initial examination may not reoccur at the same work load during subsequent examinations. Similar data on tests performed in the clinic are not available but are needed. In addition, it is clear that study of the effects of repetition on progressive multistage submaximal tests is also needed.

STANDARDIZATION OF PROCEDURES FOR DETERMINING MAXIMAL OXYGEN UPTAKE

When one subjects a normal individual to intermittent work loads which are increased by a standardized increment, a linear relationship exists between work load and oxygen intake up to the point at which maximal oxygen intake is very nearly reached. Beyond this point, additional work increments do not produce the expected increment in oxygen intake. A leveling off or even a decline in oxygen intake is frequently observed. Since in practice a plateau of oxygen intake with increasing work loads is not always observed, criteria for attaining maximal oxygen intake are needed. In the Laboratory of Physiological Hygiene, this is defined as an increment of oxygen intake for a standardized increment of work load which is less than the expected increment less 2 standard deviations (18). In young men aged sixteen to twenty-four, the oxygen consumption increment for an increase in grade of 2.5 per cent was found to be 4.02 ml/kg/min $\pm$ 1.2 ml/kg/min (unpublished data).

Increments for the commonly used loads for the bicycle are available. The Scandinavian investigators frequently employ a work load increment of 300 kpms which is equivalent to 0.59 liters/min. The standard deviations of the increments are not available from the literature. Both P.O. and I. Åstrand (5, 8) have used the measurement of lactate concentration as a device to determine whether the subject has exerted himself to the point of eliciting a maximal oxygen consumption. For young men, a value of 90 mg per 100 ml of blood appears to be an acceptable figure.

The time intervals for work increments used by investigators for maximal oxygen intake determination have varied from three (59) to five (48) to six minutes (8). Methodological comparisons carried out on the same subjects have shown that the two protocols used in Minnesota (59) and Sweden (8) give the same values (29). In well-motivated subjects, Robinson's criteria of a work load which exhausts men in five minutes or less is valid. In addition, questions have been raised regarding the type of ergometer employed in the test. Investigation of this question has led to the conclusion that it makes no difference whether one uses a bicycle or a treadmill (29). It is of some interest that if one works men to their known maximal oxygen intake using a continuous progressive test such as the Balke-Ware procedure or the Bruce test, evidence of a leveling of oxygen intake is not usually seen. The explanation for this is not clear. The result is that unless one measures the lactate concentration, the investigator is faced with a self-determined end-point which raises the specter of underperformance and the accompanying underestimate of the maximal oxygen intake. In well-motivated subjects, the procedure of working a man to exhaustion is known to give adequate estimates of maximal oxygen intake. In patients of any age, older population groups and the middle-aged, the effects on motivation of discomfort associated with working to exhaustion are always in some question. In the experience of the authors and the members of the Technical Committee, motivation of a high order of magnitude can be created in volunteer subjects, normal or otherwise, who have been properly prepared for such a test by attention from the investigator group over time and the development of a high level of confidence in the competence of the investigator. Symptom-limited performance capacity is a valuable tool in both the clinic and in physiological investigation of effects of stress (16, 35).

Documented maximal oxygen intakes are not affected by (a) motivation; (b) excitement, apprehension or other emotional factors (59); (c) skill (mechanical efficiency) in performing the assigned task (59); (d) ambient temperature (59); (e) dehydration up to 5 per cent of the body weight (29); (f) variations in the concentration of red blood cells within the normal limits found in man (50); (g) variation within the normal range of lung function (29). Accordingly, documented maximal oxygen intakes define with considerable precision the upper limit of cardiovascular performance (45, 59). This measurement is indispensable for many types of investigation of the cardiovascular performance of subjects in a wide variety of research projects since it provides a frame of reference.

STANDARDIZED EVALUATION OF CARDIAC AND PERIPHERAL CIRCULATORY FUNCTION BY THE MAXIMAL OXYGEN INTAKE

The measurement of maximal oxygen intake may be critical to the evaluation of a measurement of function. In evaluating the effects of disease the clinical investigator is frequently faced with the problem of comparing "normals" who have a very large capacity for work and a large cardiac reserve with patients whose work capacity and cardiac reserve may be severely restricted. This frequently means comparing the function in normal men working at a level which produces very little stress with patients working at a level of relatively greater stress which is much closer to their true maximal work capacity and maximal oxygen intake. By setting the maximal oxygen intake at 100 per cent for both groups and plotting function against work load, expressed as oxygen intake in per cent of maximal oxygen intake, the investigator has the opportunity of comparing function at comparable cardiovascular stress levels.

ERGOMETERS

Bicycles

Von Dobeln (25) designed a simple bicycle ergometer with a mechanical brake which is easy to use and inexpensive.* Krogh de-

---

*The Monarch bicycle is for sale in the United States by Quinton Company, Seattle and in Sweden by Monark Crescent AB, Varberg, Sweden.

signed a bicycle ergometer in which the pedals turn an electric generator and the work done is recorded as watts produced. In both these
devices the work load varies with the rate of pedaling and they are
equipped with tachometers. Technicians administering tests with this
type of equipment must be alert to maintenance of a given rate and
constancy of pedaling.

Ergometers have been designed to compensate for variations in
speed with complex electrical circuits which adjust the brake resistance
according to speed of pedaling. The National Health Examination
Survey has reported the calibration (46) of two such ergometers
after an extended period of use in the field. Errors were found in the
tachometer, power output and stability. Significant drift occurred
over a ten-minute period. Deviations of the true power output from
that indicated were as high as 20 per cent. Investigators using electrical brake equipment of this type must either set up an external
calibrating system or have on hand a "calibrated" subject and the
necessary equipment to measure oxygen consumption at standard settings.

Treadmills

Treadmills are offered by several manufacturers. They vary in cost,
size and portability and in sophistication of accessory equipment and
automated control. Treadmill speed requires frequent checking by
rotation measurements based on belt length. The Harvard Fatigue
Laboratory recommended in 1928 that treadmill grades be calculated as the vertical lift in per cent of horizontal travel (17, 22).
An alternate method of calculating vertical lift as per cent of belt
travel yields differences which become important above grades of 15
per cent.

Step Tests

Single and two-step tests of prescribed height are readily available
or can be constructed simply. Step heights which can be modified
for the relative leg length of individuals have been recommended (49).
Schemes for providing a variety of steps to vary the rate of work have
also been proposed (49).

Part II
STANDARDIZATION OF EXERCISE TESTS FOR
ECG EVALUATION

Theoretical Considerations

To compare the electrocardiogram of an individual with that of "healthy" individuals of the same age and sex, for evaluating the adequacy of myocardial oxygen supply, the conditions of work should provide a constant myocardial oxygen requirement per unit weight of heart muscle. Within individuals, the oxygen requirement of submaximal work under steady-state conditions is equal to the oxygen intake per unit time. In addition, there is a linear relationship between cardiac output per unit time and the oxygen consumption per unit time. Moreover, it is known that mean blood pressure in the aorta rises slowly as the intensity of work (and oxygen consumption) increases. Furthermore, the work pulse rate of subjects accustomed to ergometric testing has a linear relationship to oxygen consumption. If we now assume that heart size and rate of ejection are constant at any given total oxygen consumption, the conditions are present for devising a work test which defines myocardial oxygen consumption. The situation changes when comparisons are made between individuals. Walking on a 5 per cent grade at 3 mph results in constant oxygen consumption per kilogram of body weight, approximately constant cardiac output, and work blood pressure systematically related to the resting pressure level. Since heart weight and body weight have almost a 1:1 relation, heart weight per kilogram of body weight will be approximately constant. Experimental measurement of cardiac diameters during work, in cases where it has been possible to attach metal clips, suggests a systematic relationship to cardiac dimensions at rest. Despite these standardizing elements, the 5 per cent, 3 mph test in middle-aged men gives work pulse rates varying from 80 to 170/min.

Work by Sarnoff *et al.* (53) and Katz and collaborators (36) showed that in experimental preparations the myocardial oxygen consumption is related to the time-tension index and to the product of systolic blood pressure and pulse rate. Experimental constraints on this relationship were, however, maintenance of a constant diastolic

heart volume, catecholamine level, constancy of calcium ion concentration and absence of drugs such as digitalis and propranolol. Nevertheless, it is clear that pulse rate is an important determinant of myocardial oxygen consumption (13). A work test which produces wide
variation in pulse rate does not fulfill requirements for standardization:
precise comparison between individuals of electrocardiographic responses.

Measurements of Coronary Blood Flow and Myocardial Oxygen Consumption in Man During Submaximal Work

Influences on coronary blood flow and myocardial oxygen consumption have been carefully and extensively investigated in various
experimental preparations. Extrapolation to man is difficult. Integrated physiological mechanisms in the intact animal tend to reduce
variability of the coronary blood flow and myocardial oxygen consumption during work. Studies of coronary blood flow and myocardial
oxygen consumption during work in man indicate their variability and
their relationship to simple peripheral indicators. A number of these
studies during supine exercise are at work intensities which require less
than 1,000 ml of oxygen per minute (41, 43, 44). These studies have
emphasized that myocardial oxygen extraction is high at rest (70 per
cent) and, in normals, does not change as a result of work. Coronary
blood flow at light work increases in direct proportion to the increase
in oxygen consumption by the myocardium. In patients with advanced
coronary disease, the oxygen extraction at rest is the same as in puta-
tively healthy individuals but extraction is greater during light work.

Heavier work loads from 300 to 900 kpm/min with work pulse rates
up to 170 beats per minute were studied by Holmberg (32). He
measured coronary blood flow and arteriovenous oxygen difference
between aorta and coronary sinus and from these data calculated
myocardial oxygen consumption. Controls were eleven subjects free
of evidence of coronary heart disease. One had hypertension and
one aortic stenosis. Nine patients with coronary heart disease were
studied, three of whom had hypertension and one, aortic stenosis. The
variability of blood flow was minimal due to careful attention to requirements for steady-state determination of regional blood flow (37)
in the administration and measurement of xenon 133. Coronary blood

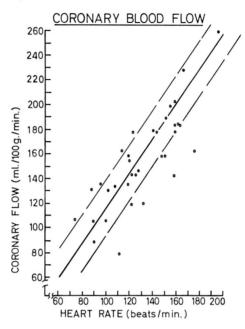

CORONARY BLOOD FLOW

FIGURE 18-2. Coronary blood flow and heart rate in patients without coronary heart disease. (Redrawn from Holmberg, reference 32.)

flow was found to be unrelated to work load, and by inference, to oxygen consumption measured at work. This confirmed, at higher work loads and pulse rates, the finding of Messer *et al.* (43, 44) that oxygen extraction was not increased during the transition from rest to work in normal individuals but was increased in C. H. D. patients. Gaos *et al.* (28) have also reported this fact but the details are not given. In Figure 18-2 Holmberg found a correlation coefficient of 0.81 between pulse rate and coronary flow rate in normals. Figure 18-3 presents the relationship of coronary blood flow to pulse rate in patients with C. H. D., plotted as a regression line along with arbitrary limits of variation from reported data in normals. Pulse rate *under*estimates coronary blood flow in normals and in patients who had hypertension or aortic stenosis. When myocardial oxygen consumption is plotted against the *product* of heart rate and mean blood pressure, underestimates of myocardial oxygen consumption are also found for patients and for the "normals" with hypertension or aortic stenosis.

These data support the concept that work pulse rate is more closely

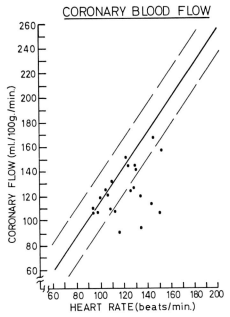

FIGURE 18-3. Coronary blood flow and heart rate in patients with coronary heart disease. (Redrawn from Holmberg, reference 32.)

correlated with coronary blood flow than with myocardial oxygen consumption. It is not known whether this apparent underestimate represents a true deficit of oxygen consumption or an error in prediction from the product of means of blood pressure and pulse rate. The correlation coefficient between the product of mean pulse rate and mean blood pressure with myocardial oxygen consumption was 0.71. This may be compared to a correlation coefficient of 0.63 between left ventricular work and myocardial oxygen consumption.

The data available lend important support to the concept that work to a constant pulse rate provides a blood flow challenge to the coronary vascular bed which is less variable from man to man than work at a constant external work load or a constant work load per unit body weight. Nevertheless, the relationship of myocardial oxygen consumption to the product of the mean blood pressure and pulse rate is not quite as good as that between pulse rate and coronary flow. This is particularly so if, as in the case of Holmberg's data, patients with valvular lesions and hypertension are included.

It appears that work to maximal oxygen consumption level results in little change in the mean aortic blood pressure from that found at rest. It follows that pulse rate is the principal contributor to the product of mean blood pressure and pulse rate during work. But classifying individuals by their resting blood pressure might be a useful method of reducing further the variability of myocardial oxygen consumption at specific target work pulse rates. More data both on normals and men whose hemodynamic characteristics at rest are not normal are required for confidence in the standardization of myocardial oxygen consumption by work to a given pulse rate.

SINGLE-STAGE TESTS VERSUS PROGRESSIVE MULTISTAGE TESTS

Comparative Prevalence of Ischemic S-T Depressions

Standard load, single-stage tests result in a large range of work pulse rates. Sheffield *et al.* (54) reported heart rates from 90 to 190/min on a double Master test in 216 men. Taylor and colleagues (38) found the range 80 to 172 beats/min in 1040 middle-age American railroad employees who walked for three minutes at 3 mph on a 5 per cent grade. If work pulse rates less than 120 are regarded as "low" then 19 per cent of men in the Master test and 45 per cent of men in that treadmill test are low. If 150 or higher is regarded as a "high" work pulse rate, then 4 per cent of the men taking this treadmill test and 5 per cent of the men taking the Master test are high. Both tests resulted in a substantial number of men who, by Holmberg's data, would have little challenge to their coronary circulation, as well as a small fraction who were perhaps "over-challenged." If one assumes that blood pressure was similarly distributed in both groups, then a similar statement can be made about myocardial oxygen consumption. It follows that a substantial number of men "negative" on a Master test would be expected to develop S-T depression with an exercise test to maximal pulse rate or to a level representing a large fraction of the expected maximal pulse rate for age.

Doan *et al.* (24) compared the Master test and a symptom-limited maximal performance test in 220 members of the YMCA. They found two with S-T depressions in the Master test versus eighteen in the "maximal" procedure. Sheffield *et al.* (54) studied 104 patients with a variety of cardiac diagnoses including uncomplicated angina, probable angina, improbable angina and old myocardial infarction with and without angina. The Master test elicited thirty-eight "positive" S-T depressions, while work to a pulse rate of 85 per cent of predicted maximal gave twelve additional "positive" cases.

ECG Response to Progressive Multistage Tests

Blomqvist (12) studied the ECG response to progressive work loads up to maximal oxygen intake, in twenty-six men, age forty-six to fifty-five years. He found that the degree of S-T depression had a straight line relationship with the per cent of aerobic work capacity up to 60 per cent of maximal oxygen intake. Thereafter, up to maximal oxygen intake the frequency of S-T responses was disproportionately larger, i.e., a curvilinear relationship. Horizontal S-T depression in one or more leads exceeded 0.5 mm in six of sixteen normal men age forty-six to fifty-five (37.5 per cent). Strandell (58) reported three cases of segmental S-T depression greater than 0.5 mm in a series of fourteen men fifty to fifty-nine years of age (21 per cent) who were worked to symptom-limited capacity. Doan and associates (24) found in a group of 226 subjects 9.4 per cent with "positive" responses in the fifth decade, 44.1 per cent in the sixth decade and 46.1 per cent in the seventh decade, after work to symptom-limited capacity. Lester *et al.* (40) have pointed out that if men with significant cardiac abnormalities were removed from the series of Doan *et al.* the incidence of "positive" S-T depression in men over the age of forty is 9 per cent and compares well with the 5 per cent "positive" S-T depressions observed in their series.

Working to 90 per cent or less of predicted maximal heart rate may result in substantially fewer "positive" S-T findings than work to maximal capacity. Lester *et al.* (40) reported only a 1 per cent frequency in 114 men who were thought to be clinically healthy and were worked to 90 per cent of predicted maximal pulse rate. Astrand (4) found three cases of segmental depression of 1 mm or more in seventy-three normotensive men age forty-eight to sixty-three (4.1 per cent) in a random sample of Stockholm men worked to pulse rates of 150 beats per minute.

SYMPTOM-LIMITED WORK CAPACITY TESTS

Multistage tests conducted to symptom-limited work capacity requires some definition. Subjects are asked to proceed with work until they can no longer continue. The subject may himself terminate the procedure because of fatigue or dyspnea. Other common complaints are weakness or discomfort in the legs. The responsible physician should be prepared to stop the test because of signs or symptoms, as described by Hornsten and Bruce (34).

The purpose of conducting this progressive procedure is to obtain a greater yield of positive ECG responses and to measure symptom-limited work capacity. This measurement is widely different between men with coronary heart disease and normals. For example, in a comparison of 130 age-matched normals with 69 A. S. H. D. patients, 55 per cent of the normals were able to perform more work on the Bruce test than 98 per cent of the patients. Median duration of the exercise occurs during stage IV for normal men while median value for patients is within stage II (34).

There are data on normals which demonstrate that peak work loads in industrial conditions which are approximately one third of the maximal oxygen intake are tolerated without fatigue. Careful studies on cardiac patients have not been carried out but this appears to be a reasonable guide in judging the work load which a patient can tolerate in industry.

Kattus (35) has used a progressive test in the evaluation of patients with angina pectoris. Work to the point of inducing characteristic angina is regarded by this investigator as the most effective method of evaluating the condition of a patient at a particular time and in documenting the course of disease or effectiveness of therapy.

In Sweden, standardized submaximal work capacity tests to a heart rate of 170, or the development of symptoms, have been widely used by cardiologists in the evaluation of cardiac patients (57).

Management and Safety Problems of Testing to Maximal Performance Compared to Near-Maximal Testing

Lester *et al.* (39) have reported that ventricular and supraventricular tachycardias are more apt to occur between 90 and 100 per cent of maximal heart rate in a maximal performance test than before or after. This phenomenon was also observed in Laboratory of Physiological Hygiene testing of middle-aged men in a pilot study on physical activity and coronary disease (18); no serious arrhythmias developed in repeated testing to heart rate 150, but two potentially serious episodes developed during the first round of tests to attain maximal oxygen uptake. These potentially life-threatening arrhythmias have been reported in approximately 0.5 per cent of men submitted to maximal testing (34). There are no reports of ventricular tachycardias developing during exercise which have required defibrillation. Three men are known to have developed a myocardial infarction within minutes *after* performing maximal tests, among the many thousands submitted to maximal symptom-limited performance and to determinations of maximal oxygen intake. Hornsten and Bruce report one infarct in 57,000 Master tests, four infarcts and two deaths in 40,000 submaximal bicycle or treadmill tests and two infarcts with one death in 5,900 maximal treadmill tests (34). Therefore there is a small risk in conducting maximal tests. Investigators should recognize this and take appropriate steps to deal with the problem if maximal tests are to be conducted in men over the age of thirty-five.

There are other problems of conducting maximal tests in middle-aged men which are important in planning experimental or clinical activities. The degree of subjective discomfort necessary to elicit a maximal oxygen intake or a maximal pulse rate is substantially greater than that required to reach a target pulse rate of 90 per cent of the expected maximum for age (18). It is during this interval between 90 percent and maximum that lactate concentration rises rapidly and the subject hyperventilates. Since the man of fifty years has lost 20 per cent of his maximal breathing capacity over the preceding twenty-five years, his threshold for dyspnea has been correspondingly reduced (27). Fatigue and dyspnea are common causes of terminating a progressive test. A proportion of middle-aged subjects experience profound weakness that may persist as long as three to five hours after a maximal exercise test (14, 18, 39). It follows that a greater degree of motivation is required to perform the maximal test and that retesting may be refused by some individuals. Nevertheless, there are situations in which it is clearly desirable to perform maximal tests. Physicians working closely with individual patients, or investigators studying small groups, create a high degree of confidence and motivation which may not be matched in a busy clinic or large epidemiological study.

Management and Safety Problems of Single-Stage Procedures

Hornsten and Bruce (34) have estimated that one myocardial infarct has occurred in 57,000 tests administered by experienced investigators. This is a very low risk. However, significant ECG changes do occur at substantially lower levels of work. In this laboratory among 130 "high coronary risk individuals" (18), three men were found who had marked S-T depressions after low level work, walking for three minutes at 3 miles per hour at zero grade. When the men were tested again for ten minutes at 3 mph on a 5 per cent grade, two cases had marked hypotension persisting at supine rest with S-T depressions for more than ten minutes after the work period. Consequently, starting at low levels of work and a gradually progressive test provides a closer estimate of the level of work at which ischemic ECG changes take place. It protects the investigator against the rare individual who may get into trouble because the pulse rate has "overresponded" to the work load, for whatever reason.

Maximal Work Pulse Rates and Their Relationship to Age

Table 18-III presents published data relating maximal work pulse rates to age. All groups were residents of either Scandinavia or the United States. Methods of selection favored relatively active individuals in the studies conducted by Robinson (48), Astrand (5) and Anderson (2). These authors are in agreement and are in general agreement with those of Bruce and his colleagues (16). Lester et al. (39) reported maximal pulse rates in the older age groups which are clearly larger than those of the other investigators. These investigators believe that their older subjects' motivation was higher and more effective than that of Robinson's subjects, resulting in better performance and higher maximal pulse rates in the older age groups. An alternative possibility is that the Birmingham group's recruitment and volunteering process resulted in a different segment of the middle-aged population. Lester and his colleagues found that men who had been conditioned by running or jogging had maximal pulse rates 7 beats per minute lower at any age. To illustrate the situation in a little more detail the mean maximal heart rates reported in Table 18-III, plus the conditioned group studied in Birmingham, and the data of Ander-

TABLE 18-III

MAXIMAL PULSE RATES BY AGE REPORTED IN THE LITERATURE

No. of Individuals Tested (N), Means and Standard Deviations (S.D.)

Age Group	I Robinson (48)		II Lester et al (39)		III Bruce et al (16)		IV I. Astrand (5)		V L. Anderson (2)	
	N	Mean S.D.	N*	Mean S.D.*	N	Mean S.D.	N	Mean S.D.	N	Mean S.D.
20-29	17	194 ± 8.0		195	81	190 ± 10	29	195 ± 11		180
30-39	10	187 ± 7.4		191	84	180 ± 10	13	181 ± 12	8	173 ± 11.2
40-49	10	177 ± 7.5		187	101	174 ± 11	9	173 ± 11	22	165 ± 14
50-59	10	170 ± 8.8		183	57	170 ± 14	66	161 ± 11	19	150 ± 12
60-69	5	160 ± 6.5		179	12	146 ± 25	8	159 ± 9	22	

*Data in column II are calculated from the equation Y = 205.02 — 0.411X, where Y is the maximal pulse rate and X is the age. The equation is based on data from 148 untrained subjects. The standard deviation from the regression line is ± 8.73.

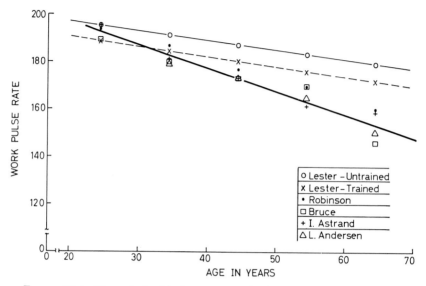

FIGURE 18-4. The relationship between maximal work pulse rate and age.

sen and the Hermansen on businessmen in Oslo, are plotted against age. Note that the Oslo businessmen age 55 had a mean maximal work pulse rate of 181 or 16 beats per minute higher than the industrial workers in the same area.

More studies with careful characterization of the individual are required. In any event, it is clear that extremely wide, 95% confidence, limits apply for any given individual. Up through the age of 60, the confidence limits vary from 15 beats per minute to 28 beats per minute above and below the sample mean. It is clear that a very substantial uncertainty exists in the prediction of maximal pulse rate from the age in the individual.

Rationale for the Target Pulse Rates Chosen as Fractions of Maximal Pulse Rate

In designing a submaximal test for ECG evaluation, it is desirable to choose a work load which imposes the same relative cardiovascular load on both the twenty- and the sixty-year-old subject. This goal is in addition to that of selecting a pulse rate which will provide reasonable protection against working men to maximal pulse rate. It is

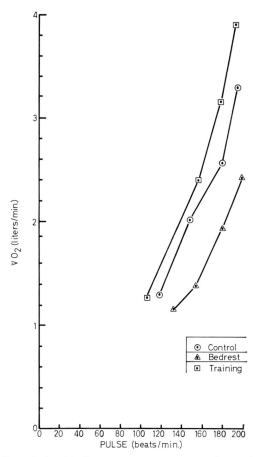

FIGURE 18-5. The relationship between oxygen consumption and pulse rate during submaximal and maximal work in 5 young men submitted to observations before, immediately following bed rest and after a conditioning period. (Redrawn from Saltin, et al., reference 52).

generally agreed that the degree of vasoconstriction in the periphery and organs not involved in exercise is related to the oxygen consumption of submaximal work loads expressed as per cent of maximal oxygen intake. It follows that the work load expressed in this way is a measure of the circulatory stress imposed on the system.

Figure 18-5 presents the pulse rate and oxygen consumption data from the study of Saltin and his colleagues (52) of five young men who were studied during a control period, immediately after bed rest

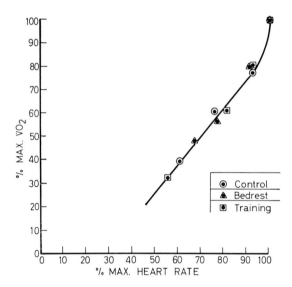

FIGURE 18-6. The relationship between oxygen consumption as percent of maximal oxygen consumption and pulse rate as percent of maximal heart rate in 5 young men observed during submaximal and maximal work before, immediately following bed rest and after a conditioning period. (Redrawn from Saltin *et al.*, reference 52.)

of three weeks and after a period of intensive physical conditioning. The maximal oxygen intake varies from approximately 2.4 liters a minute to almost 4 liters a minute with large variations in the work pulse for any level of work except maximal. The data are presented in Figure 18-6 as per cent of maximal pulse and oxygen intake.

The figure illustrates the principle that relative work loads can be estimated with considerable accuracy from pulse rate expressed as fractions of maximal in men with widely divergent maximal oxygen intakes. Figure 18-7 presents the group means of data collected on several age groups by Robinson, who used treadmill techniques, and P. -O. and I. Åstrand, who used bicycle procedures. The data from these investigators have been plotted on the same graph to show that the agreement is excellent regardless of technique, country in which the work was done, or the uncertainties of sample selection. Again it is seen that the relative work load is predicted with precision from pulse rate measurements.

When the maximal heart rate is predicted from age-pulse rate data,

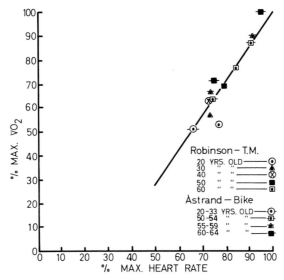

FIGURE 18-7. The relationship of submaximal oxygen consumption expressed as percent of maximal, and simultaneously measured pulse rate as percent of maximal pulse rate, in men of various ages resident in the United States and Sweden.

it is clear that a fair degree of uncertainty enters the picture. The variability has not as yet been precisely determined by application of estimated maximal pulse rates to populations which have not been previously studied. It is emphasized again that the first experience with ergometer testing with ECG recording is likely to result in over-responses of pulse rate with its consequent underestimation of fractional maximal oxygen intake loading.

Target Pulse Rates Used for ECG Work Tests

The Birmingham group (40, 54) has recommended target pulse rates for their final stage in the graded exercise test (GxT) at 90 per cent of the maximal pulse rates determined in their investigations of sedentary and trained men. The Scandinavian committee of experts recommended target pulse rates of 170 in the age group twenty to twenty-nine years, 160 in the group thirty to thirty-nine, 150 in the group forty to forty-nine, 140 in the group fifty to fifty-nine and 130 in the group sixty to sixty-nine (62). These pulse rates are approximately 85 per cent of the Swedish standards for maximal. The

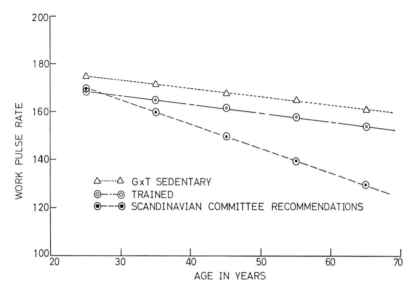

FIGURE 18-8. Target pulse rates recommended by a Scandinavian Committee (Åstrand *et al.*, reference 62) and in the graded exercise test (g × t of Lester *et al.*, reference 39).

recommendations of both groups are plotted against age in Figure 18-8.

Any target pulse rate chosen for clinical work is based in part on avoiding work to a maximal pulse rate. At age fifty the calculated 90 per cent of maximum rate for sedentary Americans is *166*, using the figures of Lester *et al.* (40), and is *18* beats per minute less than the mean maximum pulse rate for that age. The pooled standard deviation of maximum pulse rates is 10 beats per minute. If 188 beats per minute is the correct figure for maximal work pulse rate of the population of men aged fifty, only 2.5 per cent of this population will have a maximal pulse rate less than the target pulse rate of *166* (2 beats per minute lower than the 90 per cent level). But if the true maximal pulse rate for the population is closer to the estimate obtained by Bruce *et al.*, the number of men increases whose maximal pulse rate will in fact be less than the Lester *et al.* target pulse rate. If the investigator working with a population of sedentary Americans wishes to protect himself from working men at their maximal pulse rate, 80 per cent of maximal Birmingham figure or the target pulse rates recommended by the Scandinavian group, may be used (62).

The recommendation of the Scandinavian group may prove a little *low* for sedentary American males.

Currently the Birmingham group is recommending a stepwise procedure in which the work load is increased every thirty seconds according to the schedule provided below* until the desired target pulse is reached. Five separate tests are carried out to each target pulse rate of 60, 70, 80, 90 and 100 per cent of predicted maximal. When the target rate is achieved, the grade is adjusted to produce a steady-state pulse rate which is then maintained for two to three minutes while electrocardiograms are recorded. At the end of the steady-state period is a five-minute recovery period with post-exercise ECG recording. This intermittent design is believed to be particularly useful for initial examinations of unknown subjects, to accustom them to testing and occasionally to disclose S-T depressions occurring late, two to three minutes after work has been stopped.

A continuous test with uninterrupted increments of work to 85 per cent of predicted maximal pulse rate appears suitable to men whose individual work capacity and ECG responses are known. Testing to maximal pulse rate or oxygen consumption might be considered for airline pilots, heavy machine operators and others whose lives, and those of others, might be endangered by assumed integrity of their coronary circulation (30).

SUMMARY

1. Multistage work capacity procedures provide a measurement of the work intensity that a patient is able to tolerate without symptoms or electrocardiographic abnormalities.

2. Evidence is available which supports the concept that the oxygen consumption per unit weight of the individual is unrelated to the myocardial oxygen consumption. The work pulse rate is thought to be the best currently available basis for standardization of myocardial oxygen consumption during work.

3. Single-stage tests, whether they provide a constant external work load or a constant work load per unit weight, are characterized by a wide range of pulse rates which are likely to result in false negatives and overstressing a small fraction of the population.

4. For the investigator who is willing to accept the small but

---

*Protocols for this and other testing procedures will be provided upon request.

definite risk involved, multistage tests carried to symptom-limited or maximal capacity provide the clearest differentiation between normals and coronary heart disease patients. Repeated multistage tests give an excellent measure of progress. The best available estimate of the work level which a patient can tolerate in a full work day is 30 per cent of the symptom-limited work capacity.

5. Since the maximal work pulse rate declines with age, constant fraction of the maximal work pulse rate for the age of the individual is thought to be the most suitable target pulse rate for standardization of multistage submaximal tests. Conservative target pulse rates for terminating multistage tests are proposed by the Scandinavian Committee on ECG Classification as 170/min for men age twenty to twenty-nine, 160 for thirty to thirty-nine, 150 for forty to forty-nine, 140 for fifty to fifty-nine and 130 for those sixty to sixty-nine.

6. Work to higher levels than have been used in the past, particularly to symptom-limited capacity, yields an increase in the number of positive S-T depressions. The prognostic significance of such findings is unknown and systematic follow-up studies should be undertaken.

REFERENCES

1. ALLARD, C.: Commentary on current levels of fitness. *Canad Med Assoc J, 96*:879, 1967.
2. ANDERSEN, K.L.: Physical fitness—studies of healthy men and women in Norway. *International Research in Sport and Physical Education.* Jokl, E., and Simon, E. (Eds.), Springfield, Thomas, 1964, p. 489.
3. ANDERSEN, K.L., and HERMANSEN, L.: Aerobic work capacity in middle-aged Norwegian men. *J Appl Physiol, 20*:432, 1965.
4. ASTRAND, I.: Exercise electrocardiograms recorded twice with an 8-year interval in a group of 204 women and men 48-63 years old. *Acta Med Scand, 178*:27, 1965.
5. ASTRAND, I.: Aerobic capacity in men and women with special reference to age. *Acta Physiol Scand, 169* (suppl.):47-48, 1960.
6. ASTRAND, I.: The physical work capacity of workers 50-64 years old. *Acta Physiol Scand, 42*:73, 1958.
7. ASTRAND, I.; ASTRAND, P.-O., and RODAHL, K.: Maximal heart rate during work in older men. *J Appl Physiol, 14*:562-566, 1959.
8. ASTRAND, P.-O.: *Experimental Studies of Physical Working Capacity in Relation to Sex and Age.* Copenhagen, Ejnar Munksgaard, 1952, pp. 19-20.
9. BALKE, B., and WARE, R.W.: An experimental study of "physical fitness" of Air Force personnel. *US Armed Forces Med J, 10*:675, 1959.

10. BINKHORST, R.A., and VAN LEEUWEN, P.: A rapid method for the determination of aerobic capacity. *Int Z Angew Physiol, 19*:459, 1963.

11. BLACKBURN, H.; HAMRELL, B.; WINCKLER, G.; VILANDRE, J.; HODGSON, J., and TAYLOR, H.L.: (1) Comparison of the energy cost and heart rate response to five commonly-used, single-stage, non-steady state, submaximal work procedures. (2) Comparison of the energy cost and heart rate response to a continuous versus intermittent work test procedure. *International Research in Sport and Physical Education.* Jokl, E. (Ed.), Springfield, Thomas, 1969.

12. BLOMQVIST, G.: The Frank lead exercise electrocardiogram. A quantitative study based on averaging technique and digital computer analysis. *Acta Med Scand, 178* (suppl.):440, 1965.

13. BRAUNWALD, E.; SONNENBLICK, E.H.; ROSS, J., JR.; GLICK, G., and EPSTEIN, S.E.: An analysis of the cardiac response to exercise. *Circ Res, 20*(suppl.) and *21*(suppl.):44, 1967.

14. BRUCE, R.A., personal communication.

15. BRUCE, R.A.; BLACKMON, J.R.; JONES, J.W., and STRAIT, G.: Exercise testing in adult normal subjects and cardiac patients. *Pediatrics, 32* (suppl.) (4):742, 1963.

16. BRUCE, R.A.; ROWELL, L.B.; BLACKMON, J.R., and DOAN, A.: Cardiovascular function tests. *Heart Bull, 14*:9, 1965.

17. CONSOLAZIO, C.F.; JOHNSON, R.E., and PECORA, L.J.: *Physiological Measurements of Metabolic Functions in Man.* New York, McGraw, 1963.

18. Cooperative Pilot Studies on the Feasibility of Large Scale Studies of Physical Activity and Coronary Heart Disease at the Universities of Minnesota. Wisconsin and Penn State. A report.

19. CURETON, T.K.: *Physical Fitness Appraisal and Guidance.* St. Louis, Mosby, 1947, p. 566.

20. DAHLSTROM, HANS: Reliability and validity of some fitness tests. *International Research in Sport and Physical Education.* Jokl, E., and Simon, E. (Eds.), Springfield, Thomas, 1964, p. 560.

21. DENOLIN, H.; MESSIN, R., and DEGRE, S.: Testing of the working capacity of cardiac patients. *Physical Activity and the Heart.* Karvonen, M.J., and Barry, A.J. (Eds.), Springfield, Thomas, 1967, pp. 27-31.

22. DILL, D.B.; EDWARDS, H.T., and TALBOTT, J.H.: Studies in muscular activity. VII. Factors limiting the capacity for work. *J Physiol, 77*:49-62, 1932.

23. DILL, D.B.; TALBOTT, J.H., and EDWARDS, H.T.: Response of several individuals to a fixed task. *J Physiol, 69*:267-305, 1930.

24. DOAN, A.E.; PETERSON, D.R.; BLACKMON, J.R., and BRUCE, R.A.: Myocardial ischemia after maximal exercise in healthy men. *Amer Heart J, 69*:11, 1965.

25. VON DOBELN, W.: A simple bicycle ergometer. *J Appl Physiol, 7*:222-224, 1954.

26. FRICK, M.H.: Significance of bradycardia in relation to physical training.

Physical Activity and the Heart. Karvonen, M.J., and Barry, A.J. (Eds.), Springfield, Thomas, 1967, pp. 35-41.

27. GAENSLER, E.A., and WRIGHT, G.W.: Evaluation of respiratory impairment. *Arch Environ Health, 12*:146, 1966.

28. GAOS, C.; THOMAS, H.D.; JONES, W.B., and REEVES, T.J.: The effect of moderate and severe exercise on the pattern of myocardial oxygen extraction. Unpublished observations quoted by Harrison and Reeves. *Principles and Problems of Ischemic Heart Disease.* Chicago, Year B., 1968, p. 92.

29. GRANDE, F., and TAYLOR, H.L.: Adaptive changes in the heart, vessels, and patterns of control under chronically high loads. *Handbook of Physiology, Section 2: Circulation V. III.* Washington, D.C., American Physiological Society, 1965, pp. 2615-2677.

30. HARRISON, T.R., and REEVES, T.J.: *Principles and Problems of Ischemic Heart Disease.* Chicago, Year B., 1968, p. 230.

31. HELLERSTEIN, H., and HORNSTEN, T.: Assessing and preparing the patient for return to a meaningful and productive life. *J Rehab, 32*:48, 1966.

32. HOLMBERG, S.: Effect of severe muscular work on total and coronary circulation in man in relation to findings in the coronary arteriogram. *Coronary Circulation and Energetics of the Myocardium.* Marchetti, G., and Taccardi, B. (Eds.), New York, Karger, 1967.

33. HOLMGREN, A.; JONSSON, B., and SJÖSTRAND, T.: Circulatory data in normal subjects at rest and during exercise in the recumbent position with special reference to stroke volume at different intensities. *Acta Physiol Scand, 49*:343, 1960.

34. HORNSTEN, T.R., and BRUCE, R.A.: Stress testing, safety precautions and cardiovascular health. Presented at the 1968 American Industrial Health Conference, San Francisco, Calif., April 23, 1968.

35. KATTUS, A.A.: Physical training and beta-adrenergic blocking drugs in modifying coronary insufficiency. *Coronary Circulation and Energetics of the Myocardium.* Marchetti, G., and Toccardi, B. (Eds.), New York, Karger, 1967.

36. KATZ, L.N., and FEINBERG, H.: The relation of cardiac effort to myocardial oxygen consumption and coronary flow. *Circ Res, 6*:656, 1958.

37. KETY, S., and SCHMIDT, C.F.: The determination of cerebral blood flow in man by use of nitrous oxide in low concentrations. *Amer J Physiol, 143*:53, 1945.

38. KEYS, A., *et al.*: Epidemiological studies related to coronary heart disease: characteristics of men aged 40-59 in seven countries. *Acta Med Scand, 460*(suppl.):48, 1966.

39. LESTER, F.M.; SHEFFIELD, L.T.; TRAMMELL, P., and REEVES, T.J.: Effect of age and athletic training on maximal heart rate during muscular exercise. *Amer Heart J, 76*:370-376, 1968.

40. LESTER, F.M.; SHEFFIELD, L.T., and REEVES, T.J.: Electrocardiographic

changes in clinically normal older men following near maximal and maximal exercise. *Circulation, 36*:5, 1967.

41. LOMBARDO, T.A.; ROSE, L.; TAESCHLER, M.; TULUY, S., and BING, R.J.: The effect of exercise on coronary blood flow, myocardial oxygen consumption and cardiac efficiency in man. *Circulation, 7*:71, 1953.

42. MASTER, A.M., and ROSENFELD, I.: Two-step test: current status after twenty-five years. *Mod Conc Cardiovasc Dis, 36*:4, 19, 1967.

43. MESSER, J.V.; WAGMAN, R.J.; LEVINE, H.J.; NEILL, W.A.; KRASNOW, N., and GORLIN, R.: Patterns of human myocardial oxygen extraction during rest and exercise. *J Clin Invest, 41*:725, 1962.

44. MESSER, J.V.; LEVINE, H.J.; WAGMAN, R.J., and GORLIN, R.: Effects of exercise in cardiac performance in human subjects with coronary artery disease. *Circulation, 28*:404, 1963.

45. MITCHELL, J.H.; SPROULE, B.J., and CHAPMAN, C.B.: The physiological meaning of the maximal oxygen intake test. *J Clin Invest, 37*:538, 1958.

46. National Center for Health Statistics: Calibration of Two Bicycle Ergometers Used by the Health Examination Survey. Washington, D.C., Public Health Service, 1967, Series 2, No. 21.

47. NAUGHTON, J.; BALKE, B., and NAGLE, F.: Refinements in method of evaluation and physical conditioning before and after myocardial infarction. *Amer J Cardiol, 14*:837-43, 1964.

48. ROBINSON, S.: Experimental studies on physical fitness in relation to age. *Arbeitsphysiol, 10*:251, 1938.

49. RODAHL, K., and ISSEKUTZ, B., JR.: Physical performance capacity of the older individual. *Muscle as a Tissue.* Rodahl and Horvath (Eds.), New York, McGraw, 1962.

50. ROWELL, L.B.; TAYLOR, H.L., and WANG, Y.: Limitations of maximal oxygen intake. *J Appl Physiol, 19*:919, 1964.

51. ROWELL, L.B.; TAYLOR, H.L.; SIMONSON, E., and CARLSON, W.S.: The physiologic fallacy of adjusting for body weight in performance of the master two-step test. *Amer Heart J, 70*:4, 461-465, 1965.

52. SALTIN, B.; BLOMQVIST, G.; MITCHELL, J.H.; JOHNSON, R.L.; WILDENTHAL, K., and CHAPMAN, C.: Responses to exercise after bed rest and training. *Circ Res* (suppl.), Suppl. 7 to Circulation, Vols. 37 & 38, 1968.

53. SARNOFF, S.T.; BRAUNWALD, E.; WELCH, G.H.; CASE, R.B.; STAINSBY, W.N., and MACRUZ, R.: Hemodynamic determinants of oxygen consumption of the heart with special reference to the tension-time index. *Amer J Physiol, 192*:148, 1958.

54. SHEFFIELD, L.T.; HOLT, J.H., and REEVES, T.J.: Exercise graded by heart rate in electrocardiographic testing for angina pectoris. *Circulation, 32*: 622, 1965.

55. SHEPHARD, R.J.: Commentary on measurement of maximal aerobic capacity. *Canad Med Assoc J, 96*:744, 1967.

56. SIMONSON, E.: Use of the electrocardiogram in exercise tests. *Amer Heart J, 66*:4,552, 1966.

57. SJÖSTRAND, T.: Changes in the respiratory organs of workmen at an ore smelting works. *Acta Med Scand 196* (suppl.):687, 1947.

58. STRANDELL, T.: Electrocardiographic findings at rest, during and after exercise in healthy old men compared with young men. *Acta Med Scand, 174*:479-499, 1963.

59. TAYLOR, H.L.; BUSKIRK, E., and HENSCHEL, A.: Maximum oxygen intake as an objective measure of cardio-respiratory performance. *J Appl Physiol, 8*:73, 1958.

60. TAYLOR, H.L.; HENSCHEL, A.; BROZEK, J., and KEYS, A.: The effects of bed rest on cardioavscular function and work performance. *J Appl Physiol, 2*:223, 1949.

61. TAYLOR, H.L.; WANG, Y.; ROWELL, L., and BLOMQVIST, G.: The standardization and interpretation of submaximal and maximal tests of working capacity. *Pediatrics, 32*:(II)4, 1963.

62. The Scandinavian Committee on ECG Classification: *Acta Med Scand,* 1967, Suppl. 481.

63. TORNVALL, G.: Assessment of physical capabilities. *Acta Physiol Scand, 58*(suppl.):201, 1963.

64. WAHLUND, H.: Determination of the physical working capacity. *Acta Med, 215*(suppl.):9, 1948.

65. WESTURA, E.E., and RONAN, J.A.: Rate of application of work as a determinant of the ECG response to exercise in stress testing of normal subjects. *Circulation, 34*:(4) (suppl. III):238, 1966.

66. WYNDHAM, C.H.: Studies of the maximum capacity for physical effort. Part I: A comparison of methods for assessing the maximum oxygen intake. *Int Z Angew Physiol, 22*:285, 1966.

DISCUSSION

Dr. Bruce: I find myself pretty much in accord with these hypotheses you have formulated. The answer is coming closer and may be closing in somewhere around 70 to 75 per cent of maximum as an effective discriminant level of performance. That is very easy. The only catch is we need to know the maximum performance to adjust the workload at 75 per cent of it. There is only speculation trying to predict it in certain patients. This becomes almost ridiculous when our business in cardiac patients is to know and to find out. That's all I have to say.

Dr. Taylor: Dr. Bruce votes then for doing a maximal oxygen intake on all patients, so that in terms of the parameters that we were discussing he will obviously get some very useful data. From the point of view of an epidemiologist or of the practitioner, a maximal oxygen intake procedure turns out to be very time consuming and one has neither the hospital facilities nor back-up right at hand. I believe that Dr. Sheffield has some advice concerning this problem.

Dr. Sheffield: I think Dr. Åstrand brought out a very important point this morning when she mentioned the necessity of performing a test inside twenty to twenty-five minutes. I think we have to distinguish between a test that can be done in that time and a more meticulous and certainly more accurate test that would require a great deal longer and a great deal more investment of professional and technician time. We have found that predicting the maximal myocardium oxygen demand on the basis of age, this is taking the age-predicted maximum heart rate and then getting a certain high fraction of this, to be clinically very effective. It is not highly accurate since getting 85 per cent, 75 per cent, or any given per cent, and choosing a particular heart rate, such as 165 beats a minute for a fifty-year-old, the result will not be exactly 85 per cent of maximal for everyone. We can only say that it is the best choice we have available for getting the best standardization in a brief test. If you find a person with a negative exercise electrocardiographic test, the first thing I'd want to know is how hard had he to work to get this negative test. In other words, what fraction of total coronary perfusion has he proved able to furnish to the myocardium and still have a normal electrocardiogram?

Dr. Taylor: Dr. Åstrand, do you have anything to say about testing at 50 per cent versus 75 per cent or 100 per cent of maximal oxygen uptake?

Dr. Astrand: I think that 50 per cent is too low to make a decent prediction and the values I picked this morning were a heart rate of 170 for a twenty-five-year-old and so on. It means around eighty to eighty-five per cent of predicted maximal heart rate for age.

Dr. Taylor: Dr. Sheffield, were you using 85 per cent?

Dr. Sheffield: 85 to 90 per cent.

Dr. Taylor: Everybody seems to agree that you get more information if you go to higher work loads. Dr. Westura, do you have any comments on this?

Dr. Westura: I might say that we plotted our data in terms of

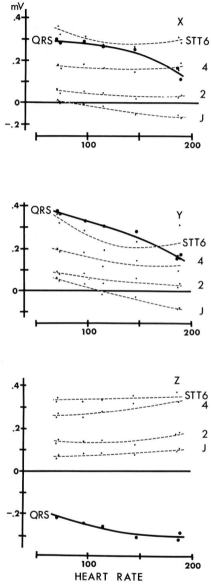

FIGURE 18-9. Mean QRS and STT amplitudes in relation to heart rate at rest and during submaximal and maximal exercise in young normal men (n = 11).

Mean QRS vector components determined from integration of scalar leads (values in mv sec × 10). STT 2, 4 and 6 correspond to mean amplitude at 2/8, 4/8 and 6/8 of the interval end of QRS (J)—end of T.

PWC 170, and we found that for many of our subjects, they came quite close to the prediction line, that slope which is available. Looked at from the point of view of the nomograms used to determine the per cent of maximal, the well subjects achieved 94 to 104 per cent of maximal predicted for upright work, whereas those who had cardiac disease or other abnormalities rarely went above 84 per cent. The mean was between 80 and 84 per cent of the value.

Dr. Blomqvist: We have collected some data on the relation between SST amplitudes during exercise and relative work-load in terms of heart rate. Frank's orthogonal lead system was used in all studies. The ECG was recorded on magnetic tape, averaged, and processed in a digital computer. The records were normalized with respect to time. PR, QRS and STT intervals were each divided into eight subsegments (e.g. STT 1, 2, . . . 8) of equal duration, and mean X, Y and Z amplitudes were calculated for points defining the end of each subsegment. Subsegment QRS 8 corresponds to the QRS-STT junction, STT 1-3 to the ST segment, and STT 5-6 to the peak of the T wave.

Figure 18-9 demonstrates the findings in a group of eleven twenty to twenty-five-year-old healthy men at rest and during submaximal and maximal exercise. X, Y and Z coordinates of the mean QRS vector were determined from integration of the scalar leads (values in mv sec X 10). During exercise at progressively higher loads, the mean QRS vector shows displacement to the right, upwards and posteriorly, while there was little change in STT vectors 4 and 6, i.e., in T wave amplitude. Frontal plane STT-junction (J) amplitudes showed a progressive decrease and a mean junctional depression of 0.1 mv in lead X and of 0.2 mv in lead Y during maximal work.

Figure 18-10 shows mean STT 4 (the point halfway between end of QRS and end of T) and QRS-STT junction amplitudes at rest and during exercise in three experimental groups: (a) The same group of eleven young normal men as illustrated in Figure 18-9; (b) a group of sixteen forty-five to fifty-five-year-old men apparently free from cardiovascular disease and (c) ten patients with classical angina pectoris not complicated by myocardial infarction or hypertension. Groups (a) and (b) were exercised to a maximal level, group (c) to a level provoking slight anginal pain.

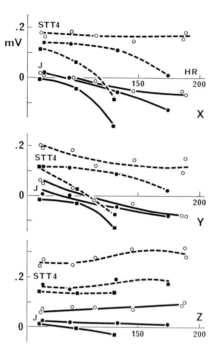

Figure 18-10. Mean STT 4 (*broken lines*) and QRS-ST (*continuous lines*) junction X, Y and Z amplitudes at rest and during submaximal and maximal exercise in (a) young normal men (*open circles,* n = 11); (b) apparently healthy middle-aged men (*filled circles,* n = 16); and (c) patients with typical, uncomplicated angina pectoris (*filled squares,* n = 10).

STT 4 corresponds to the amplitudes at half the distance end of QRS—end of T.

The response to submaximal exercise was similar in groups (a) and (b), but the middle-aged men showed a much larger ST deviation during maximal work. The patients with angina did not differ significantly from the middle-aged control group (b) at rest, but showed as a group marked changes already at the first level of exercise (below the threshold of anginal pain). The nonlinear response in the middle-aged group suggests that a small change of relative workload in the range between 60 and 100 per cent of maximum will to a great extent influence the yield of positive responses.

Dr. Taylor: There have been suggestions that something happens to myocardial performance in the area of 70 to 80 per cent of maxi-

mal, but I believe this will be covered later. We haven't said anything
about the several protocols for increasing the work load. I think you
are probably getting the feeling now that we in general aren't too wor-
ried about this; that some day we are going to start making detailed
comparisons. The differences in protocol are probably minor relative
to the problem of how hard are you going to work the subjects. I
don't know whether everybody agrees with me on this. Dr. Westura
gave us a very good example that working on your back isn't as
profitable as working upright. I think that is very important. It both-
ers me a little bit, because if anybody wants to do myocardial oxygen
consumptions, they're going to want to do it on their back, and everybody after that will say well, it really isn't what you want to measure.

Dr. Blackburn: Well, that's probably true; but they didn't give
us the results of differences in S-T depression between body positions
in terms of comparable heart rates.

Dr. Taylor: Yes, give us the scoop.

Dr. Blomqvist: I think that in answer to Dr. Blackburn's question
we found that the treadmill gave us a higher heart rate and higher
oxygen consumption. What I tried to point out in my last slide was
that using the Quinton treadmill program, using a fixed external
work load, we apply a different slope to get more information about
this problem. One thing is clear, the more the individual works, the
more apt he is to have other changes, but I have no acceleration data
along at all. I think that may be very important.

I would like to throw out a question that has been bothering me
as a clinician; we want to go out and begin to do other things besides
looking at the test itself; in other words, the clinician is chafing at the
bit to use the test; if the purpose of the test is going to be to detect
ischemic change. If I could be permitted to be pragmatic; if what
we've all been talking about is true and there doesn't seem to be any
great disagreement, why don't we go ahead then and begin to use
this approach.

Dr. Taylor: Well, I think the answer to that is that very many investigators have been accumulating data in their laboratories for many
years with a particular kind of a test. Almost everybody would agree
that this new approach would be useful, but nobody is going to throw
all his data away. As far as I'm concerned, unless you bring very pow-

erful arguments together, I think it is sore of butting your head against a stone wall, but you can always try it.

Dr. Blomqvist: I think in a way that your own research gives a very good reason why we don't have to stick to one test, as long as you measure the heart rate, it doesn't matter too much which type of work you do.

Dr. Westura: This is the point I am making that we can begin to look at some of the clinical and epidemiological problems with a test, or with the results of any test relative to what we now know about response in general, in terms of at least these parameters, even though this is not optimally satisfactory.

Dr. Taylor: Right. This is certainly the case, and we hope very much that this will be done. Does anybody else in the room want to be controversial?

Mr. Berson: We heard a couple of possibly conflicting remarks about whether or not the ECG changes one sees *during* exercise are not there after exercise. Is this true, and if so, it might have some bearing on problems you have in procedure and analysis.

Dr. Taylor: Dr. Bruce, what's your experience on this? Do you see a lot of things in exercise you don't see after exercise?

Dr. Bruce: I will talk about this later.

Dr. Taylor: Dr. Bruce has a presentation coming up. Dr. Sheffield?

Dr. Sheffield: What we do sometimes see in exercise, and I think most laboratories have found, is ST depression in the latter part of exercise extending only a few seconds into recovery. I am not sure anybody knows exactly what this means in a person with no other sign of coronary disease.

Dr. Blomqvist: For purposes of standardization I think it is preferable to use electrocardiograms recorded *during* rather than after exercise. Recordings during exercise will at least be made at a relatively steady state. A number of physiological variables are changing rapidly in the period immediately after exercise.

With respect to criteria for positive response and selection of measurements for comparative studies I would like to emphasize that we cannot take for granted that the criteria used for evaluation of the ECG after a standard step test also apply to the ECG recorded during heavy exercise at a much higher heart rate. Techniques of measurement for standard scalar records become difficult as soon as one attempts to measure amplitudes during the later parts of the ST segment, primarily because it is difficult to find proper reference points for timing.

Comment: I think in reply to Dr. Berson's question about ECG changes *during* versus postexercise that there are distinct differences between techniques. First of all, here we use V leads and not CR leads. Secondly, we don't really have a lead that is directly looking at the posterior wall, and that may be why Dr. Åstrand sees more ST during exercise than we do. I think the changes may well be present during exercise and that because of the shortening and changes of the ECG curve due to exercise alone, in the mild cases of ischemia, we don't see it, whereas in those individuals who have marked degrees of ischemia they have overcome the normal change of exercise and have become apparent.

Dr. Hamrell: I would like to make one comment about maximum testing, and this relative to Dr. Bruce's comment. I think that the kind of population with which we are dealing, in Minneapolis, a group of middle-aged men gathered, as well as possible, randomly from the population, makes maximum testing at the outset difficult, both from the standpoint of safety and also from what the individual will tolerate when he is placed in the situation of having volunteered out of a previously quite sedentary existence. As far as what we see of ST response to exercise, in our population, we excluded prominent ST responders from our study early and in the remaining with some instances of ST depression in exercise, this depression persisted into the postexercise period.

Dr. Astrand: It seems as if we all agree that we should go on with a specified increase in work load until a certain heart rate is reached. I would like to ask how long an interval of work for each load. In Sweden we always take five- or six-minute-periods because we have two purposes with our test. One of them is the revealing of the ST depressions, and the other is the evaluation of the circulatory capacity of the individual with regard to his or her occupation and activity. I think that this last purpose is as important as the first one.

Dr. Taylor: I'm willing to agree with that. Gunnar Blomqvist, do you have any comment on that?

Dr. Blomqvist: Of course I've grown up in the same environment as Dr. Åstrand, so I am biased to using the longer test periods, but I think you defend it from the point of view of standardization, too. "Steady state" is a dirty word, but it seems to me that it is easier to standardize a test if you have a methodology that gives you at least a relatively steady condition with each work level.

Dr. Taylor: If we're going to average a number of complexes, taken during progressive work intervals only two minutes long, as in our present test, and the heart rate is going up continuously, what is going to happen to the average ECG response, what's the ST depression going to look like?

Dr. Blomqvist: That's an additional reason why we use five, six-minute periods.

Dr. Taylor: I think that if we use five- or six-minute-periods on some of our ex-TV viewers that we might have to employ the services of some kind of a muscle specialist afterwards.

Dr. Simonson: I have a question. I was very much impressed with Dr. Åstrand's demonstration of the good correlation of heart rate and oxygen consumption, but what is the error for the individual? We have to consider that bicycling is better standardized so far as the work performance than treadmill work. In treadmill we have the speed and the grade but do not control the gait or frequency of steps so we have considerable variation. Dr. Åstrand and others apparently have found that variability is indeed greater with treadmills than with bicycle load. I think we have to consider these factors.

Dr. Astrand: You can make a prediction of the maximal oxygen uptake with a standard deviation of plus-minus 10 to 15 per cent. I think that is enough for the purpose of your evaluation of the individual, with regard to his occupation and activity. I think it helps a great deal if you know whether the person has a capacity of 4 liters, or if he has only two liters.

Dr. Taylor: I think that if I could summarize—a word I wish nobody had invented—electrocardiography and work testing is going on to more work and higher work loads. The concept of working middle-aged people from 75 to 100 per cent of their maximum has been with us for only a relatively short time. It results in a much larger number of recognizable abnormalities, and if research continues at its present pace the uncertainties that have been expressed here are going to resolve themselves within a few years.

Dr. Bruce said he was going to answer somebody's question later, and I think he is going to do it now in a paper entitled "The Frequency Relationships of Quantitated Electrocardiographic Response to Work to Maximal Capacity in U.S. and Oriental Populations." Dr. Bruce.

PART FIVE

PHYSIOLOGICAL SOURCES OF VARIABILITY AND HUMAN EXPERIMENTS IN THE EXERCISE ELECTROCARDIOGRAPHIC RESPONSE

19

Electrocardiographic Changes in Relation to the Type of Exercise, the Work Load, Age and Sex

IRMA ÅSTRAND

I WANT TO CONSIDER the prerequisites for comparing the results and conclusions of one study of the exercise electrocardiographic response with another.

The first consideration is the work load. Three different types of exercise with the legs are being used as tests, walking or running on a treadmill, cycling on a bicycle ergometer, and step tests. All three of these methods are employed to increase the cardiac output and thereby provoke changes in the ECG and/or subjective symptoms. The discussion will include only those methods of exercise involving the large muscle groups of the legs, while other exercise techniques, such as arm exercise, are excluded. The degree of ST-depression in the electrocardiogram is related to the circulatory load upon the individual in such a way that the ST-depression increases gradually with the work load or the heart rate and reaches the most pronounced depression at maximal load. This has been shown by Blomqvist among others (7). In order to be able to compare results from different studies the work tests must accordingly be carried out so that a well defined work load is reached. The work load should be defined both with regard to absolute load, for instance in kpm/min, watts, or O_2 uptake, and in relation to the maximal work capacity of the tested subject.

For many different reasons we often prefer to test the subject only on a submaximal load. Two principally different procedures are used to produce a standardization of this submaximal level. One way is to load all subjects equally, for instance to a certain multiple of the basal metabolic rate. Another way is to load the subject in proportion to his own work capacity.

The first method can be used if the work load is chosen so that a certain predicted oxygen uptake is reached, which, for instance, might be eight times the basal metabolic rate. The best result of this method would be expected with a technique that gives the least variation in mechanical efficiency. The coefficient of variation for oxygen uptake per kg body weight on fixed submaximal loads on the treadmill is about 10 to 15 per cent. The coefficient of variation for mechanical efficiency on the bicycle ergometer is 6 to 8 per cent. In order to load the subject to a certain multiple of the basal metabolic rate with a step test both the step frequency and the relative bench height of the step must be varied from person to person. For practical reasons such a step procedure is impossible to handle and the mechanical efficiency would certainly have even greater variation than the tread-mill test. Therefore to load the subject in relation to the basal metabolic rate the bicycle ergometer test is preferred, as the error in prediction of the oxygen uptake is least.

However, there are several drawbacks with a test performed in

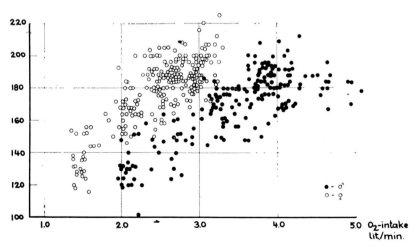

FIGURE 19-1. Heart rate in relation to oxygen uptake for adult, comparatively well trained female and male subjects (n = 86). Maximal as well as sub-maximal values are represented (4).

this way: (a) Many subjects will be tested at a comparatively low load while others will not be able to perform the task (Fig. 19-1). The standard deviation for heart rate at submaximal oxygen uptakes is about ±15 beats/min in normal man (Fig. 19-2). (b) The test cannot be used for a prediction of the circulatory capacity in many individuals because the value for heart rate might be so low that such a prediction is impossible. (c) The work load will not cover the demands of all different occupational jobs. One requirement of the test ought to be that the person is tested at an intensity at least as high as that attained during his occupational activity or during his leisure time.

The second procedure implies the choice of a load that is related to the capacity of the individual. The body weight has often been

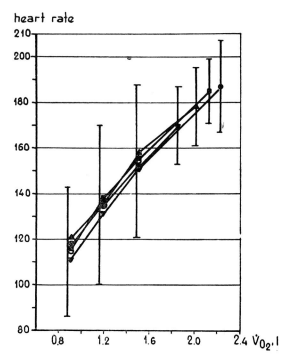

FIGURE 19-2. Heart rate in relation to oxygen uptake for different female age groups (n = 44). = 20-29; = 30-39; = 40-49 and = 50-65 years. = mean value ± 2 x SD, unfilled dots represent all subjects, filled dots the different age groups (2).

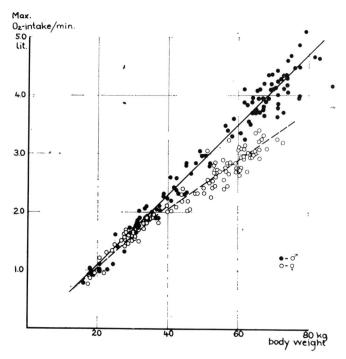

FIGURE 19-3. Maximal oxygen uptake in relation to body weight for 227 healthy female and male subjects, four to thirty years of age (4).

used in this prediction. If the intention is to validate the individual's ability to move himself it is important to take the body weight into consideration. A step test or treadmill test are then logical methods of choice. However it ought to be noted that the bicycle ergometer also can be used for such a test. The work load can be chosen in relation to the body weight, for instance 10 kpm/min per kg of body weight. Since the intensity should be related to the circulatory capacity of the individual it is, however, important to investigate the correlation between body weight and this capacity. In children and in young, healthy lean subjects there is a good correlation between body weight on one hand and maximal oxygen uptake or cardiac output, total hemoglobin, etc. on the other (Fig. 19-3). However, in subjects thirty to seventy years old the correlation between body weight and max VO_2 is low (Fig. 19-4). The reason is partly that the degree of obesity varies to a greater extent and partly that ageing is accompanied

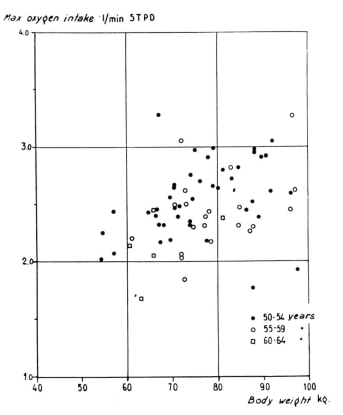

FIGURE 19-4. Maximal oxygen uptake in relation to body weight for seventy-two male truck drivers fifty to sixty-four years old (1).

by a deterioration of the oxygen transporting function that is not reflected in the dimensions of the individual.

Let us take some examples: (a) An adult who increases his body weight by forty pounds does not increase his circulatory capacity a corresponding amount. This means that when obese he will be tested on a level that is closer to his maximal level if the load is chosen in relation to the body weight. (b) If an ordinary thirty-year-old man and an ordinary seventy-year-old man who have the same body weight walk on the treadmill with the same speed and grade, they will reach the same oxygen uptake and the same heart rate but the relative load will be very different. The reason for this is the decrease in maximal cardiac output, maximal oxygen uptake and maximal heart rate with

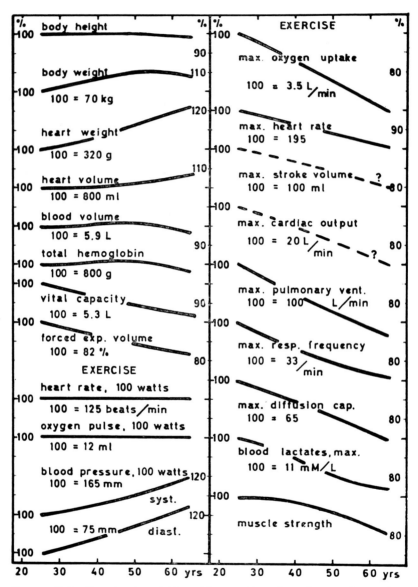

FIGURE 19-5. Functional variables with age. Data have been collected from various subjects, including healthy men. For data on the same function, only one study has been consulted. The values for the twenty-five-year-old subjects = 100 per cent; for the older ages the mean values are expressed in percentage of the twenty-five-year-old individuals' values. The values should not be

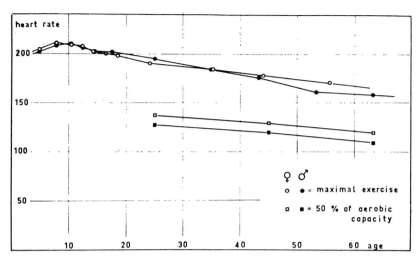

FIGURE 19-6. Heart rate during maximal exercise (*upper curves*) and during a work load in which oxygen uptake was at 50 per cent of the maximum (*lower curves*) for 350 female and male subjects four to sixty-five years of age (5).

increasing age (Fig. 19-5). On the other hand the mechanical efficiency and the heart rate at a given submaximal load do not change, in any case not in normal subjects (Fig. 19-5). The simplest way of producing a load that is related to the capacity of the individual with regard to the circulatory system is to force the test to a heart rate that is related to a maximal heart rate that is typical for the age of the individual (Fig. 19-6). If the limit for young persons twenty to twenty-nine years old is set at a heart rate of 170 beats/min, it ought to be 160/min for thirty to thirty-nine years old, 150/min for forty to forty-nine years old, 140/min for fifty to fifty-nine years old and 130/min for sixty to sixty-nine years old. It appears therefore that the best submaximal test available would be one in which work loads on either the bicycle or treadmill are carried out for five- to six-minute periods, starting with very low loads and increasing the load in stepwise fashion until the desired heart rate is reached.

considered "normal values," but they illustrate the effect of ageing. Note that heart rate and oxygen pulse at a given work load (100 watts or 600 kpm/min, oxygen uptake about 1.5 liters/min) are identical throughout the age range covered, but the maximal oxygen uptake, heart rate, cardiac output, etc., decline with age. The data on cardiac output and stroke volume are based on few observations and are therefore uncertain.

A test made in this way allows a classification of the ECG both at a fixed load independent of the individual's capacity and at a load related to the individual's circulatory capacity. Other advantages with this procedure are as follows: (a) the test will be easy to make from a practical point of view, and (b) the physical demands during different occupational activities and during different activities in leisure time can be reproduced. (c) The capacity for oxygen uptake of the individual can be predicted. It is self-evident that the exercise is only continued until the heart rates mentioned are reached, and in those subjects where the exercise is not interrupted earlier from other reasons of safety. One category by which the relative load cannot be judged in this way is in patients with atrial fibrillation.

Another condition for the comparability of results with different testing methods is that the time during the exercise or recovery period of the ECGs should be the same. From Blomqvist's thesis (7) it is evident that an ST-depression during work is not always accompanied by a change after work and from Furberg's studies in Sweden (9) it is clear that an ST-depression that appears *only* after work might be of a sympathicotonic type. Consequently the ST-changes during work are the most essential to record.

An additional condition for the comparability of studies is that the same criteria for an electrocardiographic change are used and that the different ECG lead systems give equivalent results. In the Scandinavian countries a committee has been working on these problems and some recommendations have been made. We have adapted "The Minnesota code" (11), and there are now a lot of studies at least in Sweden and Finland in which its well-documented principles have been used. It has, however, been necessary to make certain modifications to meet our conditions, including adaptation to CR leads and the addition of another category in classification of ST-changes (12). During work to relatively high heart rates three types of segmental ST-depressions appear: (a and b) horizontal or downward sloping ST-depression which exist in the Minnesota code; (c) ST-junction depression in which the ST segment is straight and slowly ascends but does not reach the baseline before the T wave. This third type is an addition to the code. The categories are divided into subclasses according to the severity of ST-segment depression (Fig. 19-7). The

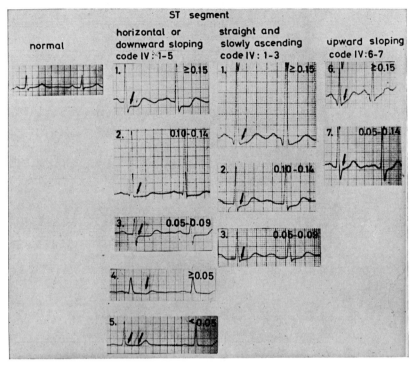

FIGURE 19-7. Different types and degrees of ST-J changes in CR and CH (H = head) leads (12).

classification has been tested by Punsar and co-authors in the interpretation of postexercise ECGs of 1300 policemen. The same authors have tested the prognostic significance of the various categories in a follow-up study of about 1,600 middle-aged men (10). The third category with a straight, slowly ascending ST segment gave a significantly worse prognostic figure than normal ECGs or strictly junctional ST changes. Figure 19-8 is an example of an ECG where we can find all these changes.

In the choice between different ECG lead systems there are two important questions that must be taken into consideration. I will limit discussion to CR and V leads, since we have modified "The Minnesota code" for CR leads. The first question deals with the number of false positive and false negative diagnoses that are made. There is nothing that speaks in favor of the V lead system compared with the CR lead

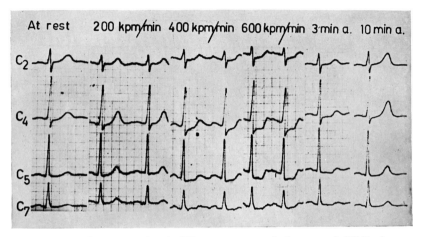

Figure 19-8. One example of different types and degrees of ST-J changes in a man fifty-four years of age at rest, three and ten minutes after exercise (CR leads) and during three exercise loads on a bicycle ergometer (CH leads).

system in that respect. The other question deals with the sensitivity of the system, it means the ability of the system to reveal and display ST changes. The difference between the two lead systems in these chest positions in question are that the CR leads give 25 to 30 per cent greater amplitudes. In other words, CR leads have a greater ability to reveal ST changes. There is another point in favor of the CR leads. When using CR leads the electrodes are usually placed in position 2, 4, 5 and 7 and when using V leads in position 2, 4, 5 and 6. It is felt that CR_6 rarely reveals any information that is not present in CR_5, while CR_7 provides an optimal lead axis for display of ECG changes originating in the lateral wall of the left ventricle. Amplitudes in lead V_7 are generally small, but this disadvantage does not apply to CR_7. For these reasons and traditional ones we prefer CR and CH leads to V leads.

Consider some results from work tests made according to the previously mentioned procedure with a stepwise increase in work load until a certain heart rate is reached, and results of classification of the ECGs recorded during and after work with conventional methods. In these studies there were few ECGs with segmental ST depression during work which disappeared one and three minutes after work, or with ST depression after work that could not be revealed during

ST depression type IV:1-4

Men		Women	
Age	*Per cent*	*Age*	*Per cent*
<40	10		
40-50	15	40-45	20
55	20	50-55	30
60	35	>55	50

Figure 19-9. The frequency of type IV: 1-4 S-T changes (12) in Swedish men and women (3).

work. The results are based on a combination of data from different studies.

The results in the older ages are based mainly on my own follow-up studies in health examination of seventy-five truck drivers fifty-five to seventy years old and eighty-seven men and 117 women forty-eight to sixty-three years old (Fig. 19-9) (3). The frequency of segmental ST depressions type IV:1-4 which usually mean changes that have a prognostic significance, was lower than 10 per cent in men below forty years of age, about 15 per cent at forty to fifty, 20 per cent at fifty-five years and about 35 per cent at sixty years of age. For women the rate at forty to forty-five years is about 20 per cent, at fifty to fifty-five years 30 per cent and over fifty-five years about 50 per cent. With regard to females, there are actually few data available. It is notable that in the Framingham study (8) a higher frequency of angina pectoris was found among females than among males, while mortality and morbidity from myocardial infarction showed the expected preponderance among males. All of my subjects were asked about subjective symptoms during the actual test and only 3 per cent complained of chest pain.

From my own studies it can also be mentioned that segmental ST changes of the minimal type observed at the first examination often progressed into a more marked type at an examination five to eight years later. The frequency of subjects with an initially completely normal ECG, who eight years later exhibited segmental changes was about 20 per cent. The frequency of subjects with isolated J depression at the first examination who had developed segmental ST depression eight years later was also about 20 per cent. Thus there was no tendency toward more frequent development of ST segment depressions in subjects who had previously had isolated J depressions compared with those exhibiting no changes.

SUMMARY

Probably the best procedure for a work test is to increase the load stepwise until a certain heart rate is reached which is related to the maximal performance of the individual for that age.

The ECG ought to be recorded both during and after exercise. The ECGs should be classified according to an objective system which makes possible a separation of different changes and a quantitative analysis of these changes.

In my opinion CR and CH leads are preferable to V leads for exercise testing.

With the procedure outlined here the frequency of segmental ST depressions in ordinary men in Sweden sixty years of age is about 35 per cent and in women of the same age about 50 per cent.

REFERENCES

1. ÅSTRAND, IRMA: The physical work capacity of workers 50-64 years old. *Acta Physiol Scand, 42*:73, 1958.
2. ÅSTRAND, IRMA: Aerobic work capacity in men and women with special reference to age. *Acta Physiol Scand, 49* (suppl.):169, 1960.
3. ÅSTRAND, IRMA: Exercise electrocardiograms recorded twice with an 8-year interval in a group of 204 women and men 48-63 years old. *Acta Med Scand, 178*:27, 1965.
4. ÅSTRAND, P.-O.: *Experimental Studies of Physical Work Capacity in Relation to Sex and Age.* Copenhagen, Munksgaard, 1952.
5. ÅSTRAND, P.-O., and CRISTENSEN, E.H.: Aerobic work capacity. In *Oxygen in the Animal Organism. Proceedings of a Symposium held in London, 1963.* Dickens, F., and Neil, E. (Eds.), Oxford, Pergamon, 1964 p. 298.
6. ÅSTRAND, P.-O. and RODAHL, K.: Textbook of Work Physiology. (to be published).
7. BLOMQVIST, G.: The Frank lead exercise electrocardiogram. A quantitative study based on averaging technic and digital computer analysis. *Acta Med Scand, 178* (suppl.):440, 1965.
8. DAWBER, T.R.; MOORE, F.E., and MANN, G.V.: Coronary heart disease in the Framingham study. *Amer J Public Health, 47* (No. 4) (2):4, 1957.
9. FURBERG, C.: Adrenergic beta-blockade and electrocardiographical ST-T changes. *Acta Med Scand, 181*:21, 1967.
10. PUNSAR, S.; PYÖRÄLÄ, K., and SILTANEN, P.: Classification of electrocardiographic ST segment changes in epidemiological studies of coronary heart disease. *Scand J Clin Lab Invest,* 19 (suppl.):95, 1967, (Annual Meeting of Finnish Medical Societies).

11. Rose, G., and Blackburn, H.: *Cardiovascular survey methods. WHO* Press, Geneva, 1968.
12. The Scandinavian Committee on ECG Classification: The "Minnesota code" for ECG classification. Adaption to CR leads and modification of the code for ECG's recorded during and after exercise. *Acta Med Scand*, 1967, suppl. 481.

DISCUSSION

Dr. Blackburn: I think it should be noted that this work of Dr. Åstrand is sound confirmation of an ancient suspicion that there are indeed qualitative differences between men and women. Why are there these differences in ischemic-like exercise ECG responses when most other factors related to coronary disease are much less frequent in women? Interestingly enough, women found in working general populations have, at certain ages, also a higher prevalence of angina pectoris. This difference in ST depression is quite significant, from one and one-half to three times in women than men of the same age. This is confirmed by resting ECG findings of Tecumseh, and could indicate in part that coronary disease is less fatal in women, the residual population containing more women with coronary artery disease and myocardial ischemia, whereas the men have been removed by sudden deaths. It could indicate other differences, largely unknown, such as autonomic neurohumoral differences. The findings I don't believe are corrected for heart rate or for body size. Both heart rate and oxygen consumption are higher in women, for a given external work-load. I would welcome comments on these interesting findings.

Dr. Bruce: These are very interesting observations. I would like to ask you about blood pressure in the sixty-year age group of women. Is it higher than the average in men?

Dr. Astrand: Not in the group I am reporting.

Dr. Simonson: Dr. Lepeschkin, this is a confirmation of your findings that the incidence of ST depression is greater in women. Would you comment?

Dr. Lepeschkin: We did find a much greater incidence of T wave changes in women, and also with the so-called positive exercise tests there was a greater percentage of women, in the later age groups, than men. I think one of the explanations could be that there seems to be differences in the potassium content of the myocardial cells in women and men, and it may be that for the same degree of myocardial ischemia, repolarization changes in men are different than in women.

Dr. Simonson: Dr. Åstrand, I would like to ask a question. You did an excellent study showing good correlation of oxygen consumption versus heart rate during work. However, there was a very large standard deviation. How is your correlation and standard deviation on other items which can be quite easily measured; for instance, pulmonary ventilation or CO_2? Is the standard deviation less than that for heart rate versus oxygen consumption?

Dr. Astrand: The standard deviation for pulmonary ventilation and heart rate during a certain fixed submaximal load is of about the same size, or about 15 per cent of the mean.

Dr. Simonson: I have still another question, Dr. Åstrand. You propose to make a correction for body weight—that is, to standardize the load per kilogram of body weight? There are theoretical considerations for bicycle work—that the load should be related to muscle cross-section, rather than to body weight. Then you could try other correlations. I am thinking of McDonald's work, who found that in level walking and straight walking the relationship between body weight and oxygen consumption is actually logarithmic. Did you ever try any of those correlations?

Dr. Astrand: No we have not tried those correlations in older people. However, one would expect a good correlation between lean body mass and maximal oxygen uptake capacity. But since this method should be used in the routine examination of patients we cannot include time-consuming methods. We must do them simply enough to be made in twenty or twenty-five minutes.

Dr. Simonson: Any other questions? If not, we will go to the next paper.

20

Variations of the Electrocardiographic Response to Exercise under Different Experimental Conditions; Deconditioning, Reconditioning and High Altitude

C. GUNNAR BLOMQVIST

VARIATIONS IN THE electrocardiographic response to exercise after large induced changes in maximal oxygen uptake and circulatory dynamics were studied in a group of five nineteen to twenty-one-year-old healthy male college students during the course of a multidisciplinary study focusing on oxygen transport. Data have been reported in full elsewhere (1, 2).

METHODS AND PROCEDURE

The study included four phases. Measurements of oxygen uptake, cardiac output (dye dilution technique), and intra-arterial pressures during submaximal and maximal work were obtained during each phase. Baseline determinations were made during early June, 1966. The subjects were confined to bed for three weeks, restudied, and subjected to an intensive physical training program lasting fifty-five days. Four of the five subjects also took part in a later study on the adaptation to high altitude during which they had their fourth set of measurements during early September after two and one-half weeks' stay at an altitude of 14,000 feet (Mt. Evans, Colorado). The study at the end of the training period provided baseline data for the altitude experiment.

Note: This study was supported in part by grants by the United States Public Health Service (HE 06296) and the United States Air Force (HE 07744).

Electrocardiographic methods have been detailed in a previous publication (3). Frank lead orthogonal electrocardiograms were recorded on magnetic tape, averaged and digitized in a computer of average transients, and processed in a digital computer. The analog-to-digital conversion rate was 200 samples per second and lead, i.e., each sampling interval corresponded to 5 msec. The wave recognition program was based on an approximation of the spatial velocity function:

$$SV_n = 200 \sqrt{(X_{n+1} - X_n)^2 + (Y_{n+1} - Y_n)^2 + (Z_{n+1} - Z_n)^2}$$

where SV is spatial velocity in $\mu v/msec$, n the sampling interval, and X, Y and Z Frank lead amplitudes in mv. The program identified peak QRS amplitude and then scanned the spatial velocity function. The onset of QRS was defined as the first sampling interval prior to peak QRS where $SV \leqslant 7\mu V/msec$. The limit value for determination of the end of the T wave was set equal to the average spatial velocity, $\overline{SV}$, over the interval end of QRS — estimated end of T. Estimated end of T was computed according to the following formula, modified from Simonson (4)

$$n = 2880/\text{heart rate} + QRS_{start} + 29.$$

The formula tends to overestimate QT intervals at low heart rates. The rate was, therefore, set equal to actual heart rate at values of 60 beats/min and above, but considered equal to 60 at lower rates. To define end of T the computer started scanning the spatial velocity function at a sampling interval equal to estimated end of T + 85 msec and proceeded stepwise in the direction of the QRS until it found a sampling interval with $SV < \overline{SV}$ where during at least two of the three preceding intervals $SV > \overline{SV}$.

Each P-R, QRS and ST-T segment was divided into eight subsegments of equal duration, and X, Y and Z amplitudes at the end of each subsegment were analyzed in terms of mean values and range.

RESULTS

Bedrest and Physical Training

Figure 20-1 demonstrates changes in maximal oxygen uptake induced by bedrest and training. Three of the subjects were sedentary

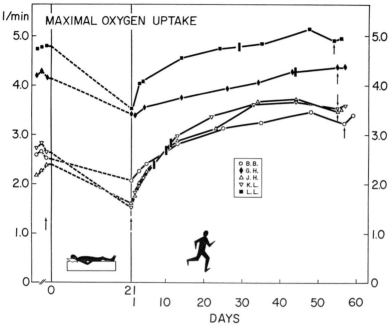

FIGURE 20-1. Changes in maximal oxygen uptake with bedrest and training. Individual data before and after bedrest and at various intervals during training. *Arrows* indicate circulatory studies. *Heavy bars* mark the time during the training period at which the maximal oxygen uptake had returned to the control value before bedrest.

TABLE 20-I

MEASUREMENTS DURING MAXIMAL WORK BEFORE AND
AFTER BEDREST
(n = 5)

	Before *(mean)*	*After* *(mean)*	*Change, %* *(mean and range)*
Oxygen Uptake liters/min	3.30	2.43	—26.4 —17.8, —42.1
Cardiac Output liters/min	20.0	14.8	—26.0 —4.9, —47.4
Heart Rate beats/min	193	197	+2.1 ±0, +5.9
Stroke Volume ml	104	74	—28.8 —5.4, —48.8
AV—O_2 Diff. vol %	16.5	16.4	—.6 +1.7, —1.8

at the beginning of the study, and had maximal oxygen uptakes between 2.4 and 2.8 liters/min; two were physically active and had maximal oxygen uptakes of 4.3 and 4.8 liters/min. The range in ml/kg was 33 to 59. Maximal oxygen uptake fell from a mean of 3.3 liters/min before bedrest to 2.4 liters/min after bedrest, or by 26 per cent. The largest relative decrease was 42 per cent and the smallest 18 per cent. There was no difference between the active and the sedentary subjects with respect to the magnitude of the decrease.

The results of the cardiovascular measurements during maximal work are summarized in Table 20-I. The decrease in maximal oxygen uptake was primarily due to a fall in stroke volume and cardiac output. There was little change in maximal heart rate and in A-V O_2 difference.

The stroke volume was reduced to the same degree during maximal and submaximal treadmill exercise. A somewhat smaller but still significant decrease was seen during submaximal supine exercise, or from 116 to 88 ml at a load of 600 kpm/min. Heart rate and A-V O_2 difference were higher after bedrest at any given level of oxygen uptake, but the relationship to relative workload (relative workload calculated as oxygen uptake in per cent of maximal oxygen uptake) did not change. Arterial pressures at rest (both positions) and during supine exercise did not change, but mean pressures during upright exercise were 10 to 20 mm Hg lower after bedrest. Total peripheral resistance did not change significantly. Total heart volume as measured from biplane radiographs taken simultaneously with the x-ray tubes at 90° angle and the subject in the prone position decreased by 10 per cent.

The three sedentary subjects responded rapidly to the training program and reached their pre-bedrest values of maximal oxygen uptake after about ten days (Fig. 20-1). Recovery was much slower in the two active subjects who required thirty and forty-five days to return to their control values. At the end of the training program they showed only a very small increase in maximal oxygen uptake, 4 per cent. By contrast, the sedentary subjects showed an increase by 33 per cent of their control values before bedrest.

Table 20-II summarizes circulatory changes induced by training. Measurements made before bedrest serve as control data. Maximal heart rate did not change. The large increase in maximal oxygen uptake in the sedentary group can be attributed equally to an increase in stroke volume and in A-V O_2 difference. Blood pressure and peripheral resistance did not change significantly. Total heart volume increased by 10 per cent compared to the value before bedrest.

Electrocardiographic results are presented in Figures 20-2 and 20-3. Figure 20-2 displays mean X, Y and Z amplitudes and range at rest and during submaximal and maximal treadmill exercise at the control study (C), after bedrest (B), and after training (T). The analysis of the ECG during exercise was limited to one level of supine exercise (300 or 600 kpm/min), two levels of submaximal treadmill exercise (40 per cent and 60 to 80 per cent of maximum), and maximal exer-

TABLE 20-II

MEASUREMENTS DURING MAXIMAL WORK BEFORE AND
AFTER TRAINING

A. PREVIOUSLY SEDENTARY MEN (n = 3)

	Before (mean)	*After* (mean)	*Change, %* (mean and range)
Oxygen Uptake			
liter/min	2.52	3.41	+33
ml/kg x min	36	48	22 — 42
Cardiac Output	17.2	20.0	+16.5
liter/min			13 — 20
Heart Rate	192	191	—0.5
beats/min			—3 —2
Stroke Volume	90	105	+17
ml			11 — 19
AV-O₂ Diff.	14.6	17.0	+16.5
vol %			11 — 24

B. PREVIOUSLY ACTIVE MEN

	Subject G.H. Before	After	*Subject L.L.* Before	After
Oxygen Uptake				
liter/min	4.15	4.38	4.80	4.91
ml/kg x min	59	62	47	49
Cardiac Output				
liter/min	22.8	27.3	25.8	26.4
Heart Rate				
beats/min.	201	193	187	187
Stroke Volume				
ml	113	141	138	141
AV-O₂ Diff.				
vol %	18.2	16.1	18.6	18.6

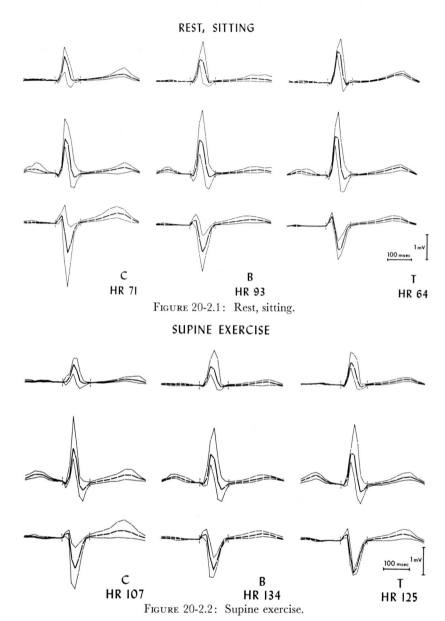

REST, SITTING

C
HR 71

B
HR 93

T
HR 64

FIGURE 20-2.1: Rest, sitting.

SUPINE EXERCISE

C
HR 107

B
HR 134

T
HR 125

FIGURE 20-2.2: Supine exercise.

FIGURE 20-2. Frank lead electrocardiogram at rest and during submaximal and maximal exercise at the control study (*C*), after bedrest (*B*), and after training (*T*). Each individual PR, QRS and STT segment has been divided into eight subsegments of equal duration. Group mean amplitudes (*heavy lines*) and range (*thin lines*) are given for the onset of the P wave and the point at the end of each subsegment in the X or transversal (*top*), Y or vertical (*middle*) and Z or sagittal (*bottom*) lead. Vertical lines mark the onset and offset of QRS.

SUBMAXIMAL TREADMILL EXERCISE

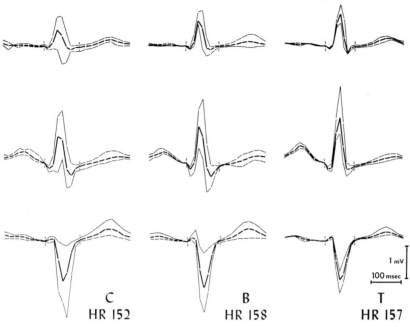

C
HR 152

B
HR 158

T
HR 157

FIGURE 20-2.3: Submaximal treadmill exercise.

MAXIMAL EXERCISE

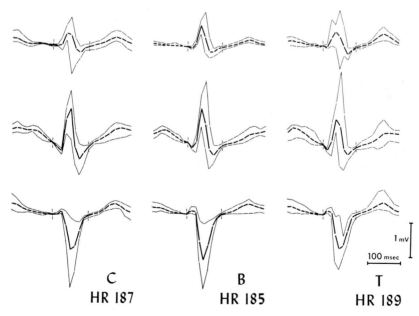

C
HR 187

B
HR 185

T
HR 189

FIGURE 20-2.4: Maximal exercise.

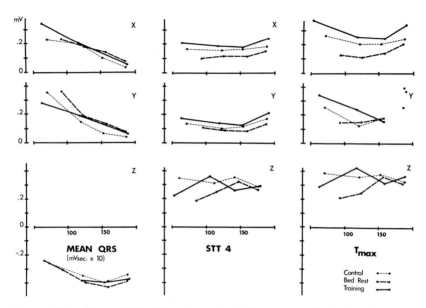

FIGURE 20-3. Mean QRS, ST and maximal T wave amplitude in relation to heart rate at rest and during submaximal and maximal exercise at the control study, after bedrest, and after training.

STT 4 represents the amplitude at half the distance between end of QRS and end of T. T maximal amplitudes during maximal work in lead Y are to a significant degree determined by the amplitude of the atrial T wave. The baseline is defined as the level of the PR segment immediately before the onset of QRS.

cise to minimize the effect of inter- and intra-individual variations in heart rate. Figure 20-3 gives mean QRS area vectors, and ST and T amplitudes at rest and during exercise related to heart rate.

Mean maximal QRS, X, Y and Z vector components (QRS 4) at rest in the sitting position at the control study were 0.56, 1.13 and -1.15 mv with a spatial magnitude of 1.88 mv. Corresponding figures for maximum T vector (STT 5 or 6, whichever largest) components and spatial magnitude were 0.26, 0.25, 0.39 and 0.55 mv. QRS changes with increasing workloads and heart rates included displacement of the initial vectors upwards and to the right, decrease of the maximal spatial magnitude, and displacement of the terminal vectors to the right, upwards, and anteriorly. The mean QRS vector (determined from integration of the QRS complex in the scalar X,

Y and Z leads) showed a progressive decrease in spatial magnitude during exercise at increasing loads and a more strictly posterior orientation (Figure 20-3). ST-junction and STT amplitudes during the early part of the segment (STT 1, 2, 3) also showed a progressive decrease with increasing workloads while there was little change in X and Z amplitudes during the latter part of the STT segment. STT changes in the Y lead were difficult to evaluate due to the marked effect of atrial repolarization on the baseline at high heart rates. ST-junction X, Y and Z amplitudes during maximal work at a heart rate of 187 beats/min were -0.03, -0.10, and -0.02 mv. Corresponding figures for the largest negative amplitudes seen in any subject were -0.14, -0.20 and -0.09 mv. STT amplitudes at half the distance between the end of QRS and the end of T (STT 4) were always positive in all subjects and all leads; there were no instances of horizontal or near-horizontal ST segment depression.

There were no QRS changes after bedrest but a decrease in spatial magnitude of the maximal T vector at rest both in the supine and the sitting position. Mean values at the control study were 0.65 and 0.55 mv compared to 0.54 and 0.32 mv after bedrest. All five subjects showed a decreased T amplitude in the sitting position. Heart rates in the supine position was 61 before and 60 beats/min after bedrest. Corresponding figures for the sitting position were 71 and 93 beats/min.

The relationship between QRS, ST-junction and STT 1, 2 and 3 amplitudes during exercise and heart rate did not change. STT amplitudes 4, 5 and 6 tended to be lower after bedrest. A decrease in spatial magnitude of the maximal T vector during light treadmill exercise was seen in all subjects. Mean spatial magnitude and heart rate were 0.45 mv and 122 beats/min at the control study compared to 0.34 and 125 after bedrest. The spatial magnitude of the T vector during supine submaximal exercise was also smaller after bedrest. One subject even showed a rightward T vector both during treadmill and supine bicycle ergometer work but reverted to a normal leftward direction during maximal work. Mean maximal T vector components and spatial magnitudes during moderately heavy and maximal treadmill exercise did not change with bedrest.

Training did not influence QRS or STT 1-3 amplitudes at rest, but there was a small increase in mean spatial magnitude for STT vectors 4-6. Mean spatial magnitude for the maximal T vector at rest in the sitting position was 0.04 mv higher after training than at the control study, or 0.59 mv. Differences of similar magnitude with respect to mean maximal T vector and STT 4-6 were present also during exercise, but there was considerable intraindividual variation. QRS amplitudes during exercise were similar to those at the control study.

High Altitude

Maximal oxygen uptake was reduced to 70 per cent of the sea level value after three days at altitude. This reduction persisted throughout the two weeks with no tendency to improve. Mean maximal oxygen uptake was 2.72 liters/min after two weeks at altitude compared to 3.83 at sea level. Acute elevation of the alveolar oxygen tension to approximately 100 mm Hg at high altitude resulted in an increase in maximal oxygen uptake only to near sea level values despite an increased oxygen carrying capacity of the blood due to an increase in hemoglobin concentration. Mean values for arterial pO_2, pCO_2, and pH during maximal exercise at sea level were 90 and 33 mm Hg and 7.26. Corresponding values after two weeks at altitude were 45 and 23 mm Hg and 7.42 during maximal exercise and 51 and 23 mm Hg and 7.45 during submaximal exercise.

The maximal cardiac output decreased by 22 per cent or from 22.4 to 17.7 liters/min (n = 3). In addition, two of the subjects showed a fall in maximal heart rate of 20 beats/min. Hemodynamic data could not be obtained in one of these subjects. The stroke volume was about 20 per cent lower at altitude at rest and during both submaximal and maximal work. Mean values during maximal work (n = 3) were 121 ml at sea level and 99 ml after two weeks at altitude. Arterial pressures tended to be higher at altitude.

The efficiency of the alveolar capillary gas exchange as reflected by alveolar-arterial oxygen tension differences did not change, nor did the relationship between oxygen transported and oxygen utilized by the peripheral tissues. The A-V O_2 difference did not change. Blood gas measurements showed the expected changes with arterial oxygen tensions of 50 and below (mean value of 51 during submaximal and

REST

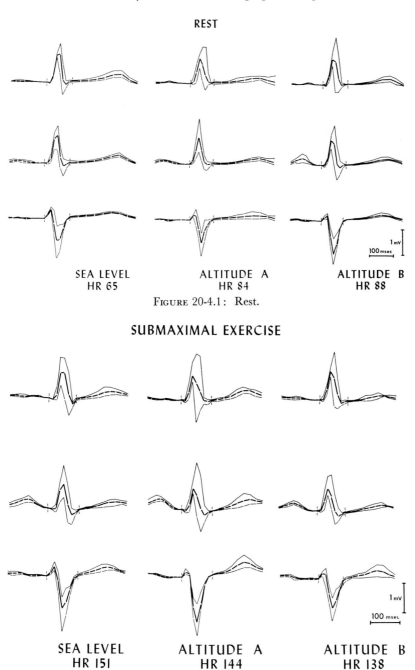

SEA LEVEL
HR 65

ALTITUDE A
HR 84

ALTITUDE B
HR 88

FIGURE 20-4.1: Rest.

SUBMAXIMAL EXERCISE

SEA LEVEL
HR 151

ALTITUDE A
HR 144

ALTITUDE B
HR 138

FIGURE 20-4.2: Submaximal exercise.

MAXIMAL EXERCISE

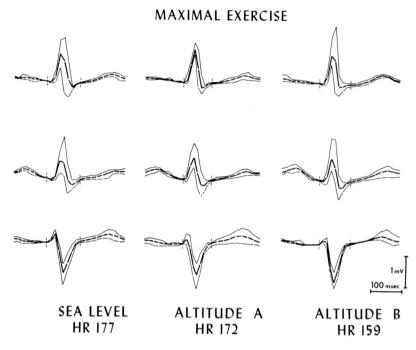

SEA LEVEL	ALTITUDE A	ALTITUDE B
HR 177	HR 172	HR 159

FIGURE 20-4.3: Maximal exercise.

FIGURE 20-4. X, Y and Z lead amplitudes (mean and range) at rest and during submaximal and maximal exercise at sea level, after two days at 14,000 feet (*Altitude A*) and after twelve days (*Altitude B*).

45 during maximal work) and relative alkalosis with pH values about 7.40 during maximal work.

Electrocardiographic changes during adaptation to high altitude are presented in Figures 20-4 and 20-5.

Figure 20-5 shows group mean amplitudes and range at sea level, one to two days after ascent to 14,000 feet, and after twelve days at altitude as well as mean QRS and ST amplitudes at rest and during exercise related to heart rate.

The maximal spatial P vector at rest showed a small but progressive increase in magnitude. Mean values were 0.15, 0.21, and 0.26 mv after two, eight and twelve days at altitude at heart rates 84, 89 and 88 beats/min. A displacement of the mean QRS vector toward a more strictly posterior position was seen in all subjects both at rest

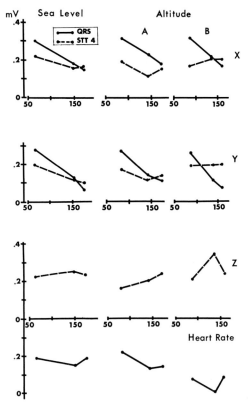

FIGURE 20-5. Mean QRS and X, Y and Z lead ST amplitudes in relation to heart rate at rest and during submaximal and maximal exercise at sea level and at altitude after two days (*A*) and twelve days (*B*).

and during exercise after twelve days at altitude. The magnitude of the maximal spatial QRS vector at rest did not change significantly but was slightly lower than the control value after two days at altitude, 1.56 compared to 1.83 mv, and somewhat higher after twelve days, 2.00 mv. There was no increase in initial anterior or terminal rightward vector components. There were only minor changes in STT amplitudes at rest if the higher heart rate at altitude is taken into consideration. Differences during exercise were also small and statistically nonsignificant. Some reduction of STT amplitudes, excluding the ST junction, was seen during submaximal exercise after two days at altitude. Differences during maximal exercise and during both submaximal and maximal exercise after twelve days were small. The relation between RR and PR and RR and QT intervals was similar at altitude and at sea level.

DISCUSSION

Electrocardiographic measurements during and after exercise were included in the present study primarily to define sources of variability in young normal male subjects. As expected, large changes in cardiovascular dynamics over relatively short periods of time were reflected in the electrocardiogram only to a limited extent.

A three-week period of bedrest resulted in a large decrease in maximal oxygen uptake. The large decrease in cardiac output and stroke volume during upright exercise after bedrest is compatible with venous pooling and impaired venous return. However, the reduction in cardiac output and stroke volume also during supine leg exercise with the working extremities well above the heart level makes it difficult to invoke deficient control of capacitance vessels as the sole explanation for the reduction in stroke volume.

There was no fall in total peripheral resistance and maximal A-V O_2 difference after bedrest which indicates an efficient distribution of a reduced cardiac output and implies that there was no loss of arterial control. Furthermore, there was no change in maximal heart rate, and the relationship between heart rate and relative workload at submaximal levels also remained unchanged. These findings and the failure of the supine position to abolish hemodynamic and electrocardiographic changes in this series suggests an effect on the myocardial level, e.g., in the muscle cell itself, or perhaps in the myocardial response to sympathetic outflow rather than a defective central regulation of the circulation. The electrocardiographic changes by themselves do not provide any clue to any specific mechanism responsible for the decrease in stroke volume and cardiac output.

Patients with syndromes attributed to alterations of sympathetic outflow differ from our subjects after bedrest in several respects. A decreased sympathetic outflow is probably present in patients with postural hypotension associated with central nervous system damage. These patients tend to have an impaired control of both resistance and capacitance vessels, a reduced heart rate response both to exercise and to changes in body position, and a low cardiac output and stroke volume in the upright position (5, 6). However, during supine exercise they usually have a normal cardiac output and a normal or high stroke volume, and a low arterial pressure. On the other hand, Holmgren *et al.* (7) have postulated an increased sympathetic outflow in a group of patients with clinical findings compatible with neuro-circulatory asthenia. They were characterized by a high cardiac output and a low arteriovenous oxygen difference both at rest and during exercise, a low physical working capacity and STT wave changes, particularly in the standing position and during upright exercise. The ECG at rest in the supine position was usually, but not always, within normal limits. The ECG response during exercise was similar to that in our subjects after bedrest in that the STT changes did not become more marked with increasing workloads and in that they disappeared after a period of physical training. Furberg (8) has later studied a group of patients similar to those included in Holmgren's *et al.* series and shown that the abnormal response to exercise can be abolished by adrenergic beta-receptor blockade.

It is well established that well-trained athletes frequently show QRS changes suggesting right or left ventricular hypertrophy and large T wave amplitudes with essentially normal orientation of the T vector (9). There is evidence that the spatial angle between the QRS and T vectors is decreased in athletes with large QRS magnitudes while the QRS-T angle characteristically increased in patients with hypertrophy secondary to hypertension. Recent data suggest that younger athletes may show predominantly right and older athletes left ventricular preponderance (10). Longitudinal data are scarce, but Hugenholtz (11) has reported significant increases in spatial QRS magnitude in most members of a group of young college students during an eight-month training program for competitive rowing. The absence of significant QRS changes after training in the present series combined with some increase in STT amplitude could reflect a true difference between the effects of long-term and short-term physical training.

Acute exposure to high altitude leads to a decrease in maximal oxygen intake of a magnitude corresponding to the reduction in oxygen tension of the inspired air and the decrease in oxygen content of arterial blood. Maximal cardiac output and stroke volume do not change

(12). Adaptation to altitude includes an increase of pulmonary ventilation causing the alveolar oxygen pressure return toward sea level values and an increase in hemoglobin concentration and oxygen carrying capacity of the blood. However, most studies performed at an altitude of 3,000 meters (10,500 feet) and above have failed to demonstrate a progressive increase in maximal oxygen uptake with acclimatization (2). Our data seem to indicate that a decrease in maximal cardiac output due to a decrease in stroke volume and, in some cases, also a decrease in maximal heart rate, explains the failure of the increase in oxygen content of the arterial blood to improve maximal oxygen uptake during prolonged stay at altitude. There were no findings suggesting an impairment of the gas exchange in lungs or tissues.

The ECG findings at altitude were essentially negative. The small change in STT amplitudes cannot be considered an indication of a discrepancy between myocardial oxygen demand and supply. The subjects most likely had some elevation of pulmonary arterial pressures, but there were no ECG changes that could be interpreted as indicating RVH or RV strain at rest or during exercise. The absence of major ST changes during exercise in young male subjects at a high altitude is in agreement with findings in a previous study on acute exposure to the same altitude in a similar group studied by the same technique (13).

Changes in the ECG at rest with adaptation to high altitude have recently been studied and reviewed by Harris *et al.* (14, 15). Reports based on standard leads indicate a decrease in QRS amplitudes at altitude which has been interpreted as a sign of myocardial ischemia. The present results suggest that the apparent changes in conventional leads may be due at least to some extent to a change toward a more strictly posterior orientation of the QRS.

A common feature of both the bedrest training study and the altitude study is that while there were some changes in STT amplitudes during the course of the experiment, the relationship between workload or heart rate and ECG response did not change significantly. If anything, there was a trend during maximal work toward less discrepancy between amplitude values before and after intervention. The results of measurements of arterial potassium concentrations dur-

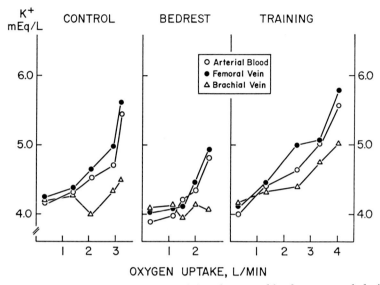

FIGURE 20-6. Serum potassium in arterial and venous blood at rest and during submaximal and maximal exercise at the control study, after bedrest, and after training.

ing exercise (Figure 20-6) at various workload levels suggest that hyperkalemia may at least partially explain the trend toward normalization of the STT amplitudes during heavy and maximal exercise. The preservation of a normal dynamic response is in sharp contrast to the results of multilevel exercise tests in middle-aged men and in patients with angina pectoris. In these groups increasing workloads are associated with increasingly large deviations from the typical response in young healthy subjects studied under normal conditions.

REFERENCES

1. SALTIN, B.; BLOMQVIST, G.; MITCHELL, J.H.; JOHNSON, R.L., JR.; WILDEN-THAL, K., and CHAPMAN, C.B.: Response to exercise after bedrest and training. A longitudinal study of adaptive changes in oxygen transport and body composition. Suppl. 7 to Circulation, Vols. 37 & 38, 1968.

2. SALTIN, B.; GROVER, R.F.; BLOMQVIST, G.; HARTLEY, H., and JOHNSON, R.L., JR.: Maximal oxygen uptake and cardiac output after two weeks at 4,300 meters. *J. Appl. Physiol.* 25:400-409, 1968.

3. BLOMQVIST, G.: The Frank lead exercise electrocardiogram. A quantitative study based on averaging technic and digital computer analysis. *Acta Med Scand, 178* (Suppl 440):9-39, 1965.

4. SIMONSON, E.: *Differentiation Between Normal and Abnormal in Electro-cardiography.* St. Louis, Mosby, 1961.
5. BEVEGÅRD, S.; JONSSON, B., and KARLÖF, I.: Circulatory response to recombent exercise and head-up tilting in patients with disturbed sympathetic cardiovascuar control (postural hypotension). Observations on the effect of norepinephrine infusion and antigravity suit inflation in the head-up tilted position. *Acta Med Scand, 172*:623-636, 1962.
6. MARSHALL, R.J.; SCHIRGER, A., and SHEPHERD, J.T.: Blood pressure during supine exercise in idiopathic orthostatic hypotension. *Circulation, 24*: 76-81, 1961.
7. HOLMGREN, A.; JONSON, B.; LINDERHOLM, H.; SJÖSTRAND, T., and STRÖM, G.: ECG changes in vasoregulatory asthenia and the effect of training. *Acta Med Scand, 165*:259-271, 1959.
8. FURBERG, C.: Adrenergic beta-blockade and electrocardiographic ST-T changes. *Acta Med Scand, 181*:21-32, 1967.
9. ARSTILA, M., and KOIVIKKO, A.: Electrocardiographic and vectorcardiographic signs of left and right hypertrophy in athletes. *J Sports Med, 6*: 166-175, 1966.
10. RAUTAHARJU, P.M., and KARVONEN, M.J.: Physiological consequences of the adaptive dilatation of the heart. In *Physical Activity and the Heart. Proceedings of a Symposium, Helsinki, Finland.* Karvonen, M.J., and Barry, A.J. (Eds.), Springfield, Thomas, 1967, pp. 159-183.
11. HUGENHOLTZ, P.G.: The accuracy of vectorcardiographic criteria as related to the hemodynamic state. In *Vectorcardiography.* Hoffman, I., and Taymor, R.C. (Eds.), Philadelphia, Lippincott, 1966, pp. 163-168.
12. STENBERG, J.; EKBLOM, B., and MESSIN, R.: Hemodynamic response to work at simulated altitude 4,000 m. *J Appl Physiol, 21*:1589-1594, 1966.
13. BLOMQVIST, G., and STENBERG, J.: The electrocardiographic response to submaximal and maximal work during acute hypoxia. *Acta Med Scand, 178* (suppl. 440):82-89, 1965.
14. HARRIS, C.W., and HANSEN, J.E.: Electrocardiographic changes during exposure to high altitude. *Amer J Cardiol, 18*:183-190, 1966.
15. HARRIS, C.W.; SHIELDS, J.L., and HANNON, J.P.: Electrocardiographic and radiographic heart changes in women at high altitude. *Amer J Cardiol, 18*:847-854, 1966.

DISCUSSION

Dr. Simonson: Thank you very much. Are there any questions?

Dr. Bruce: That was a splendid presentation. I was very much intrigued by your finding a decrease in cardiac output and maximal oxygen consumption after bedrest. Were there any changes in lean body weight and total blood volume?

Dr. Blomqvist: There was no change in total body weight, but a small decrease in lean body mass and blood volume.

Question: What was the efficiency of work after bedrest?

Dr. Blomqvist: Mechanical efficiency did not change with bedrest or training.

Question: Will you tell me, please, what amount of training these people had after bedrest. Was it the same for all subjects?

Dr. Blomqvist: We tried to regulate intensity of training according to each individual's maximal capacity. They were exposed to interval training during a one-hour morning session every day with repeated short runs during which they usually reached a maximal heart rate. They then had afternoon sessions of prolonged work at 70 to 80 per cent of maximal capacity. External work loads were modified and increased during the training period to keep the relative work load constant.

Dr. Simonson: How long was the bedrest period?

Dr. Blomqvist: Three weeks.

Dr. Simonson: Did you try to find out for how long it would be before you would notice any deterioration—is it five days, eight days? It would be interesting.

Dr. Blomqvist: It would be interesting to know, but the only way of finding out would be to take similar groups and expose them to periods of various lengths. As soon as you bring your subjects up once, you have ended your experiment.

21

Comparison of Heart Rate, Oxygen Consumption and Electrocardiographic Responses to Submaximal Step Exercise and Near Maximal Exercise on a Treadmill and Bicycle Ergometer

Edwin E. Westura *and* James A. Ronan, *with the technical assistance of* Norma J. Pitts *and* C. Ray White

INTRODUCTION

The prevention of cardiovascular disease is a major goal of the Heart Disease and Stroke Control Program. Special urgency exists for programs to control coronary heart disease because of its prevalence in our society at this time, especially in those at the peak of social and economic productivity. The current adverse effect of this disease upon morbidity rates and longevity is widely appreciated. Before such programs of prevention can be undertaken, however, we should have effective standard methods of detecting the disease and of controlling its progression. The requirement for standard detection and health evaluation techniques is of particular importance because these will be the reference standards against which the effectiveness and value of specific preventive measures and programs will be evaluated. These standard detection and evaluation techniques should be available before any large preventive program is undertaken. The difficulties in research programs of this type have been reviewed by Taylor and most recently by Cady (1, 2).

The purpose of this report is to present the results of research comparing test methods for detecting latent ischemic heart disease which are now in common use. This research is directed toward developing

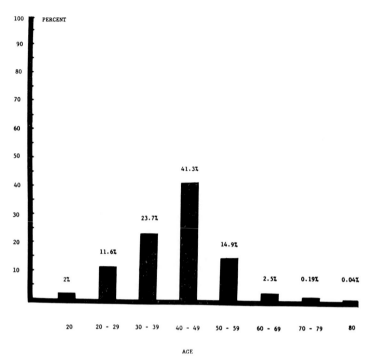

FIGURE 21-1. Age distribution of available study population by decade. The preponderance of subjects are in the fifth decade.

guidelines for a standard and quantitative detection method for coronary heart disease employing physical exercise and the electrocardiogram.

The population available for study consists of 2,289 adult male subjects. The majority of this population consists of normal, healthy volunteers. Some subjects are referred because of definite or suspected cardiovascular disease. The age distribution of the entire population by decade is presented in Figure 21-1. This report consists of studies conducted on sixty-six subjects as part of a clinical research program providing general health evaluations to participating volunteers with special emphasis on the determination of cardiovascular health status. The mean age of these subjects was forty-two years. Twenty-four of the subjects had known cardiovascular disease. The remaining forty-two subjects were free of cardiovascular disease and otherwise healthy as determined by clinical evaluation. This included complete history and physical examination, CBC, urine analysis, lipid profile, blood sugar, resting electrocardiogram and chest x-ray. The purpose of this study was to compare methods of stress testing by the parameters of heart rate and oxygen consumption response and the frequency of ischemic electrocardiographic changes to submaximal step exercise (double Master's test) and near maximal exercise on a bicycle ergometer and treadmill. Since we are concerned only with comparing the three test methods no reference will be made to the clinical subgroups.

METHODS

After complete medical history was recorded and physical examination performed, fasting blood was obtained for complete blood count, blood sugar, cholesterol, triglyceride and uric acid. Lean body mass was determined by isotope dilution technique (3). A resting supine electrocardiogram was recorded on a direct writing electrocardiograph machine.* Silver plated electrodes† were attached to the precordium in conventional V lead positions and an additional electrode was placed in the fifth right intercostal space in the anterior axillary line. This latter electrode served as the indifferent electrode for a transthoracic, bi-polar lead which was monitored and recorded during exercise and which was considered equivalent to conventional lead V_5. A control tracing of this lead was obtained at rest supine, sitting and standing before upright exercise in order to evaluate stability of the electrocardiographic trace and any postural alterations in the ST segment or T wave. The frequency modulated electrocardiogram* was monitored during exercise on an oscilloscope of a multichannel photographic recorder† and recorded on a direct writing electrocardiograph machine, at thirty-second intervals and continuously on magnetic tape.‡ Expired air was collected in Douglas bags and analyzed

---

*Model 100, Sanborn Division, Hewlett-Packard Co., Palo Alto, California.

†Telemedic's Electrodes, Telemedics, Vector Division, United Aircraft Corp., South Hampton, Pennsylvania. Beckman Electrodes, Beckman Instrument Co., Fullerton, California.

*RKG 100, Telemedics, Vector Division, United Aircraft Corp., South Hampton, Pennsylvania. TCC Transmitter-Receiver, Onyx, Lexington Instrument Co., Waltham, Massachusetts.

†DR-16, Electronics for Medicine, White Plains, New York.

‡FR 1100, Ampex Corp., Redwood City, California.

for oxygen[§] and carbon dioxide,[¶] and total volume. Oxygen consumption was determined from the standard gas equations and reported as volume at standard temperature and pressure dry (STPD).

A physician was in constant attendance during the exercise stress procedures. All subjects initially performed a double Master two-step test according to published specifications (4). Expired air was collected at rest before exercise and during the third minute of the test. Electrocardiograms were obtained before and during exercise as described.

Following exercise, leads I, II, III AVL, AVF, V_4, V_5 and V_6 were obtained immediately and at two and five minutes. All subjects then exercised in the supine position on a bicycle ergometer[*] and in the erect position on a treadmill.[†] The test sequence was randomized. Supine bicycle exercise was performed for a total of seven minutes. There was an initial warm-up period at 50 watts of work for one minute and this was immediately followed by two continuous external work loads of 100 and 200 watts for three minutes each. The treadmill test consisted of walking at a constant speed of 3.0 mph for nine minutes. After an initial warm-up, walking on the level for one minute, the subjects walked for four minutes at an 8 per cent grade and for another four minutes at a 16 per cent grade. Oxygen consumption was measured for the last minute of exercise at each level of work on both bicycle and treadmill. Electrocardiograms, during and after exercise, were monitored and recorded in the same manner and at the intervals described above for the step test. Tracings were also obtained at ten minutes after exercise and in those cases in which there was a persistent electrocardiographic change at ten minutes, electrocardiograms were taken at frequent intervals until the pre-exercise configuration returned. Two to four hours intervened between treadmill and ergometer exercise. In addition to the electrocardiogram, heart rate was continuously recorded on a cardiotachometer.

Maximum heart rate was estimated from data representing a com-

---

§ Model E2, Beckman Instrument Co., Fullerton, California.

¶ Model CG58003, Infrared Capnograph, Godart, Utrecht, Holland.

*Fleisch Bicycle, Godart, Utrecht, Holland.

† Model 18-60, Quinton Instrument Co., Seattle, Washington.

posite of published reports on age dependent changes in maximum heart rate (5). Maximum oxygen consumption was estimated from the data of Astrand (6). Electrocardiograms were interpreted independently by two cardiologists according to the criteria of Mattingly (7). Results were coded according to the classification of Blackburn (8) as modified by Åstrand (9). Aerobic cost was estimated for each level of exercise by the product of the increase in oxygen consumption per minute at a given level of work over the resting oxygen consumption and the duration of work at that level (10). The sums of aerobic cost at each level are used to represent the total aerobic cost of each test. The area under the heart rate curve was integrated and this value, expressed as heart rate minutes, was used as an index to express the aerobic cost of the test to the heart. This value is also referred to as heart rate work. Mean heart rate for each level of exercise and for each test was determined as the quotient of heart rate minutes and time. A table with anthropometric data and the responses of each subject to each test is available upon request.

RESULTS

Heart Rate

Representative cardiotachometer tracings obtained on a single subject during the double Master test, the bicycle ergometer test and on the treadmill are presented in Figure 21-2. We have repeatedly noted that heart rate reaches a plateau during the last one and one-half to one minute of this test, as shown in the Figure. The slope of heart rate increase was initially greater for both the step test and treadmill than for the bicycle. Peak heart rates, however, were comparable for both bicycle and treadmill. When the data for all three tests are compared, Figure 21-3, with heart rate expressed as either mean heart rate or heart rate minutes (heart rate work), it is clear that the heart rate was higher for a longer period of time for the treadmill test than for the bicycle test. It was higher for both of these tests than for the step test. The continuous tracings of heart rate change, Figure 21-2, also indicate that a relative plateau was reached at each stage of the bicycle test and treadmill test. This plateau was less definite on the treadmill than the bicycle and was especially difficult to obtain at the highest work loads.

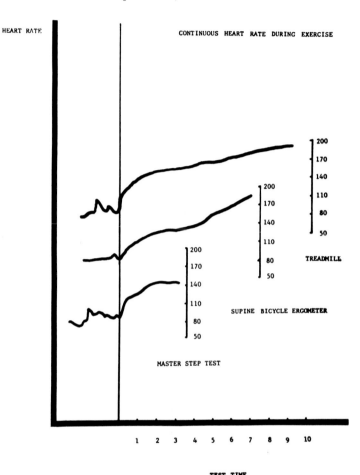

HEART RATE

CONTINUOUS HEART RATE DURING EXERCISE

200
170
140
110
80
50

TREADMILL

200
170
140
110
80
50

SUPINE BICYCLE ERGOMETER

200
170
140
110
80
50

MASTER STEP TEST

1 2 3 4 5 6 7 8 9 10

TEST TIME

FIGURE 21-2. Characteristic continuous heart rate response in a single subject to step exercise, and to near maximal exercise on a bicycle ergometer and treadmill.

Peak heart rates during the step test were consistently between 65 per cent and 75 per cent of age predicted maximum heart rates (mean = 69%; SD ± 7 per cent). Peak heart rates were slightly higher on the bicycle supine at 100 watts (mean = 73 per cent ± 6 per cent). Peak heart rate on the treadmill at 8 per cent grade and 3 mph was higher than either of these (mean = 80 per cent ± 10 per cent). Peak heart rates for the group were comparable at 200

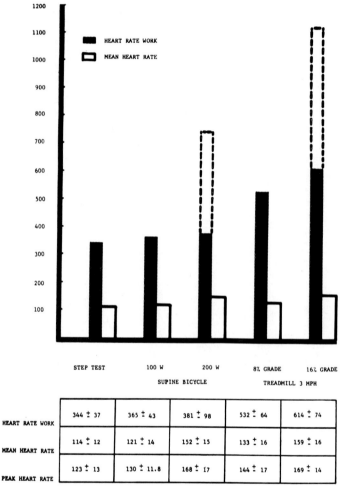

HEART RATE WORK	344 ± 37	365 ± 43	381 ± 98	532 ± 64	614 ± 74
MEAN HEART RATE	114 ± 12	121 ± 14	152 ± 15	133 ± 16	159 ± 16
PEAK HEART RATE	123 ± 13	130 ± 11.8	168 ± 17	144 ± 17	169 ± 14

FIGURE 21-3. Heart rate work (heart rate minutes), mean heart rate and peak heart rate for step test, and for each level of near maximal multistage testing on a bicycle ergometer and treadmill. Since work is cumulative for continuous testing, total heart rate work is also shown.

watts and 16 per cent grade, both eliciting a response 94 per cent or more of age predicted maximums (bicycle mean = 94 per cent ± 9 per cent; Treadmill mean = 94 per cent ± 8 per cent).

Oxygen Consumption

As might be expected from the known relationship between heart

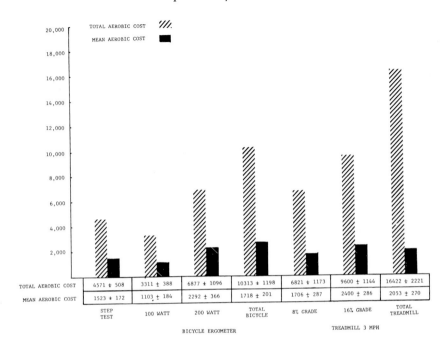

TOTAL AEROBIC COST	4571 ± 508	3311 ± 388	6877 ± 1096	10313 ± 1198	6821 ± 1173	9600 ± 1144	16422 ± 2221
MEAN AEROBIC COST	1523 ± 172	1103 ± 184	2292 ± 366	1718 ± 201	1706 ± 287	2400 ± 286	2053 ± 270
	STEP TEST	100 WATT	200 WATT	TOTAL BICYCLE	8% GRADE	16% GRADE	TOTAL TREADMILL
		BICYCLE ERGOMETER				TREADMILL 3 MPH	

FIGURE 21-4. Estimated total aerobic cost and mean aerobic cost for step test and for multistage near maximal testing on a bicycle ergometer and treadmill.

rate and oxygen consumption, the same trends found in the heart rate data for each test were also found in the oxygen consumption data. Oxygen consumption was higher for the step test than for the bicycle at 100 watts. Aerobic cost of the treadmill test was higher at each level of treadmill testing and for the total test than for the bicycle test used in these studies, Figure 21-4.

Maximum oxygen consumption was predicted from the data of Åstrand. The difficulties in making such estimations have been noted by Rowell (11). The mean values for per cent of maximum oxygen consumption for each test and level of exercise used in this study are presented in Figure 21-5. The treadmill test procedure produced the highest aerobic cost of the three test methods, both for each level of work and for the total test. The same data is presented in cubic centimeter oxygen consumed per minute per kilogram of body weight, in Figure 21-6.

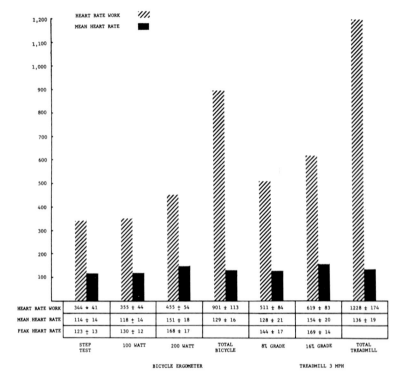

	STEP TEST	100 WATT	200 WATT	TOTAL BICYCLE	8% GRADE	16% GRADE	TOTAL TREADMILL
HEART RATE WORK	344 ± 41	355 ± 44	455 ± 54	901 ± 113	511 ± 84	619 ± 83	1228 ± 174
MEAN HEART RATE	114 ± 14	118 ± 14	151 ± 18	129 ± 16	128 ± 21	154 ± 20	136 ± 19
PEAK HEART RATE	123 ± 13	130 ± 12	168 ± 17		144 ± 17	169 ± 14	

BICYCLE ERGOMETER TREADMILL 3 MPH

FIGURE 21-5. Per cent of maximum heart rate and oxygen consumption for step test and for multistage near maximal testing on a bicycle ergometer and treadmill.

Heart Rate and Oxygen Consumption

Mean heart rates have been plotted against mean values for oxygen consumption with standard deviations for all three tests in Figure 21-7. Each step in the multistage procedures is presented separately. The linear relationship between heart rate and oxygen consumption, independent of the type of external exercise performed is clearly evident ($r = 0.98$; $y = 20.5$ x $- 1051$; $p < 0.001$).

Ischemic Responses

Horizontal or downward sloping ST segments, ischemic according to the criteria of Mattingly, were present in nineteen subjects (28.7 per cent). Seven subjects had ischemic responses after bicycle testing

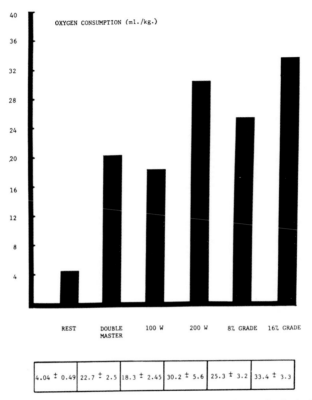

4.04 ± 0.49	22.7 ± 2.5	18.3 ± 2.45	30.2 ± 5.6	25.3 ± 3.2	33.4 ± 3.3

FIGURE 21-6. Mean oxygen consumption (cc/kg) and standard deviation for step test and multistage near maximal testing on a bicycle ergometer and treadmill.

(10.5 per cent). Eighteen subjects were positive after treadmill testing (27 per cent). Six subjects were positive on both tests (9.9 per cent). One subject was positive on the ergometer only and eleven subjects on the treadmill only. The subject who had a positive response on the bicycle but a negative response on the treadmill achieved a higher peak heart rate on the bicycle than he did on the treadmill. His values for mean heart rate and heart rate work were also higher for the bicycle than for the treadmill. All those who were positive on the treadmill had higher peak heart rates with this test than with the bicycle. Therefore, 94 per cent of the positive responses were found after the test program with the treadmill. Only 37 per cent of the positive responses were found with the bicycle program. Only one

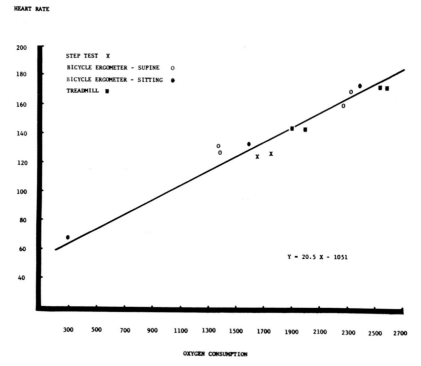

HEART RATE

FIGURE 21-7. Mean values for heart rate and oxygen consumption obtained in sixty-six adult male subjects to step test and near maximal exercise, supine and sitting on a bicycle ergometer and walking on a treadmill.

of these subjects had a positive Master's step test. Most ischemic responses noted were coded as IV-2. Examples of normal and positive electrocardiographic responses are shown in Figures 21-8 and 21-9.

While these changes are typical of the positive and negative responses found either during or after exercise, positive changes during exercise are uncommon in our experience. In over 5000 Master tests and over 200 near maximal exercise tests on the bicycle ergometer or tread-mill in this laboratory, only one subject was found to demonstrate ischemic changes during and not following exercise. Ninety-eight per cent of the positive responses have occurred after exercise alone. The most common situation is for ischemic changes to be found at two minutes following the step test and at five minutes after near maximal work, whether on the bicycle or treadmill, using our time

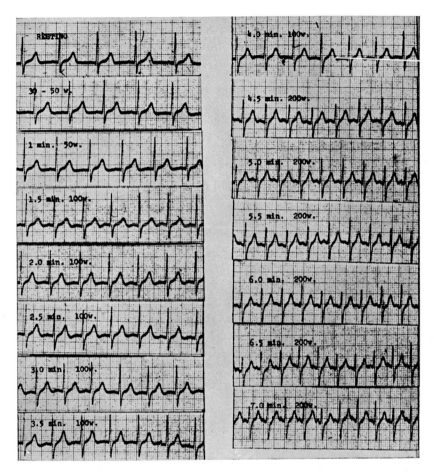

FIGURE 21-8. Normal electrocardiographic response to near maximal exercise.

intervals for sampling. Of the multiple leads taken post exercise, V_4 and V_5 most often demonstrate these ischemic changes. Lead III has been most difficult to interpret following exercise since it frequently has an "ischemic" configuration at rest. In subjects with this type of lead III pattern in the resting electrocardiogram, lead III often exhibits an iso-electric or "square wave" response after exercise when a truly ischemic pattern is not present in other leads. For these reasons, we have not considered a test positive when the ischemic changes in the postexercise period are limited to lead III.

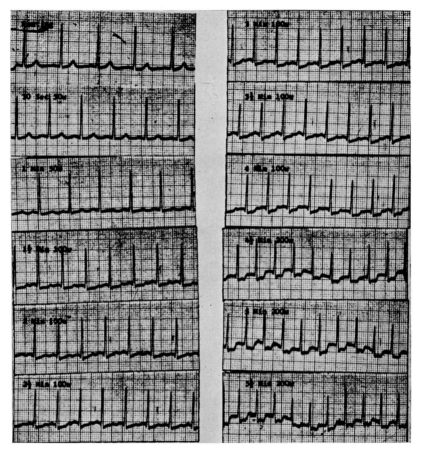

Figure 21-9. Ischemic electrocardiographic response to near maximal exercise.

DISCUSSION

The accepted electrocardiographic endpoint during or after exercise stress testing is the horizontal or downward sloping ST segment. Depressions of this type greater than 0.5 millimeter following the step test proposed by Master are considered significant. They have been associated with an increased risk for subsequent clinical coronary events (7, 12, 13, 14) and equated "for all practical purposes with coronary heart disease" (15). The relationship of positive or ischemic responses after higher levels of exercise to coronary artery disease is not yet clear although evidence has been presented which indicates that such changes are not found in normal subjects with normal hearts (16). Available correlation studies between the step test and coronary arteriography have shown that males with a history of infarction or classical angina and positive exercise responses usually have multiple coronary artery involvement (17). On the other hand, similar studies in females with angina, in patients with neurasthenia, and in males with classical angina have indicated that a classical ischemic response may be present on the electrocardiogram with no demonstrable anatomic disease by current angiographic techniques (18, 19). Similar "false positive" responses have been noted in severe anemic states, in thyrotoxicosis, in cardiomyopathies and in patients on digitalis. A good correlation between coronary arteriographic findings of atherosclerosis and ischemic responses after higher levels of exercise have recently been reported by Mason (20).

Clearly, a decision on an optimal method of stress testing demands that precise data on the sensitivity and specificity of any method proposed for detecting coronary heart disease be available. This type of data can only be obtained in one of two ways: first, by conducting tests in a large sample and then determining the fate of all cases tested; second, by extensive correlation studies using the best available reference standards for coronary artery disease to evaluate test specificity.

The data presented in this study do not bear directly on either test sensitivity or specificity. However, they may be helpful in determining the optimal test method that should be used in embarking upon either of the two programs noted above, either or both of which are required to determine the ultimate utility of a test method. Factors of importance in test selection are listed in Table 21-I.

Personal and Physician Acceptance

Experience in our laboratory with the three test methods discussed in this paper indicate that no subject refused to accept any of the test methods. The subject or patient will usually accept a test which a physician he trusts deems indicated or helpful in his care. This particular aspect of stress testing therefore quickly becomes a question of what test method is safe for the subject and morally, ethically and professionally sound. There is no quick and easy answer to this question. Our own experience indicates that most normal subjects can

TABLE 21-I

FACTORS OF IMPORTANCE IN ELECTROCARDIOGRAPHIC
TEST DESIGN

1. Personal and Physician Acceptance
2. Exercise Loads and Intensities
3. Near Identical Physiologic Loads for All Subjects
4. Intervals of Work
5. Initial Warm-up
6. What, if any, Intervals of Rest or Near Rest
7. What Speeds Walking, Stepping or RPM
8. What Terminal Position and/or Activity
9. Cost-Benefit Ratios

be tested to the levels used in this study without any adverse reaction or effects except for a feeling of muscle fatigue. However, the elaborate prescreening employed in processing our subjects before testing and the elaborate precautions taken during testing suggest that stress testing to these levels is not adaptable to many multiphasic screening programs now in existence. Moreover, until data are available to indicate that individuals detected by these high levels of stress are, in fact, in the early stages of their disease, such testing may not be practical or useful. There is little question, both from these data and from published reports, that the frequency of positive responses increases as the level of stress testing increases.

From an examination of duration of exercise accomplished by the subjects in these three test procedures and on the sitting bicycle at comparable external work loads in more recent studies, we have seen that all subjects completed the step test, unless severely ill. The mean time on the supine bicycle was 6.0 minutes (mean = 5.9 min ± 1.1) with only 65 per cent completing the test protocol. Sitting on the bicycle, 85 per cent completed the seven-minute protocol, but most subjects complained of some degree of leg muscle fatigue.

Subjects have completed the treadmill protocol in 96 per cent of the tests with only moderate tachypnea and light sweating. Our experience indicates that our untrained middle-aged subjects accept and easily tolerate testing which elicits a response between 70 per cent and 80 per cent of their predicted maximum physiologic tolerance and that while either the bicycle, sitting or supine, or the treadmill is acceptable, the treadmill is the most acceptable. We have also found that the subjects have accepted and tolerated even higher levels of stress on the treadmill than with any other method, usually between 90 per cent and 95 per cent of predicted maximums.

Mode of Exercise

Disagreements continue to arise over the most suitable method of testing the subject. The Master's test has been critized because it does not permit a steady state of exercise and because it tends to bias the amount of work against the young subject and for the overweight subject (21). Similar bias has been pointed out by Haskell (22) for tests which employ age predicted maximums for either heart rate or oxygen consumption to determine the amount of work to be accomplished. On a practical basis, these considerations may not be valid objections to any method if the end-point is ischemic electrocardiographic change rather than to evaluate physical fitness.

The data presented here clearly indicate that the frequency of ischemic responses is not contingent upon the mode of exercise. Rather, the frequency of ischemic responses is greatest with the mode of external exercise which permits the subject to do the most work.

Exercise Loads or Intensities

The tests employed in this study were multistage tests. Intermittent tests appear to be too time consuming to be of value in a screening program and single stage tests are more suited for endurance testing and fitness evaluations. We have had no experience with the latter procedures. Our test design has been based upon the premise that the optimal procedure should not exceed fifteen minutes and optimally ten minutes in view of the ancillary procedures involved in testing. The total duration of our current treadmill or ergometer method is thirty minutes from start to finish, including patient preparation, testing and postexercise tracings. A multistage test was chosen because most physiologic literature indicates that such a method permits near steady state conditions to exist if three minutes or more are allowed at each stage and that this technique is well tolerated by the subject. The requirement for a ten-minute procedure therefore, with near steady state at each level enforced a two or three phase multistage test.

Intervals of Work

The intervals of work selected for the bicycle protocol and for the treadmill were again determined by practical considerations and constraints. Inasmuch as the frequency of ischemic responses was dependent, at least in part, upon the level of work, a high level of work appeared to be optimum. We also were concerned, for purposes of evaluating the test methods, with selecting levels of work which would permit all our untrained subjects to complete each test. Our data indicate that the 100 watt level for the bicycle ergometer is approximately equivalent in physiologic work, both in terms of heart rate and aerobic cost, to the Master test. It would be unlikely, therefore, that this level of work would be more sensitive for ischemic responses than the step test. This level of work was easily completed by all subjects. The 200 watt level, however, was too much work for these subjects supine, and for a significant percentage sitting. Our data suggest that a peak work load of approximately 150 watts may be optimal in this untrained group. Early experience with the treadmill indicated a fact known to all those experienced in its use. At a speed of approximately 4.0 mph the subject becomes very uncomfortable because of confusion over whether he should walk or trot or, occasionally, run. A speed of 3.0 mph has obviated this difficulty by inducing a brisk walk in the subject but no desire to trot or run. Increases in work load and heart rate then, appeared to be best induced by increasing the steepness of the grade. A review of published data indicated that at this speed, grade steps of 8 per cent and 16 per cent should induce heart rates and oxygen consumption levels comparable to those which we had obtained on the bicycle supine at 100 and 200 watts (24). However, this did not prove to be the case in our population, probably due to the older age of our subjects (mean = 42 vs. mean = 30). At 16 per cent grade and 3.0 mph, almost all subjects completed the test and peak heart rates were consistently in the range of 95 per cent of age predicted maximum. In those who demonstrated an ischemic response, the value was frequently above 100 per cent of predicted maximum by 5 to 10 per cent. Our most recent experience with changes in technique based upon previous studies, is that an intermediate level of 12 per cent grade for three minutes together with three-minute intervals at 8 per cent and 16 per cent is optimal.

Terminal Position and/or Activity

For purposes of comparison, all postexercise tracings in this study were obtained with the same system that had been used during exercise and the patient remained in the supine position. Following treadmill testing, the subject stepped from the treadmill and was assisted to the bed, immediately adjacent to it. No postural difficulties have been encountered with this procedure. In addition, electrocardiograms obtained in this manner have been free of artifacts and other noise frequently encountered in tracings obtained either upright or sitting, especially those related to motion of the thorax with respiration. The frequency-modulated electrocardiogram is monitored continuously during this transfer from treadmill to bed so that adverse changes are not missed and monitoring of the subject is constant.

Development of a standard test for use in research studies to determine the effectiveness of exercise stress testing in terms of test sensitivity and specificity requires additional investigation of test methods now in common use and close cooperation between groups interested in establishing such a standard technique. A number of factors must be considered when evaluating test methods. Agreement on a standard method may depend upon a combination of practical, scientific and ethical considerations. Implementation of a large research effort to test the sensitivity and specificity of a given method need not await the availability of proven methods of secondary prevention of coronary heart disease but does require agreement on the optimal technique. Research in both areas should go hand in hand. This is especially true because, while it is impossible to change some of the factors which predispose individuals to coronary heart disease, such as heredity, and difficult or inconvenient to change others, such as personality and geographic location, some "risk factors," such as cigarette smoking, hypertension and hyperlipidermia can be modified.

While the data presented do not permit any final conclusions, they suggest some tentative conclusions regarding which test method would be optimal for a larger program to detect latent coronary heart disease.

Some prescreening of subjects before stress testing is essential. Subjects with overt evidence of cardiovascular disease have no place in a detection program using stress evaluations. The tests should be physician monitored or monitored by para-professional personnel who can interpret the findings and can make the necessary judgements to terminate the procedure or handle emergency situations should they arise.

In conclusion, of the methods evaluated, the treadmill has decided advantages. It permits work against body weight. It permits untrained subjects to execute high levels of work, where sensitivity for early disease may be optimal, safely and with a minimum of muscle fatigue. It involves large muscle groups in meeting the stress of exercise, employs an activity natural to man and is well accepted and tolerated, even by those with known cardiovascular disease. It has been limited in application because of the size of the apparatus and high initial cost, but these limitations are minimal especially if such testing is performed in hospitals or other centers for community health services which will service many subjects or physicians. Current data indicate that other external methods of testing can be used satisfactorily but will undoubtedly have less sensitivity. Our data suggest that an initial test should be done at the physiologic cost level of the Master's test before testing at higher levels (heart rate 130, VO_2 1700 cc). If positive responses are noted at this level of work, only more definite changes will be found at higher levels and such additional testing is superfluous.

Experience at this level of exercise in the normal subjects in our population indicates a positive rate of 0.4 per cent. Prescreening of this small group, however, may be important in that available data indicate these subjects are most likely to have extensive disease. Heavy stress testing in this group could be extremely dangerous.

SUMMARY

Heart rate, oxygen consumption and the frequency of ischemic electrocardiographic responses were compared in sixty-six subjects in response to standard step testing and to near maximal exercise stress testing on a treadmill and supine on a bicycle ergometer. The relationship between heart rate and oxygen consumption was linear in these subjects and was independent of the mode of external work. The frequency of ischemic responses was highest with the treadmill and appears related to the fact that with this technique, higher amounts of aerobic cost and heart rate work were experienced by the subject. That ischemic responses are dependent upon these factors is also suggested by the findings in one subject who was positive on the ergometer but negative on the treadmill. The implications of these data for developing a standard test for the detection of latent coronary heart disease are discussed.

REFERENCES

1. TAYLOR, H.L.; PARLIN, R.W.; BLACKBURN, H., and KEYS, A.: Problems in the analysis of the relationship of coronary heart disease to physical activity or its lack with special reference to sample size and occupational withdrawal. In *Physical Activity in Health and Disease*. Proceedings of the Bertostolen Symposium. Baltimore, William's & Wilkins, 1966.
2. CADY, L.D., JR.: Epidemiology of coronary heart disease. *Amer J Cardiol, 20*:5, 692, 1967.
3. WERBIN, H.; CHAIKOFF, I.L., and IMADA, M.A.: Rapid sensitive method for determining tridium water in body fluids by liquid scintillation spectrometry. *Proc Soc Exp Biol Med, 102*:8, 1959.
4. MASTER, A.M.; FRIEDMAN, R., and DACK, S.: Electrocardiogram after standard exercise as functional test of the heart. *Amer Heart J, 24*:777, 1942.
5. HASKELL, W.L., personal communication.
6. ASTRAND, I.: In Physiology of Muscular Exercise. AHA Monograph. No. 15: 1-212, 1967.
7. MATTINGLY, W.: The post exercise electrocardiogram. Its value in the diagnosis and prognosis of coronary arterial disease. *Amer J Cardiol, 9*: 355, 1962.
8. BLACKBURN, H.; KEYS, A.; SIMONSON, E.; RAUTAHARJU, P., and PUNSAR, S.: The electrocardiogram in population studies. *Circulation, 21*:1160, 1960.
9. ÅSTRAND, I.: Exercise electrocardiogram recorded twice with an eight year interval in a group of 204 women and men 48-63 years old. *Acta Med Scand, 178*:27, 1965.
10. ASSMUSSEN, E.: Muscular exercise. In *Handbook of Physiology*. Amer Physiological Soc., 1965, Vol. II, sect. 3, p. 939.
11. ROWELL, L.B.; TAYLOR, H.L., and WANG, Y.: Limitations to prediction of maximal oxygen uptake. *J Appl Physiol, 19*:919, 1964.
12. BRODY, A.J.: Master two step exercise test in clinically selected patients. *JAMA, 171*:1195, 1959.
13. RUMBALL, C.A., and ACHESON, E.C.: Latent coronary heart disease detected by electrocardiogram before and after exercise. *Brit Med J, 5328*:423, 1963.
14. ROBB, G.P., and MARKS, H.H.: Latent coronary artery disease; determination of its presence and severity by the exercise electrocardiogram. *Amer J Cardiol, 13*:603, 1964.

15. Robb, G.P., and Marks, H.H.: Post exercise electrocardiogram in arteriosclerotic heart disease. Its value in diagnosis and prognosis. *JAMA, 200*:918, 1967.

16. Simonson, E.: Use of the electrocardiogram in exercise tests. *Amer Heart J, 66*:552, 1963.

17. Cohen, L.S.; Elliott, W.C.; Klein, M.D., and Gorlin, R.: Coronary heart disease. Clinical cinearteriographic and metabolic correlations. *Amer J Cardiol, 17*:153, 1966.

18. Likoff, W.; Segal, B.L., and Kasparian, H.: Paradox of normal selective coronary arteriograms in patients considered to have unmistakable coronary heart disease. *Circulation, XXXIV* (suppl. III):157, 1966.

19. Friesinger, G.C.; Likar, I.; Biern, R.O., and Mason, R.E.: Vasoregulatory asthenia. A cause for false positive exercise electrocardiograms. *Circulation, XXXII* (suppl. II):90, 1965.

20. Mason, R.E.; Likar, I.; Biern, R.O., and Ross, R.S.: Multiple lead exercise electrocardiography. *Circulation, 36*:517, 1967.

21. Rowell, L.B.; Taylor, H.L.; Simonson, C.E., and Carlson, W.S.: The physiologic fallacy of adjusting for body weight in performance of the Master two step test. *Amer Heart J, 70*:461, 1965.

22. Haskell, W.L.: Unpublished data.

23. Damato, A.N.; Galante, J.G., and Smith, W.M.: Hemodynamic response to treadmill exercise in normal subjects. *J Appl Physiol, 21*(3):959, 1966.

22

Physiological Factors Influencing the Electrocardiographic Response to Exercise

Eugene Lepeschkin

THE PURPOSE OF THE electrocardiographic exercise test is to obtain objective documentation of a deficiency in the coronary circulation which is not possible by simple means at rest. Of the electrocardiographic changes which may be caused by such a coronary insufficiency (disproportion between coronary flow and the blood demands of the myocardium), changes due to aberrant myocardial repolarization (abnormalities of the S-T segment and the T wave) are more common and specific than those due to aberrant conduction (abnormalities of the P wave, P-R interval or QRS complex), and the present report will deal primarily with the repolarization abnormalities.

According to the most recent work of Kato and co-workers (12) in experimental animals, slight constriction of one of the major branches of the left coronary artery causes slight depression of the S-T segment only in direct leads from the periphery of the epicardial area supplied by this branch; as the degree of constriction increases the S-T depression becomes greater in the periphery and spreads toward the center of this region, but with severe constriction the S-T depression in the central region disappears and is transformed into an elevation while the depression in the peripheral regions increases in magnitude. As leads from the left ventricular cavity and intramural leads from the subendocardial layers of the affected region showed S-T elevation during all degrees of narrowing, the S-T depression in sur-

Note: This investigation was supported by the United States Public Health Service Grant HE-01486 and by a Research Career Award HE-K6-440 from the National Heart Institute to Dr. Lepeschkin.

[363]

face leads is considered reciprocal to this elevation, and due to predominant ischemic injury of the subendocardial ventricular muscle layers, as can be demonstrated with experimental subendocardial injury (38). The reason why the subendocardial layers are the first to suffer injury is (15) because of the systolic transmural pressure gradient. The coronary flow during systole is channeled entirely to the subepicardial layers whenever the pressure in a main coronary branch shows a moderate reduction. When the narrowing is severe, the entire region supplied by the branch shows ischemic injury, the transmural systolic potential gradient which was responsible for the S-T depression disappears and the entire region is now positive in systole with respect to the adjoining normal regions. S-T elevation without S-T depression results also from narrowing of the smaller coronary artery branches which do not extend to the subendocardial layers (28, 29).

In a region of acute ischemic injury, the decreased amplitude of the action potential which is responsible for the elevation of S-T in surface leads from this region is preceded and accompanied by accelerated repolarization, and this latter is responsible for increased positive polarity of the T wave in these leads (16, 28, 29). The same process, confined to the subendocardial layers, is probably responsible for the inversion of T in surface leads which is sometimes observed during mild injury of the subendocardial layers (38). If T wave changes are caused by an acceleration of repolarization, the inversion of T should be preceded by a diphasic T with an initial negative phase, and the total corrected Q-T interval should be short or normal; this is usually true of T wave changes in the early phases of myocardial ischemia. On the contrary, after myocardial ischemia has been present for many minutes or hours, a late inversion of the T wave usually appears where diphasic T waves have a terminal negative phase and the total corrected Q-T interval is prolonged; this is usually true of the T wave inversion appearing during healing of transmural myocardial infarction (16). The inverted T waves caused by repolarization delay in leads from the borders of the infarction can be due in part to the cooling of these regions resulting from reduced metabolism (37) but have been attributed, together with the slight S-T depression (27, 30), mainly to an increased intracellular potassium concentration in the slightly ischemic regions surrounding the region of intense injury.

We shall now try to apply our basic knowledge concerning the electrocardiogram in experimental myocardial ischemia to the interpretation of the exercise test.

The first step in the recognition of an S-T depression caused by absolute or relative myocardial ischemia (coronary insufficiency) is to rule out an instrumentation artifact as a possible cause. With the almost universal use of direct-writing electrocardiographs one of the most common artifacts is caused by over-damping of the stylus, which can be due to too much stylus pressure, too little paper tension (resulting in a wider contact surface between stylus and paper) or too much stylus heat (resulting in increased friction because of tackiness of the plastic paper coating). The result of over-damping is a slow return of the trace to the baseline following the S wave which can simulate a junctional depression of the S-T segment; this can usually be recognized by the slow ascent and return of the square calibration pulse. An important observation of Bradlow's (5) is that such distortion due to over-damping can be present only at the upper, middle or lower level of the record (his Fig. 63), and this is probably due to variations of the stylus pressure or magnetic damping with different positions of the writing arm. This condition may accordingly not become apparent in the calibration unless this is carried out at all levels of the paper or throughout the operating range of the stylus. Appearance of such artifacts only during or after exercise can be the result of a different position of the baseline due to change in skin potentials, of the gradual heating-up of the stylus during longer periods of registration but especially if the paper tension becomes considerably less as the end of the paper roll approaches. Such a false S-T depression can develop during exercise without any change in damping if the voltage of the S wave increases as a result of positional changes; when the heart rate increases and the Q-T interval becomes shorter a false junctional S-T depression can seem to involve the entire S-T segment. It would be therefore of value to insert a calibration periodically throughout the exercise test.

One important artifact which can appear at the end of the paper roll in some machines, due to decrease of paper tension, is slight movement of the paper by the stylus; this results in obliteration of all small electrocardiographic waves (such as P and U waves) and a horizontal course of the S-T segment terminating in a sharp angle with the T wave, without much influence on the larger deflections such as the QRS complex and the calibration pulse. This finding therefore cannot be recognized from the appearance of the calibration pulse. It can, however, be recognized by a blurred appearance of the QRS deflections and by inspection of the paper drive.

Additional artifacts can be introduced by the equipment used to transmit exercise electrocardiograms by means of radio frequency waves (radiocardiogram). Most of this equipment was designed especially for telemetry during exercise, where it is desirable to suppress baseline wandering. The ECG is reproduced with a noncompensated time constant of less than one second. This results in a gradually decaying negative baseline displacement after every positive wave, and therefore in an ascending "false" S-T depression, the magnitude of which is proportional to the area of the previous R wave (16, 21). An increase in the voltage or width of the R wave during exercise will therefore automatically cause a greater "false" S-T depression, and acceleration of the heart will make it appear to extend further into the T wave. In addition, transmitters with automatic frequency control may cause periodic displacement of the S-T segment after each R wave, especially if the "tuning" control is slightly off balance, and the amount of this displacement can change as the transmitter warms up (21, 32). It is therefore very important to adjust the tuning if these artifacts appear (33), and to register the calibration square pulse during exercise periodically by having the patient push the button on the transmitter (not on the receiver or on the electrocardiograph, as is sometimes done). In general, telemetry is invaluable if exercise under natural conditions is being studied, but the additional source of artifacts which it introduces makes a direct electrocardiographic connection preferable if exercise can be carried out at the same location (21).

The baseline wandering which accompanies the violent body movements during exercise makes evaluation of the S-T segment very difficult, and any attempts to filter it out must necessarily filter some components of the S-T segments which have the same frequency spectrum. This is especially important if areas of S-T and T or the ventricular gradient are to be studied. On the other hand, averaging fifteen to

one-hundred consecutive complexes (6, 8), while reducing the artifacts nonsynchronous with the heartbeat, may reduce or even ob-
literate rapid changes in the configuration of T and S-T (in some
patients diagnostic changes may be present only during 5 to 10 beats)
(1). It is much preferable to attempt to reduce this wandering. Part
of this is caused by variations of contact of the patient with regions
of the electrode surface having a different potential. These inhomo-
geneities can be avoided best by using pure silver electrodes after cleaning with virgin sandpaper the cut edges which contain particles of
other metals and by chloriding the electrodes and leaving them connected in an electrolyte solution for several days before using, so that
any battery effects will have exhausted themselves. Another approach
is to keep the resistance between skin and various regions of the electrode as constant as possible even if the electrode should move; this
can be done by avoiding direct contact between electrodes and skin
("liquid junction electrodes") (10). The electrode movement can
also be reduced by attaching the electrodes to the surrounding skin
with plaster or spray cement, to make the wires leading to the electrodes as flexible as possible, and the electrodes themselves as light as
possible. However, even if movement artifacts can be eliminated, the
slow active variations of skin potential which form part of the psycho-
galvanic reflex still remain; these can be reduced by removing as much
as possible of the horn layer of the skin by means of a clean emery
wheel and anesthetizing the skin with Xylocaine®.

The small size of the liquid junction electrodes has the disadvantage
that because of decreased total skin capacity and increased electrode
resistance even with the recommended high input impedance of the
electrocardiographs (100,000 ohms) (13) there may be distortion of
the ECG because of the skin capacity and electrode polarization. This
distortion manifests itself by reduction in size of the R wave and especially the T wave, and initial S-T depression (16, 21). With a 1
cm diameter electrode the input impedence must be greater than 2
megaohms if such distortion is to be avoided (10). Of course, this
effect can always be noticed as it will affect a calibration pulse introduced in series with the patient in the same way as it will the ECG.
These effects can be avoided completely if separate so-called buffer
amplifiers are used at each electrode.

Mechanical artifacts may appear due to skin potentials synchronous with the heartbeat if one or more of the precordial electrodes are placed in the region of the apex beat or jugular or subclavian pulsation, or if any of the limb electrodes are placed in the proximity of the radial artery (16). These artifacts appear in the form of a junctional depression or a sudden change of slope of the S-T segment, and also as a terminal deflection resembling the U wave. The increased force of precordial pulsation during exercise is likely to accentuate these artifacts temporarily. Usually these artifacts appear when the electrode contact is poor or the electrode paste has begun to dry out and there are also other fluctuations of the baseline.

The U wave itself can be considered as a mechanical artifact since this wave, as well as the "after-potentials" appearing in intracellular tracings synchronous with the U wave, seem to correspond to mechanical events during ventricular relaxation (17). The inversion of the U wave during angina, which usually accompanies S-T depression but sometimes may be the only abnormal finding, is probably also related to the sequence of relaxation; in several cases where this isolated U wave inversion appeared after exercise this was accompanied by a late outward movement in the precordial pulsation curve. Under the influence of epinephrine, low external potassium, digitalis or quinidine, the U wave becomes elevated through incorporation of slow "after-potentials" which correspond to a slow terminal phase of the action potential. The U wave accordingly seems to have a rapid "mechanical" and a slow "metabolic" component. Sjöstrand (36) considers only the rapid component as the U wave proper, and the small slow terminal component as an "after-potential," but this is a matter of terminology.

The elevation of the usual positive U wave after exercise, which is probably related to the increase of stroke volume and to discharge of epinephrine, can lead to an elevation of the diastolic T-P interval. This, in turn, will result in a false diagnosis of an S-T depression if the S-T segment is measured from this "false" baseline (line 1 of Fig. 22-1). As the U wave does not show the same degree of shortening with increased heart rate as the Q-T interval (17) it extends into the following P-R segment and QRS complex so that even a line drawn through the initial points of successive QRS complexes (line 2 in Fig. 22-1) cannot be considered the "true" baseline.

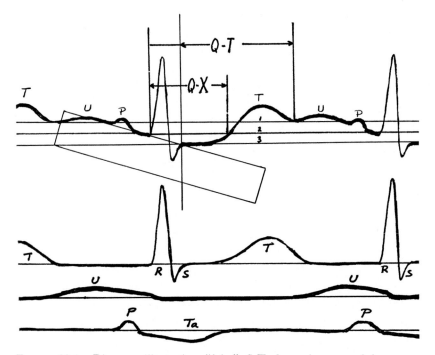

FIGURE 22-1. Diagram illustrating "false" S-T depression caused by super-position of T and P on a high U wave and continuation of a depressed P-Ta segment into the S-T segment. The true form of S-T and T, as well as of the U wave and the atrial P and P-Ta waves, is shown separately below. Using baseline 1, (connecting the points of origin of the P waves), would cause a false diagnosis of marked S-T depression. Using baseline 2, (connecting points of origin of QRS), would still give a sizeable S-T depression, with a Q-X/Q-T over ½. The true baseline can be approximated by holding the edge of a strip of cellophane tape parallel to the last portion of the P-R segment and measuring S-T from the level of the intersection of this edge with the time line corresponding to the end of QRS.

Another factor which makes quantitative evaluation of S-T segment depression difficult is the superposition of the atrial repolarization wave (Ta) on the S-T segment (Fig. 22-1). The Ta wave is usually of opposite polarity to the P wave and the P-Ta segment shows slight displacement in the same direction as Ta. The duration of the P-Ta interval is similar in humans to that of the Q-T interval at the same heart rate (6, 16). The identity of the Ta wave is clearly apparent in esophageal or atrial intracardiac leads, but in the normal resting surface electrocardiogram with upright P waves the P-Ta segment causes only a slight normal depression of the P-R segment while the Ta wave is so low in amplitude that it makes only an inconspicuous dent in the S-T segment or is completely buried in it (15). However, the sympathetic effects of exercise almost always lead to increased P wave amplitude and the tachycardia causes the P-Ta segment to be displaced more strongly and opposite in direction to the P wave. In leads with upright P waves, this causes more marked depression of the P-R segment which continues downward through the QRS complex and causes a "false" depression of the S-T segment even with respect to the P-R level at the beginning of QRS (Fig. 22-1). If the P-R interval is considerably shortened, the ascending phase of the inverted Ta wave contributes to an ascending configuration of the S-T segment. If P-R is longer, the apparently depressed S-T segment has an initial downward slope. One practical method of avoiding interference of atrial repolarization with the S-T segment would be to utilize leads where the P wave is very low, iso-electric or diphasic; this is more often true of leads from the precordial region to the back or the central terminal than of leads to the head or the right arm.

To approximate the true baseline from which the S-T level could be measured, the author (18) proposed to measure the amplitude of S-T segment displacement from the intersection of a tangent to the last portion of the P-R segment and a vertical line at the end of the QRS complex (Fig. 22-1). Using the edge of a transparent plastic ruler as the tangent, the distance of the S-T segment from this intersection can be estimated in units of a quarter of a millimeter (0.025 mv). With practice this estimate can be made to within 0.1 mm (0.01 mv). Care must be taken not to consider a horizontal or ascending initial portion of QRS as the end of the P-R segment. If the P-R interval is so short that there is no clearcut P-R segment, a straight line between the beginning and end of P must be used as the nearest approach to the P-R tangent.

When this method of S-T measurement was used, thirty (12.5 per cent) of 243 apparently normal students showed a depression of the S-T segment junction exceeding 0.5 mm immediately after the double Master two-step exercise test (55 or 23 per cent showed such a depression if the P-R level at the beginning of QRS was used as the reference). Only twenty (8 per cent) showed a depression of ¾ or more mm and this was proposed as a diagnostic criterion. Hellerstein (10a) found this latter value too restrictive when applied to cases with rheumatic heart disease.

The method of extending the P-R segment into QRS probably causes a slight overcompensation for the negative Ta wave amplitude since the P-Ta segment is curved. However, it does not compensate for the elevation of the T-P and P-R segments by the descending branch of a tall U wave. Theoretically, residual depolarization after the action potential does not extend into the following action potential but is cut short by it; in other words, a U wave should not extend into the following S-T segment. Sjöstrand (36) found that in young, healthy persons there was a direct relationship between the level of S-T segment and the heart rate which was constant for the same person whether the changes of heart rate were caused by exercise, vagolytic or sympathomimetic drugs. Compared to the P-R level, S-T was slightly elevated at rates below 70 to 80 but became iso-electric at a rate of 100 to 110 and showed a depression of up to 2 mm at higher rates. When the S-T displacement at a given heart rate was subtracted algebraically from its displacement at the lowest heart rate and the result plotted against the corresponding time interval between QRS and the previous T wave, the curve had the form of the U wave with a slow terminal portion ("after-potential"). Some of the S-T segment depression observed in Sjöstrand's studies may have been caused by continuation of the Ta segment but his conclusions are correct in general, and should certainly be taken into consideration in any evaluation of the electrocardiogram at high heart rates. One practical approach to compensation for the effect of the U wave in exercise tracings would be to measure the distance from the end of QRS to the apex of the preceeding U wave (which can be identified easily even at very high heart rates) and to subtract the amplitude of the U wave in the resting tracing at this distance from its apex from the observed exercise S-T depression. Another approach is to produce a momentary slowing of the heart after exercise by means of carotid pressure or the Valsalva maneuver sufficient to bring the QRS complex out of range of the U wave.

After excluding "false" depressions of the S-T segment after exercise we must consider "true" S-T depression appearing as a normal

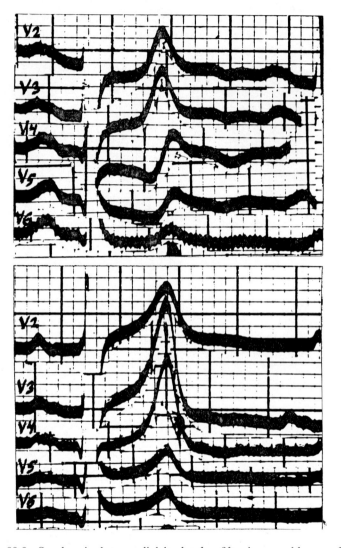

FIGURE 22-2. Synchronized precordial leads of a fifty-six-year-old man. Upper
half, during an anginal attack induced by exercise. The upper tracing shows true
ascending S-T depression in V_{2-3}, descending S-T depression and diphasic T
waves in V_{4-5} and only minimal S-T depression in V_6. U waves are also
inverted in V_2 through V_5. Apparently in this case only a small region of
subendocardial ischemia was present in the antero-septal region. In the lower
tracing, taken after all pain had disappeared, the T waves are peaked but
still within normal limits. The U wave is still inverted in leads V_3 and V_4.

result of tachycardia and the consequent steeper slope of the "plateau" or initial repolarization ("phase 2") of the action potential (16) (Fig. 22-2). This depression usually is greatest at the beginning of the S-T segment. It is proportional to the QRS voltage and to the ratio of QRS duration to Q-T duration (both show shortening with rise of heart rate but there are indiviual differences). This relationship has been found for the amplitude of the T wave (*see later*). All factors which cause an increased slope of the plateau accentuate this effect. This is probably why significant S-T depression after exercise can appear in persons with nonischemic hearts in the presence of digitalis medication or hypokalemia (19). As in bundle branch block, this type of S-T depression occurs only in leads with a positive value of QRS area while in leads with a negative QRS area the S-T segment shows upward displacement (16). Perhaps the total area of QRST (19), or the algebraic sum of the QRS area and the area of the first half of the S-T segment and T wave, as have been determined by computer (35), could, when related to the heart rate, differentiate between this type of S-T depression and that due to myocardial ischemia. Another method of differentiation might derive from the fact that S-T displacement due to early repolarization is not accompanied by change in the diastolic baseline while that due to myocardial ischemia is caused largely by an opposite shift of the diastolic baseline due to injury potentials which disappear in systole (16, 28, 34). However, a practical differentiation would be difficult even with use of D-C amplifiers since the changes of skin potentials during exercise usually exceed any changes due to cardiac injury currents.

We have seen that most "normal" S-T depressions during exercise involve only the initial portion of the S-T segment. They are due either to artifacts arising at the electrodes, or in the transmitting, amplifying or registering systems, or to superposition of atrial Ta waves or accelerated repolarization. In contrast, injury currents caused by myocardial ischemia involve the entire S-T segment. It is not surprising that from an empirical point of view, ascending or "junctional" S-T segment depression has been considered harmless while the horizontal or descending S-T depression, called "ischemic" by P. Wood, corresponded better to clinical angina (4, 7, 25, 26) and to a mortality rate 4.3 times that expected for age and sex (19, 31). This relates to the observation (8) that S-T voltages sampled at a greater distance from the nadir of the S waves gave more satisfactory differentiation between the responses of normal persons and angina patients. The horizontal or descending course was originally defined (31) as one involving at least the first 0.08 seconds or more of the S-T segment. However, as the Q-T interval and the S-T segment are shorter at high than at low heart rates, an absolute duration criterion was considered misleading and a relative criterion, the Q-X/Q-T ratio, was introduced (18). This ratio expressed the duration of the portion of the S-T segment below the line connecting successive ends of the P-R intervals. Only nine (3.3 per cent) of the 272 apparently normal persons showed "true" S-T depression over 0.75 mm and a QX/Q-T ratio over 50 per cent (18). Other quantitative methods used for diagnostic differentiation are measurement of the area of the depressed portion of S-T (19), the area of the first half of the interval from end of QRS to the end of T (35), and the slope of the S-T segment in relation to the amount of junctional depression (23).

While most laboratories consider an "ischemic" S-T depression as abnormal or "significant" if it exceeds 0.5 mm (0.05 mv) (4, 7, 10a, 19, 25), the values of 0.75 mm (18) and 1 mm (1, 6, 31) have been employed to exclude as many apparently normal persons as possible. However, this also excludes an increasing number of patients with typical clinical angina. It is clear that any quantitative criterion based on the voltage of S-T should take into consideration general factors which modify electrocardiographic voltages such as the distance of the electrodes from the heart, the configuration of the chest and the conductivity of tissues surrounding the heart as well as hypertrophy of ventricular muscle fibers. All these factors modify the voltage of QRS in the same direction, and it should increase diagnostic accuracy if the amount of S-T depression were related to the voltage of QRS in that lead. For example, the "normal" and abnormal S-T depression as well as the QRS voltage are greater in the unipolar left precordial leads than in the limb leads, and greater still in bipolar chest leads used for monitoring and radiocardiography (1, 2, 4, 6, 8, 7, 24, 32, 39).

In recent statistical studies of Mattingly (31), persons showing junctional type S-T depression after exercise were found to have the same or even lower mortality rates than those without S-T depression. However, in this study no differentiation was made between "false" junctional S-T depression which is likely to occur in young, vigorous persons and "true" deep junctional S-T depression. Most observers consider a junctional depression of 1-1.5 mm or more as pathological (1, 4) and in many cases such a depression is found to precede deep ischemic S-T depression (1, 2, 8). Perhaps in these cases the elevation of T appearing toward the end of exercise and attributed to a rise of serum potassium (*see later*) masks the end of a true "ischemic" S-T depression. In most cases junctional depression is present in some leads while "ischemic" depression is seen in others (Fig. 22-3). In the latest statistics of Master (25, 26) all patients with junctional depression showing a Q-X/Q-T ratio over 50 per cent had clinical angina. It must be emphasized, however, that this ratio includes "false" together with "true" S-T depression. More significant values could be obtained perhaps if this ratio were determined with respect to a straight line connecting the point of intersection of the continuation of P-R with the time line at the end of QRS and the T-U junction, but new criteria would have to be established for this measurement.

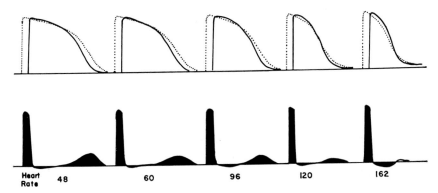

| Heart Rate | 48 | 60 | 96 | 120 | 162 |

Figure 22-3. Effect of heart on the configuration of the action potential of human subepicardial ventricular muscle (from W. Trautwein, D. G. Kassenbaum, R. M. Nelson and H. H. Hecht, Electrophysiological study of human heart muscle. *Circulation Res.*, 10:306, 1962) and on the constructed electrocardiogram (22) (*see text*).

We now consider factors which modify the T wave during and after exercise. Increased heart rate in itself displaces the T wave in a direction opposite to that of the QRS complex (16) as illustrated in Figure 22-3. The continuous line tracings of the action potential in this figure are actual epicardial action potentials from excised human ventricular muscle recorded at different rates of stimulation. The dotted curves are endocardial action potentials constructed on the assumption that they begin 0.04 seconds earlier and have the same form but a total duration 15 per cent longer than their epicardial counterparts. (The longer duration is related mainly to the lower temperature [37] and higher potassium content [30] of these layers.) The surface electrocardiogram, constructed as the difference between the two action potentials (16) shows only minimal S-T depression at low heart rates. As the rate approaches 100 this depression increases while the amplitude of the positive T wave decreases until at a rate of 160 frank S-T depression and a diphasic configuration of the T wave appears. We have studied the effect of heart rate changes under the influence of atropine in normal volunteers (22) and found that there is a straight-line relationship between the heart rate and the voltage of the T wave; the slope of this line was on the average 0.037 mv for every 10-beat change in rate in lead II, but it differed for each individual. The slope showed a positive correlation to the amplitude of the T wave at rest, to the amplitude of R and R+S, to the QRS area and to the decrease of Q-T and Q-T/QRS with rising heart rate. At heart rates ranging from 100 to 260 (on the average, 186) all the lines intersected the isoelectric line and at higher rates the T waves became diphasic or inverted.

During exercise many other factors than tachycardia are known to cause T wave inversion in apparently normal persons. Among these are postural change, i.e., assumption of the upright position, sympathetic stimulation with discharge of epinephrine, and hyperventilation. To study these inter-relationships a group of young women, in whom the effect of epinephrine infusions had been studied previously (20), were given a Master double two-step test. The electrocardiogram was also registered immediately after standing up just prior to the exercise test. In Figure 22-4 the amplitude of the T wave in lead II was plotted against the heart rate and the value at rest for each person

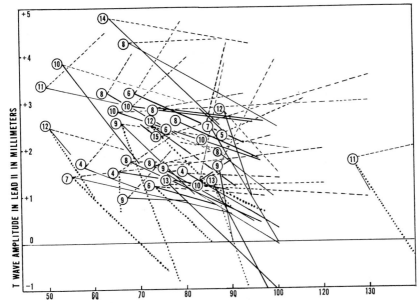

Figure 22-4. Relation of the T wave amplitude in lead II to the heart rate in thirty-five normal young women at rest (*circles*), after standing up (*heavy line* terminating in "S"), immediately after the double Master two-step exercise test (*interrupted line*) and after a five-minute infusion of 2 μg epinephrine per minute (*plain heavy line*). The numbers in the circles indicate the mean potential of QRS in lead II in millimeters.

was connected by means of straight lines to the corresponding values after standing up, one minute after termination of exercise (recumbent) and one minute after beginning of an infusion of epinephrine (recumbent). As was previously found for atropine, epinephrine and standing up caused the T wave to become lower as the heart rate increased; the lines connecting the T wave amplitudes show a downward slope, but this slope is steeper for epinephrine and especially the upright position than for atropine. In both cases the lines intersect the O-line, i.e., the T wave tends to become iso-electric and then inverted as a certain heart rate is reached, but the rate for T inversion is faster for epinephrine than for the upright posture. On the contrary, the lines connecting the amplitude at rest with that after exercise are horizontal or slope upward, i.e., the T wave remains the same or increases in amplitude although much higher heart rates are reached. In general, the angle between the exercise and epinephrine lines tends to be similar between individuals. That is, persons who show marked T wave elevation after exercise usually show a smaller-than-average decrease of T amplitude under postural change or epinephrine at comparable heart rates.

One of the causes of the relative elevation of T amplitude immediately after exercise is undoubtedly the elevation of serum potassium liberated from the working muscles (see the paper of G. Blomqvist in this volume). Another mechanism studied only in animals (37) is increased heat production in the ventricular myocardium, combined with relative cooling of the subendocardial muscle layers because of the increased heart output. This accentuates the transmural temperature gradient which is in part responsible for the positive polarity of T waves. These factors are probably responsible also for the "normalization" after exercise of "functional" T wave inversion, sometimes seen in apparently normal persons.

In an attempt to determine the relative contribution to postexercise electrocardiographic changes of acceleration of the heart rate, sympathetic nervous influence and persistence postexercise of hyperventilation, all exercise tests carried out in this center during the last ten years were preceded by a multiple-lead electrocardiogram taken after thirty seconds of intense hyperventilation and another taken immediately after standing up and just prior to the exercise. Analysis of the findings in 346 consecutive exercise tests (164 of these were analyzed together with Dr. B. Surawicz) are presented in Table 22-I. In ninety-two of these patients the response of the S-T segment was considered abnormal on the basis of the criteria previously developed (depression of the S-T segment junction 0.75 mm or more below the projected reference from the P-R interval, a simultaneous Q-X/Q-T ratio exceeding 50 per cent, *and* a depression of 0.5 mm or more lasting two or more minutes beyond the end of exercise). In 252 persons the response was less than these normal limits. The age of the patients with an abnormal response was higher than of those showing a normal response, but the surprising finding was that the percentage of women in the group with abnormal responses was much higher than in the group with normal responses. This finding is emphasized by other speakers at this conference and may be related to the fact that women

TABLE 22-I

INCIDENCE OF NORMAL (N) AND ABNORMAL (A)

T WAVE RESPONSE TO EXERCISE (E), ORTHOSTATIC POSITION (O)

AND 30-SECOND HYPERVENTILATION (H) IN 346 PATIENTS WITH NORMAL

OR ABNORMAL S-T RESPONSE TO EXERCISE

S-T	T-wave O	H	No.	%	% ♀	Age	% Ve	% Ho	F_o	F_H	Rest T (mm) II	V	Abnormal T (%) E	E>OH	F<
N	N	N	207	82	27	47	30	35	89	95	1.89	4.69	3.2	3.2	0.5
	A	N	14	5.5	29	45	37	7	93	94	1.18	2.80	34	7	0
	N	A	12	4.5	33	43	33	58	88	115	1.38	3.27	50	16	8
	A	A	19	7.5	47	48	32	26	101	105	0.88	2.01	41	5.3	5.3
Total			252	100	29	47	31	32					10	3.8	1.3
A	N	N	76	81	39	53	25	37	87	93	1.49	4.04	45	45	32
	A	N	9	9.5	56	54	11	55	87	89	1.06	2.72	79	44	0
	N	A	4	4.3	50	56	25	50	84	104	1.50	3.10	100	50	50
	A	A	5	5.3	20	53	40	40	99	109	0.65	3.50	80	40	0
Total			94	100	40	53	30	39					52	45	28

Ve = vertical, Ho = Horizontal electric heart position. F = heart rate; E>OH = T wave abnormality is greater after exercise than after standing up or hyperventilation. F< = same as E>OH, but heart rate at this time is smaller than or equal to that after H or O.

have, in general, a more horizontal S-T segment and lower T waves than men. The same amount of "ischemic" S-T depression may more easily make the electrocardiogram abnormal in women than in men. An alternate explanation could be that, because of the well-known predominance of coronary disease among men, physicians may tend to order an exercise test for women only if typical clinical symptoms of angina are present, but such selection factors are difficult to demonstrate objectively.

In 82 per cent of the nomal and 81 per cent of the abnormal exercise responses based on S-T response, there were no T wave abnormalities (defined as inverted or iso-electric T in any of leads I, II, V_2, V_4, V_5 or V_6) either in the upright position of the orthostatic test or after hyperventilation. In 18 per cent of the normal and 19 per cent of the abnormal S-T responses to exercise the T wave became inverted during hyperventilation, or on standing, or both, and there was no significant difference in the age of these persons compared to those with a normal T wave response. However, among persons with an abnormal response there was a significantly higher percentage of women, especially for the hyperventilation response. Persons with normal S-T exercise response but showing orthostatic T wave abnormalities were less likely to have horizontal electrical heart positions than persons not showing them. The greatest differences between the groups with normal and abnormal T concerned the maximal heart rates reached during hyperventilation or orthostatic position. Heart rates were definitely higher in persons showing T wave abnormalities, and the resting T wave amplitude was lower in both limb and precordial leads. Apparently the line of the dependence of T amplitude on heart rate starts from a lower level in these people.

The comparison between T wave abnormalities during hyperventilation or standing with those after exercise is of great diagnostic value. In 3.2 per cent of normal S-T segment reactions the T wave became inverted after exercise but not after standing up or hyperventilation. In all but 0.5 per cent of these the heart rate during exercise was higher than that during the other maneuvers. Almost half of the persons showing T wave abnormalities after hyperventilation and/or standing also showed them after exercise. The T wave findings were *greater* after exercise in only about 8 per cent, and the heart rate at this time was lower in only about 5 per cent. On the contrary, almost half of the persons with abnormal S-T response showed greater T wave abnormalities after exercise than after standing or hyperventilation, and in a third this happened despite the fact that the rate after exercise was lower. In other words, in persons who have a tendency to T wave inversion at high heart rates under the influence of sympathetic stimulation, this will appear also after exercise, but the response will not be greater after exercise unless the heart rate at that time exceeds that after hyperventilation or standing. If an "ischemic" S-T response is registered after exercise the incidence of T wave inversion is much higher, and it is more pronounced than after hyperventilation or standing, although the heart rate after exercise is lower.

Master originally considered inversion of the T wave after his exercise test as an abnormal response, but lately he accepts only inversion of 1.5 mm or more as definitely abnormal (25). In his latest statistical summary, Robb (31) finds that persons with inversion of T after exercise as the only abnormality have a mortality 1.2 times higher than expected. Such a response is often the only abnormality in persons with documented pervious infarctions (10a) or abnormal coronary angiograms (2, 24, 7). Usually T wave inversion appears late after exercise, when the significant "ischemic" S-T depression is subsiding. Theoretically, it could be a counterpart of the late T wave inversion appearing in leads from the border regions of myocardial infarction (*see earlier*) and it is possible that in some cases the stage of S-T displacement which precedes it is either too transient or too small to be diagnostically significant. This form of T wave inversion is accompanied by a prolongation of the corrected Q-T interval. This may be one way to differentiate it from "harmless" T wave inversion (19, 25). We have seen that "harmless" T inversion appears only at high heart rates and in leads with a positive QRS area. An orthostatic or hyperventilation test could be a useful method of differentiation. Finally, repetition of the exercise test after pretreatment with sympatholytic drugs can eliminate apparently abnormal T wave responses due to tachycardia and sympathetic stimulation (3, 25), but since these factors can contribute to the appearance of coronary insufficiency after exercise in coronary sclerosis (29) such pretreatment can also cause true coronary disease to remain electrocardiographically silent. More experience in this regard is needed.

CONCLUSION

In conclusion I must say that the tremendous advances in data storage and computer analysis have given us the tools to develop and apply new criteria for the differentiation between a normal and abnormal electrocardiographic response. It would be a waste of resources to utilize only the criteria now in use, obtained by more cumbersome and artifact-prone means. Because of cost and space limitations the new analytical methods are now applied usually to a limited number of leads, but since the abnormal electrocardiographic responses in different parts of a diseased heart may partially neutralize each other, only application of multiple precordial leads from the entire cardiac region, or even intracardiac leads may give us the desired information in *all* subjects.

REFERENCES

1. ABARQUEZ, R.F. JR.; KINTANAR, Q.L.; VALDEZ, E.V., and DAYRIT, C.: Evaluation of some criteria for the dynamic and postexercise electrocardiogram in diagnosing coronary insufficiency. *Amer J Cardiol, 13*: 310-319; *14*:275-277, 1964.

2. ARESKOG, N.H.; BJÖRK, L.; BJÖRK, V.O.; HALLEN, A., and STRÖM, G.: Physical work capacity, ECG reaction to work tests and coronary angiogram in coronary artery disease. *Acta Med Scand, 472* (suppl.):9-35, 1967.

3. ARVEDSON, O.; FURBERG, C., and LINDERHOLM, H.: The effect of a gangionic blocking agent (chlorisondamine) on electrocardiogram, physical working capacity and hemodynamics in patients with vasoregulatory asthenia. *Acta Med Scand, 472* (suppl.): 36-53, 1967.

4. ÅSTRAND, I.: Exercise electrocardiograms in a 5-year follow-up study. *Acta Med Scand, 173*:257-268, 1963.

5. BRADLOW, B.A.: *How to Produce a Readable Electrocardiogram.* Springfield, Thomas, 1964.

6. BLOMQUIST, G.: The Frank lead exercise electrocardiogram. *Acta Med Scand, 440* (suppl.):1-98, 1965.

7. BELLET, S., and ROMAN, L.: Comparison of the double two-step test and the maximal exercise treadmill test. *Circulation, 36*:238-244, 1967.

8. BRUCE, R.A.; MAZZARELLA, J.A.; JORDAN, J.W., and GREEN, E.: Quantitation

of QRS and ST segment responses to exercise. *Amer Heart J, 71*:455-466, 1966.

9. DOAN, A.E.; PETERSON, D.R.; BLACKMON, J.R., and BRUCE, R.A.: Myocardial ischemia after maximal exercise in healthy men. *Amer J Cardiol, 17*:9-19, 1966.

10. GEDDES, L.A.; BAKER, L.E., and MOORE, A.G.: The use of liquid-junction electrodes in recording the human electrocardiogram (ECG) *J Electrocardiol, 1*:51-56, 1968.

10a. HELLERSTEIN, H.K.; PROZAN, G.B.; LIEBOW, I.M.; DOAN, A.E., and HENDERSON, J.A.: Two-step exercise test as a test of cardiac function in chronic rheumatic heart disease and in arteriosclerotic heart disease with old myocardial infarction, *Amer J Cardiol, 7*:234-252, 1961.

11. ISAACS, G.H.; WILBURNE, M.; MILLS, H.; KUHN, R.; COLE, S.L., and STAIN, H.: The ischemic T loop during and following exercise. A vectorelectrocardiographic (VECG) study. *J Electrocardiol, 1*:57-76, 1968.

12. KATO, K.; FUKUDA, H., and KOYAMA, S.: Depression of the S-T segments in the epicardial electrocardiogram associated with major coronary artery constriction. *J Electrocardiol, 1*:167-174, 1968.

13. KOSSMANN, CH. E.; BRODY, D.A.; BURCH, G.E.; HECHT, H.H.; JOHNSTON, F.D.; KAY, C.; LEPESCHKIN, E., and PIPBERGER, H.V.: Recommendations for standardization of leads and of specifications for instruments in electrocardiography and vectorcardiography. *Circulation, 25*:583-602, 1967.

14. LACHMAN, A.B.; SEMLER, H.J., and GUSTAFSON, R.H.: Postural ST-T changes in the radioelectrocardiogram simulating myocardial ischemia. *Circulation, 31*:567-583, 1965.

15. LEPESCHKIN, E.: Uber das Elektrokardiogramm bei experimenteller Koronarinsuffizienz. *Cardiologia, 2*:236-272, 1938.

16. LEPESCHKIN, E.: *Modern Electrocardiography*. Baltimore, Williams & Wilkins, 1951, Vol. I(The QRSTU Complex).

17. LEPESCHKIN, E.: The U wave of the electrocardiogram. *Arch Intern Med, 96*:600-617, 1955.

18. LEPESCHKIN, E., and SURAWICZ, B.: Characteristics of true-positive and false-positive results of electrocardiographic Master two-step exercise tests, *New Eng J Med, 268*:511-520, 1958.

19. LEPESCHKIN, E.: Exercise tests in the diagnosis of coronary heart disease. *Circulation, 22*:986-1001, 1960.

20. LEPESCHKIN, E.; MARCHET, H.; SCHROEDER, G.; WAGNER, R.; SILVA, P., and RAAB, W.: Effect of epinephrine and norepinephrine on the electrocardiogram in 100 normal subjects. *Amer J Cardiol, 5*:594-603, 1960.

21. LEPESCHKIN, E.: Electrocardiographic instrumentation. *Prog Cardiovasc Dis, 5*:498-520, 1963.

22. LEPESCHKIN, E.; NAWATA, Y., and SILVA, P.: Relation of QRS and Q-T

to the effect of heart rate on the T wave in normals. *Fed Proc, 24*:136, 1965.

23. LESTER, F.M.; SHEFFIELD, L.T., and REEVES, T.J.: Electrocardiographic changes in clinically normal older men following near maximal and maximal exercise. *Circulation, 24*:5-14, 1967.

24. MASON, R.E.; LIKAR, I.; BIERN, R.O., and ROSS, R.S.: Multiple-lead exercise electrocardiography. *Circulation, 36*:517-525, 1967.

25. MASTER, A.M., and ROSENFELD, I.: Two-step exercise test: Current status after twenty-five years. *Mod Conc Cardiovasc Dis, 36*:19-24, 1967.

26. MASTER, A.M., and ROSENFELD, I.: Current status of the two-step exercise test. *J Electrocardiol, 1*:5-6, 1968.

27. PRINZMETAL, M.; TOYOSHIMA, H.; EKMEKCI, A.; MIZUNO, Y., and NAGAYA, T.: Myocardial ischemia: Nature of ischemic electrocardiographic patterns in the mammalian ventricles as determined by intracellular and electrographic and metabolic changes. *Amer J Cardiol, 8*:493, 1961.

28. PRINZMETAL, M.; ISHIKAWA, K.; NAKASHIMA, N.; OISHI, H.; OZKAN ,E.. and BAINES, J.M.: Correlation between intracellular and surface electrograms in acute myocardial ischemia. *J Electrocardiol, 1*:(161-166), 1968.

29. RAAB, W.; VANLITH, P.; LEPESCHKIN, E., and HERRLICH, H.C.: Catecholamine-induced myocardial hypoxia in the presence of impaired coronary dilatability, independent of external cardiac work. *Amer J Cardiol, 9*:455-470, 1962.

30. RAAB, W.; KIMURA, H., and LEPESCHKIN, E.: Unpublished observations.

31. ROBB, C.G., and MARKS, H.H.: Post-exercise ECG in arteriosclerotic heart disease, *JAMA, 200*:918-926, 1967.

32. ROSENFELD, I.; MASTER, A.M., and ROSENFELD, C.: Recording of the electrocardiogram during the performance of the Master two-step test. *Circulation, 29*:204-211; 212-218, 1964.

33. SANDLER, G.: Comparison of radiocardiography and conventional electrocardiography in the exercise tolerance test. *Brit Heart J, 29*:719-724, 1967.

34. SAYEN, J.J.; PEIRCE, G.; KATCHER, A.H., and SHELDON, W.F.: Correlation of intramyocardial electrocardiograms with polarographic oxygen and contractility in the non-ischemic and regionally ischemic left ventricle. *Circ Res, 9*:1268-1279, 1961.

35. SMITH, R.F., and WHERRY, R.J., JR.: Quantitative interpretation of the exercise electrocardiogram: Use of computer techniques in the cardiac evaluation of aviation personnel, *Circulation, 34*:1044-1055, 1966.

36. SJÖSTRAND, T.: The relationship between the heart frequency and the S-T level of the electrocardiogram. *Acta Med Scand, 138*:200-210, 1950; *Acta Physiol Scand, 24*:247, 1951.

37. TAKAHASHI, N.; HERRLICH, H.C., and LEPESCHKIN, E.; Unpublished observations.

38. Zakopoulos, K.S.; Herrlich, H.C., and Lepeschkin, E.: Effects of subendocardial injury on the electrocardiogram of intact dogs. *Amer J Physiol, 213*:143-149, 1967.
39. Blackburn, H.; Taylor, H.L.; Okamoto, N.; Rautaharju, P.M.; Mitchell, P.L., and Kerkhof, A.C.: A systemic comparison of chest lead configurations employed for monitoring during exercise. *Physical Activity and the Heart*. Karvonen, M. and Barry, A. (Eds.), Springfield, Thomas, 1967, chapt. 9.

DISCUSSION

Dr. Simonson: Thank you. Are there any questions.?

Dr. Hinkle: I would like to ask a question about something we are seeing on our day-long monitoring of people under ordinary conditions and activities. There are changes in the T wave in relation to posture and to various activities. These are frequently pronounced and it is very hard for us to interpret this. Also we see, as I think many others have also, a serial change in the form of the T waves after exercise. Initially there is a loss of the T wave and sometimes inversion, but as the exercise ends there is the most peaking, so if one does not observe all the way through, one misses these things.

I'm bewildered about the relation of these T wave findings to coronary circulation. They certainly appear in many people, including young women and quite young men and children, in whom one would not expect heart disease, and yet, if one finds an inversion of the T wave sometime during the day, there may be some association with coronary heart disease.

Dr. Lepeschkin: I would say that in most cases, this inversion of the T wave of a "functional" nature can be normalized by giving oral potassium, while inversion of the T wave in a coronary patient usually becomes accentuated or it is not changed by potassium. I have summarized about 1200 cases from the literature where a potassium test was given, and I am sure that the serum potassium plays a great role in the T wave changes after epinephrine and exercise. Dr. E. Kimura, in his study of orthostatic T wave changes, found that the resting serum potassium in those persons who did show a T wave inversion was definitely lower than those who didn't show it.

Dr. Friedell: I wonder if respiration or respiratory disease would influence the change in the serum potassium in these patients?

Dr. Lepeschkin: Well, we know that anything that increases the carbon dioxide concentration also is accompanied by an elevation of serum potassium. And also we have studied the effect of temperature. We have been trying to find how much respiration has to do with the normal polarity of the T wave in the ventricular gradient, so we asked a series of persons to breathe air which has exactly the same temperature as their body temperature, and the T waves became lower under these conditions but the venticular gradient did not disappear. It became smaller but retained its normal direction, so I think that the cooling of the subendocardial regions of the heart is partly responsible for T wave changes.

Dr. Hinkle: I might mention in this connection one other phenomenon we have observed. One sees a certain number of persons who in the supine position show an inverted T wave in their ECG, but after exercise these become upright and remain upright for the rest of the day. Most of those whom we observed have been suspected of having coronary heart disease.

Dr. Lepeschkin: Persons with abnormal electrocardiograms at rest were not included in this table, but we have made a separate study of them. In most of these with "functional" T wave changes, the T wave becomes upright after exercise, and also after potassium, but in the coronaries or persons after myocardial infarction, the T waves often become *more* negative after exercise.

Dr. Simonson: Several years ago we had a small series conducted by Dr. Kahn and myself in the Laboratory of Physiological Hygiene on the effect on the electrocardiogram of strenuous exercise in army personnel. We did not find a significant individual correlation between serum potassium changes during work and T wave amplitude. Usually we are seeking to describe recovery changes in more exact physical terms, in terms of oxygen consumption or myocardial oxygen consumption, but we should be aware that exercise also has an emotional effect. Dr. Lepeschkin's approach may be very interesting in that respect. I was fascinated by the changes produced by epinephrine. I recently became interested in the stress of driving an automobile, and we do see T wave changes in this activity. There was a recent series published in England in which the author found during automobile driving approximately 30 to 40 per cent of persons showing T wave inversion. They then gave atropine and the T wave did not change. We have also just started a series taking the ECG while automobile driving, together with other variables, GSR and EEG and so on, but we have not yet any results. In any case you do see significant T wave changes of an emotional origin. This, of course, is very well known. I want to thank all speakers for excellent and fascinating presentations.

23

Quantitative Effects of Physical Conditioning on the Exercise Electrocardiogram of Middle-aged Subjects with Arteriosclerotic Heart Disease

STEPHEN H. SALZMAN, HERMAN K. HELLERSTEIN, JOHN D. RADKE, HERBERT W. MAISTELMAN *and* RAY RICKLIN

INTRODUCTION

EXERCISE ELECTROCARDIOGRAPHY is a valuable and sensitive clinical tool which may be used to identify subclinical heart disease. Proof of the clinical importance of exercise ECG abnormalities, especially of the ST-T complex, have been provided by epidemiologic and laboratory observations. Depending on the criteria used for evaluation (1), abnormalities in the exercise ECG are associated with an increased mortality rate (2, 3) and an increased rate of new coronary events (4, 5). Changes in the ST-T complex reflect inadequacy of myocardial nutrition and can be elicited by the experimental production of myocardial oxygen deficiency due to ischemia (6) or disproportionate oxygen needs.

Although impressive scientific justification now exists for the clinical and epidemiologic use of exercise tests, lack of standardization has made comparisons between the data of different investigators difficult. Some of the important variables needing standardization include the type and intensity of exercise, and methods for recording and analysis of the ECG by man or computer (7, 8).

Note: This study was supported in part by grants from United States Public Health Service RE 06304, from the Republic Steel Corporation through the Health Fund of Greater Cleveland, and from Mr. and Mrs. William H. Loveman.

[388]

Recent studies of normal and cardiac subjects have shown that the sensitivity of exercise tests is dependent on the work level performed (9-12). The number of abnormal tests and the slope and displacement of the ST segment vary quantitatively with the intensity of the exercise. Therefore in order to make meaningful comparisons the intensity of the work performed, either as external work or as a per cent of maximal aerobic power, must be identical.

The importance of the difference between normal and abnormal ECG responses to exercise has been established by the reported follow-up mortality data of Mattingly and Robb and Marks (2, 3). These authors have evaluated exercise tests as a binomial function, i.e., in terms of a population with only two kinds of responses, either normal or abnormal. Lester *et al.* (10) have reported a simple reproducible method of hand analysis of the exercise ECG which allows the option of binomial categorization and expresses the ST-T complex response to exercise as a continuous function in terms of ST-J displacement and slope of the ST segment.

The purpose of the present report is to study the quantitative effects of physical conditioning on the exercise electrocardiogram of subjects with arteriosclerotic heart disease. A modification of the method of Lester *et al.* (10) has been combined with the criteria of Robb and Marks (3) to classify the exercise ECG.

MATERIALS AND METHODS

The exercise electrocardiograms of one-hundred men, mean age 48 ± 0.72 years, with a clinical diagnosis of arteriosclerotic heart disease (ASHD) were analyzed prior to, and after an average of thirty-three months (range 6-67 months) participation in a program designed to enhance their physical fitness. Details of the Western Reserve University Physical Fitness Evaluation Program have been presented elsewhere (13, 14). The subjects were white, middle-aged, middle and upper class businessmen, executives, managers and professionals. Sixty-six subjects previously sustained a myocardial infarct of whom twenty-seven had angina pectoris. An additional fourteen subjects had typical angina pectoris and twenty subjects had atypical left anterior chest pain and abnormal exercise electrocardiograms.

The following data were obtained on each study subject: detailed cardiovascular history, physical examination, somatotype, skinfold measurements, serum cholesterol and triglycerides, estimation of obesity, resting and exercise ECG, ECG Flack Test (15) and bicycle exercise ergometry.

Submaximal exercise testing on a mechanically braked bicycle ergometer (16) (Monark, Sweden) consisted of intervals of six minutes of exercise alternating with four minutes of rest. Beginning at an initial work load of 300 kilopond meters per minute (kpm/min) work loads were progressively increased by increments of 150 kpm/min for each interval until a heart rate of 150 per minute was reached in the last two minutes of exercise. Three work loads were usually required to attain or exceed this end-point. The electrocardiogram was monitored continuously and recorded at minute intervals throughout the pre-exercise, exercise and recovery periods. Left brachial artery blood pressure was recorded by the cuff method.

In order to reduce the effects of extraneous factors on the results of the tests, the subjects entered the laboratory at least two hours after a standard light meal. They were carefully instructed in the procedures of the ergometric tests. This included a period of at least ten minutes during which they remained seated on the bicycle and repeated electrocardiograms and measurements of blood pressure were made. A warm-up period consisting of several minutes pedaling at 50 rpm with a work load of 0 kpm preceded the actual test. The temperature in the laboratory was approximately 70° F and the relative humidity between 40 and 60 per cent.

Following the completion of the above tests, the subject met with a study physician and physical educator who reviewed with him the results of all tests performed, answered any questions, and prescribed for him a specific exercise program. The exercise prescription, consisting of walking, running and calisthenics, was compounded to stress each subject at 60 to 70 per cent of his aerobic capacity (14).

Each subject was encouraged to attend exercise classes at the Jewish Community Center of Cleveland at least three times a week. The subject kept a record of his attendance and made a note of comments or reactions to the exercise program. A staff physical educator examined the records kept by the subject at monthly intervals and determined whether he was ready to progress to a more strenuous level

ST SEGMENT SLOPE
mV / sec

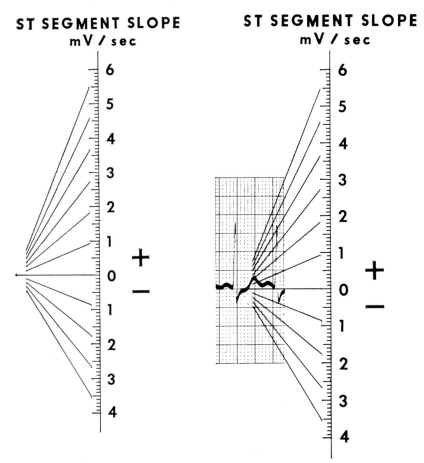

FIGURE 23-1. Method of slope analysis. Two consecutive J points are connected by the baseline of the slope analyzer. The distance between the origin of the baseline and the perpendicular line is 25 mm (one second). The origin of the baseline is placed on the first J point and the slope of the ST segment is read directly in millivolts per second.

of work. Subjects with heart disease were carefully supervised during exercise by trained physical educators. In many subjects, the ECG was telemetered during the exercise class. Scheduled reevaluations, including bicycle ergometry and psychological testing were made at six-month intervals.

Electrocardiograms were analyzed according to the method of Lester *et al.* (10), namely, in terms of the ST-J displacement and the slope of the first 0.08 seconds of the ST segment. A small transparency (Fig. 23-1) placed over the electrocardiographic record facilitated the measurements of ST J displacement (in millimeters) and slope of the ST segment (in millivolts/second).

Electrodes for electrocardiographic monitoring were arranged according to a modified system of Arbaquez *et al.* (17) with the right arm electrode placed on the forehead, the left arm electrode at the ensiform process, the left leg electrode at the V_6 position, the chest electrode at the V_4 position, and the right leg ground electrode at the V_4-R position. Electrocardiograms were taken with the unipolar leads aVR, aVL, aVF, and V and bipolar lead CR.

Standard plate electrodes were used and the recordings made on a Sanborn 500 Viso-cardiette with a time constant of three seconds. Electrocardiograms were recorded at a paper speed of 25 mm/second. The sensitivity was usually 1 cm/mv, if not, the appropriate values were corrected to that sensitivity. The leads used for analysis were the C_4V, CH_6 and C_4R leads. A single complex during exercise which was picked for analysis was typical of those complexes during a period of several seconds. On no occasion was a single unusual beat measured. The measured complex was one showing the greatest ST J displacement and the least positive ST segment slope for the given work load. This usually occurred during the last minute of exercise. The criteria for evaluating the exercise electrocardiogram are displayed in Figure 23-2. The abnormal category included a ST J displacement of 0.01 mv or more with a zero or negative slope. Each lead for every work level was categorized as being normal, borderline, or abnormal. The ECGs of follow-up tests were evaluated in the same manner and comparisons between tests were made for the same lead at identical external work loads. Improvement or deterioration of the exercise ECG was judged by a change of category.

Physical fitness was characterized by the physiological variables, heart rate, blood pressure and their derivatives HR X SBP, work load 150 (14) and predicted maximal oxygen uptake (8). Predicted maximal oxygen uptake per kilogram body weight (ml O_2/kg B.W./min) was calculated according to the method of Åstrand (8). Work load 150 per kilogram body weight (WL 150 kpm/kg B.W./min) was calculated according to methods previously described (14). A minimal

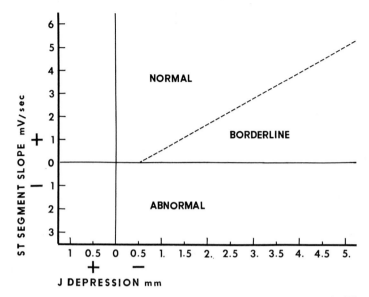

FIGURE 23-2. Criteria for categorization of ST J displacement (millimeter) and ST segment slope (millivolt per second) according to the method of Lester *et al.* (10).

heart rate of 135 was used to extrapolate to work load 150. An indirect measure of myocardial oxygen consumption was obtained from the product of heart rate (HR) and systolic blood pressure (SBP) (18, 19), HR X SBP, which was computed for the last minute of exercise at each work level and expressed in units times 10^2 power.

In the final categorization of the change in physical fitness, the HR X SBP product was used rather than the more familiar work load 150 or predicted maximal oxygen uptake because many ASHD subjects were unable to attain a heart rate of 135 beats per minute (20, 21). Fifty-eight subjects attained this required heart rate. The change in physical fitness as measured by WL 150 was concordant with the change in physical fitness measured by the HR X SBP in 88 per cent of subjects. Eighty-three subjects attained the required heart rate of 120 used to calculate the predicted maximal oxygen uptake (8). The change in physical fitness as measured by predicted maximal oxygen uptake was concordant with the change in physical fitness as measured by the HR X SBP in 83 per cent of subjects. Physical fitness was considered to have improved if HR X SBP decreased by more than

10 x 10^2 and to have worsened if it increased by more than 10 x 10^2 for the identical work level at different test dates.

Using the criteria for HR X SBP the subjects were placed into one of three groups, Improved Fitness Group (IFG) sixty-four subjects, No Change Fitness Group (NCFG), seventeen subjects, or Worse Fitness Group (WFG) nineteen subjects. Because of the small number of subjects, the last two groups were combined for comparisons with the IFG.

The three groups (IFG, NCFG and WFG) were similar in regards to the common work level 471 ± 17.6 kpm, 441 ± 45.4 kpm, and 497 ± 36.4 kpm and to initial body weights, 76.2 ± 1.1 kg, 79.8 ± 2.9 kg, and 78.9 ± 3.1 kg, respectively. There was a decrease in body weight of 0.9 kg, 1.6 kg, and 0.7 kg respectively for each group between the initial and final test.

Regression analyses were performed to correlate changes in the physiologic parameters, with changes in the electrocardiographic parameters (ST J displacement, ST segment slope). The physiological data attained on the final test was divided by the respective value on the initial test. A ratio value of 1.0 indicated that the final and initial value of either heart rate or HR X SBP were the same, above 1.0 indicated worsening and below 1.0 an improvement in physical fitness.

Adherence to the exercise plan was graded independently by the study physical educators (H.M.M. and R.R.) who reviewed the attendance records but had no knowledge of the heart rate, blood pressure or ECG responses to bicycle ergometry. Detailed attendance records were available for analysis for ninety-three subjects. Each subject was graded for adherence. Grade 1 represented minimal or no participation, whereas grade 5 represented full participation. The latter represented one or more hours of running and calisthenics, three days per week. Grades 2, 3 and 4 were various degrees of partial participation, in a progressive order. Changes in physical fitness and exercise ECG categories were compared with the adherence grade of the participants.

The sensitivity of ECG changes during exercise was determined by comparing the maximal change during exercise with the maximal change during recovery. The ECG categories of the recovery and exercise ECG response were determined at 425 separate work loads for fifty subjects.

In twenty-three ECGs the ST segment had a U shaped configuration (22) during exercise or recovery and the first 0.08 second inscription of the ST segment could not be represented by a straight line. These records were analyzed for changes in ECG categories between exercise and recovery.

Calculation of means, standard error of the means, t value for paired samples and regression analysis were performed on an Olivetti Underwood Programma 101 computer. The differences between proportions were tested for significance by calculating the standard error of the difference between two proportions (23). The reported statistics are the means ± the standard error of the mean.

RESULTS

Changes in Physical Fitness

Physical fitness improved in sixty-four, did not improve in seventeen, and worsened in nineteen subjects (Table 23-I). In the improved fitness group (IFG), the following decrements occurred: heart rate for the same work level from 129.2 ± 2.1 to 112 ± 1.9 (p < 0.001); systolic blood pressure (SBP) from 191.3 ± 3.1 to 171.6 ± 2.9 mm Hg (p < 0.001); and HR X SBP from 248.3 ± 6.4 to 192.7 ± 5.3 (p < 0.001). There was no significant change in exercise heart rate, systolic blood pressure or HR X SBP of the no change fitness group (NCFG). In the worsened fitness group (WFG), there was an increase in the systolic blood pressure from 170.5 ± 5.3 to 189.9 ± 6.5 mm Hg (p < 0.001); and in HR X SBP from 212.9 ± 11.0 to 243.8 ± 12.0 (p < 0.001). The increase in heart rate from 124.3 ± 4.4 to 127.7 ± 3.9 was not statistically significant.

The physiological parameters derived from heart rate, i.e., work load 150 and predicted maximal oxygen uptake similarly increased in the IFG. A total of fifty-eight subjects attained a heart rate of 135, and eighty-eight subjects attained heart rate of 120. The WL 150 (kpm/kg B.W./min) of the IFG increased from 8.2± 0.2 to 10.3 ± 0.3 (p <0.001). The maximal predicted oxygen uptake (ml 0_2/kg B.W./min) increased from 23.4 ± 0.5 to 28.1 ± 0.6 (p < 0.001). There were no significant changes in the WL 150 or predicted maximum oxygen uptake for the NCFG or the WFG.

The physiological parameter that worsened significantly in the WFG was the blood pressure and not the heart rate. Thus only those physio-

TABLE 23-I

EFFECT OF PHYSICAL CONDITIONING ON PHYSIOLOGICAL
PARAMETERS (HEART RATE, BLOOD PRESSURE, HR X SBP, WORK
LOAD 150, PREDICTED MAXIMAL O_2 UPTAKE) OF 100 MEN
WITH ASHD

Change in Fitness	Initial N*	Mean	S.E.**	Final Mean	S.E.	P***
HEART RATE						
Improved	64	129.2	2.1	112.0	1.9	<0.001
No Change	17	122.3	5.7	119.2	4.6	NS****
Worsened	19	124.3	4.4	127.7	3.9	NS
BLOOD PRESSURE (mm Hg)						
Improved	64	191.3	3.1	171.6	2.9	<0.001
No Change	17	181.1	8.1	184.0	9.3	NS
Worsened	19	170.5	5.3	189.9	6.5	<0.001
HR X SBP*****						
Improved	64	248.3	6.4	192.7	5.3	<0.001
No Change	17	225.4	18.2	223.9	18.1	NS
Worsened	19	212.9	11.0	243.8	12.0	<0.001
WORK LOAD 150 (kpm/kg B.W./min.)						
Improved	40	8.2	0.2	10.3	0.3	<0.001
No Change	9	7.6	0.4	8.4	0.3	NS
Worsened	9	7.8	0.6	8.9	0.6	NS
PREDICTED MAXIMUM OXYGEN UPTAKE (ml O_2/kg B.W./min)						
Improved	57	23.4	0.5	28.1	0.6	<0.001
No Change	14	24.6	1.2	24.8	1.0	NS
Worsened	12	25.0	1.5	25.6	1.4	NS

*number of subjects attaining necessary heart rate for extrapolation, i.e., 135
for calculation of Work Load 150, 120 for calculation of Predicted Maximal
Oxygen Uptake.

**Standard error of the mean

***Determined by the t test for paired samples

****Not significant

***** x 10^2

logical calculations which include the systolic blood pressure (i.e., SBP,
HR X SBP) deteriorated significantly. Those parameters calculated
only from the heart rate (WL 150, and predicted maximal oxygen uptake) did not change significantly.

The initial systolic blood pressure of the IFG was higher than that
of the WFG, 191.3 $\pm$ 3.1 mm Hg and 170.5 $\pm$ 5.3 mm Hg respectively (p < 0.005). There was no significant difference between
the initial heart rates of the two groups, 129.2 $\pm$ 2.1 and 124.3 $\pm$
4.4 respectively. Both groups were exercised to comparable work levels,

TABLE 23-II

RELATIONSHIP BETWEEN CHANGE IN PHYSICAL FITNESS AND
CHANGE IN EXERCISE ECG OF 48 MEN WITH ASHD AND
INITIAL NORMAL EXERCISE ECG

| Exercise ECG | Physical Fitness Category | | |
	Improved (IFG) (28)* per cent	No Change or Worse (NCFG + WFG) (20) per cent	p**
No Change	61	30	< 0.05
Worse	39	70	< 0.05

*Number of subjects.

**In tables II, III, IV, and VI, p is calculated from the standard error of the differences between proportions (23). Comparisons are made between the IFG and the pooled data of the NCFG and WFG.

TABLE 23-III

RELATIONSHIP BETWEEN CHANGE IN PHYSICAL FITNESS AND
CHANGE IN EXERCISE ECG OF 49 MEN WITH ASHD AND
INITIAL ABNORMAL EXERCISE ECG

| Exercise ECG | Physical Fitness Category | | |
	Improved (IFG) (33)* per cent	No Change or Worse (NCFG + WFG) (16) per cent	p
Improved	79	31	< 0.003
No Change	21	56	< 0.05
Worse	—	13	—

*Number of subjects

6.2 and 6.3 kpm/kg B.W./min respectively. Therefore by using the physiological parameters derived from heart rate, there was no significant difference between the initial physical fitness of the IFG and WFG. However, the initial physical fitness as measured by a derivative of SBP (HR X SBP), was higher in the WFG than the IFG, 248.3 ± 6.4 and 212.9 ± 11.0 (p < 0.01) respectively.

The discordance between the WL 150 and predicted maximal oxygen uptake with the heart rate in the WFG is probably due to elimination from the calculations of the more physically unfit subjects because they could not attain a heart rate of either 135 or 120.

Similar percentages of subjects improved their physical fitness whether the initial exercise ECG was normal, borderline, or abnormal. Physical fitness improved in twenty-eight of forty-eight subjects (58 per cent) with initial normal exercise ECG (Table 23-II) and in thirty-three of forty-nine subjects (67 per cent) with initial abnormal or borderline exercise ECG (Table 23-III).

CHANGES IN EXERCISE ECG CATEGORIES AND PHYSICAL FITNESS

Improvement in the exercise ECG was related to improvement in physical fitness. The initial exercise ECGs were abnormal or borderline in forty-nine subjects, normal in forty-eight subjects, and showed U shaped ST segments in three subjects.

Table 23-IV shows the relationship between the changes in physical fitness and the changes in the exercise ECG in the entire group, irrespective of the original exercise ECG category. The exercise ECG improved in thirty-one, did not change in forty-one, and deteriorated in twenty-eight subjects. This relationship between changes in the exercise ECG and physical fitness became more meaningful when the change in physical fitness was related to the initial exercise ECG category. Twenty-six of the thirty-one subjects with initial borderline or abnormal exercise ECG (84 per cent) who improved their exercise ECG also improved their physical fitness. Of the forty-nine subjects with initial abnormal or borderline exercise ECG, thirty-three subjects were in the IFG and sixteen subjects were in the NCFG-WFG. Seventy-nine per cent (26/33) of subjects in the IFG showed improvement in their exercise ECG whereas only 31 per cent (5/16) of subjects in the NCFG-WFG showed improvement ($p < 0.003$) (Table 23-III).

Table 23-II shows that deterioration of the exercise ECG was likewise related to worsening of the physical fitness. In the forty-eight subjects with initial normal exercise ECG, deterioration of the exercise oc-

TABLE 23-IV

RELATIONSHIP BETWEEN CHANGE IN PHYSICAL FITNESS AND CHANGE IN EXERCISE ECG OF 100 MEN WITH ASHD

Exercise ECG	*Physical Fitness Category*		
	Improved *(IFG)*	*No Change or Worse* *(NCFG + WFG)*	*p*
	(64)* *per cent*	*(36)* *per cent*	
Improved	41	14	< 0.003
No Change	41	42	NS
Worse	18	44	< 0.05

*Number of subjects.

TABLE 23-V

CHANGES IN EXERCISE ECG CATEGORIES IN 100 MEN WITH ASHD

Change in ECG Category	N	Initial Mean	Initial S.E.	Exercise ECG Final Mean	Final S.E.	p
			ST J Displacement (mm)			
Improved	31	1.74	0.34	0.78	0.16	<0.001
No Change	38	1.18	0.17	1.19	0.19	NS
Worsened	28	0.90	0.15	1.22	0.16	<0.025
			ST Segment Slope (mv/sec)			
Improved	31	0.16	0.18	0.91	0.13	<0.001
No Change	38	1.10	0.20	0.95	0.26	NS
Worsened	28	1.06	0.15	0.25	0.16	<0.001

curred in 70 per cent (14/20) of subjects in the NCFG-WFG and in 39 per cent (11/28) of subjects in the IFG (p < 0.05).

In the entire population irrespective of initial ECG category, electrocardiographic improvement occurred in 41 per cent (26/64) of subjects in the IFG, and in 14 per cent (5/36) of subjects in the NCFG-WFG (p < 0.003). Electrocardiographic deterioration occurred in 18 per cent (12/64) of subjects in the IFG and in 44 per cent (16/36) of subjects in the NCFG-WFG (p < 0.05) (Table 23-IV).

In the subjects with improvement of exercise ECG the mean ST J displacement decreased from 1.74 ± 0.34 mm to 0.78 ± 0.16 mm (p < 0.001). The mean slope increased from 0.16 ± 0.18 mv/sec to 0.91 ± 0.13 mv/sec (p < 0.001) (Table 23-V).

In the subjects with deterioration of exercise ECG the mean ST J displacement increased from 0.90 ± 0.15 mm to 1.22 ± 0.16 mm (p < 0.025). The mean slope decreased from 1.06 ± 0.15 mv/sec to 0.25 ± 0.16 (p < 0.001) (Table 23-V).

The three subjects with U shaped ST segments at their initial test also had U shaped ST segments at their follow-up test.

CORRELATION OF THE CHANGES IN PHYSIOLOGICAL PARAMETERS WITH THE CHANGES IN ECG PARAMETERS

Four correlations between the changes in physiological parameters (i.e., HR, HR X SBP) and the changes in ECG parameters (i.e., ST J displacement, and ST segment slope) were determined (Fig. 23-3).

Only one of these correlations, change in HR versus change in ST J displacement was significant (r = −0.226, p < 0.05). The regres-

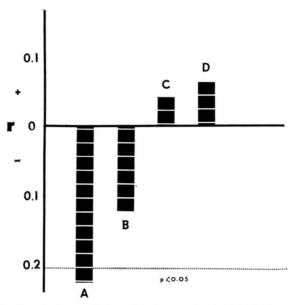

Figure 23-3. Correlation coefficients for changes in physiological versus changes in ECG parameters. *A.* Change in heart rate versus change in ST J displacement, $r = -0.226$. *B.* Change in HR X SBP versus change in ST J displacement, $r = -0.123$. *C.* Change in heart rate versus change in ST segment slope, $r = 0.046$. *D.* Change in HR X SBP versus change in ST segment slope, $r = 0.062$. The value for $p < 0.05$ level of significance is displayed by the hashed line.

sion equation is $y = 2.63 + (-0.026)X$, where $X =$ heart rate final/heart rate initial, and $y =$ change in ST J displacement (negative if ST J displacement increases). Thus, as fitness improved, the heart rate for the same work load decreased and the ST J displacement decreased. As fitness worsened the opposite occurred.

The other three correlations: change in HR versus change in ST segment slope; change in HR X SBP versus change in ST segment slope; and change in HR X SBP versus change in ST J displacement, were not statistically significant.

CHANGES IN EXERCISE ECG AND PHYSICAL FITNESS RELATED TO ADHERENCE TO THE EXERCISE PROGRAM

Improvement in physical fitness was related to adherence to the

TABLE 23-VI
RELATIONSHIP BETWEEN ADHERENCE TO TRAINING PROGRAM AND CHANGE IN PHYSICAL FITNESS AND EXERCISE ECG OF 93 SUBJECTS WITH ASHD

Physical Fitness	*N*	*Adherence Grade*				*p*
		1+2		*3+4+5*		
		number	*per cent*	*number*	*per cent*	
Improved	60	9	32	51	78	<0.003
No Change	16	11	39	5	8	<0.05
Worse	17	8	29	9	14	NS
Exercise ECG						
Improved	28	4	14	24	37	<0.05
No Change	40	14	50	26	40	NS
Worse	25	10	36	15	23	NS
Total	93	28	100	65	100	

exercise program (Table 23-VI). Improvement in physical fitness occurred in 86 per cent (30/35), 69 per cent (9/13), 71 per cent, (12/17), 27 per cent (3/11), and 35 per cent (6/17) of subjects with grades 5, 4, 3, 2 and 1 adherence respectively. The difference in improvement between adherence grade 1 and 2 versus the grade 3, 4 and 5 groups was significant ($p < 0.003$).

Improvement in the exercise ECG was similarly related to adherence to the exercise program. Of the subjects with initial abnormal or borderline exercise ECG, improvement in the exercise ECG occurred in 64 per cent (Table 23-VII) (9/14), 67 per cent (6/9), 75 per cent (9/12), 50 per cent (3/6), and 25 per cent (1/4) of subjects with grades 5, 4, 3, 2 and 1 adherence respectively. Thirty-seven per cent (24/65) of all subjects with grade 3, 4, or 5 adherence showed improvement in the exercise ECG whereas only 14 per cent (4/28) with grades 1 or 2 adherence showed improvement in the exercise ECG ($p < 0.05$) (Table 23-VI).

Deterioration of physical fitness or of the exercise ECG occurred more frequently in the low adherence groups although these differences were not statistically significant (Table 23-VI). Twenty-nine per cent (8/28) of subjects with grade 1 or 2 adherence showed worsening of their physical fitness whereas only 14 per cent (9/65) of subjects with grade 3, 4, or 5 adherence showed worsening of their physical fitness. Thirty-six per cent (10/28) of subjects with grade 1 or 2 adherence showed deterioration of the exercise ECG whereas 23 per cent (15/65)

TABLE 23-VII
RELATIONSHIP BETWEEN ADHERENCE TO TRAINING PROGRAM
AND CHANGE IN PHYSICAL FITNESS AND EXERCISE ECG OF 45
SUBJECTS WITH ASHD AND INITIAL ABNORMAL OR
BORDERLINE EXERCISE ECG

Physical Fitness	N	*Adherence Grade*			
		1+2		*3+4+5*	
		number	per cent	number	per cent
Improved	30	2	20	28	80
No Change	4	3	30	1	17
Worse	11	5	50	6	3
Exercise ECG					
Improved	28	4	40	24	68
No Change	17	6	60	11	32
Total	45	10	100	35	100

of subjects with grade 3, 4, or 5 adherence showed deterioration of their exercise ECG.

COMPARISON OF THE ECG DURING EXERCISE WITH THE ECG DURING RECOVERY

The categorical difference in ECG responses during exercise or recovery was determined in 425 records in a subsample of fifty men with ASHD. One hundred and thirty-three of the 425 records (31.3 per cent) were abnormal. ECGs recorded during exercise identified 81 per cent (108/133) as abnormal whereas those taken during recovery identified 74 per cent (99/133) as abnormal. These differences are not significant. Although neither the exercise nor the recovery ECG was superior in identifying the abnormal response, the exercise ECG was more sensitive in identifying the borderline response. The total number of abnormal and borderline ECGs was 206 of which 181 or 88 per cent were identified by exercise ECGs, and 144 or 70 per cent by recovery ECGs. These differences are significant ($p < 0.01$) and indicate that electrocardiograms taken during either exercise or recovery are of equal value in identifying abnormal ECG responses but records taken during exercise are superior in identifying borderline ECG responses.

RELATIONSHIP OF U SHAPED ST SEGMENTS TO OTHER ST SEGMENT CONFIGURATION

Twenty-three records showed a U shaped ST segment during recovery, five of which (22 per cent) were abnormal during exercise. Twenty records showed a U shaped ST segment during exercise, two of which (10 per cent) were abnormal in recovery. Therefore a U shaped ST segment is nondiagnostic, and may be present in normal or abnormal subjects.

Follow-up

The study population has been followed for a total of 305 patient years. The follow-up for the thirty-nine subjects with previous myocardial infarction without angina, twenty-seven subjects with previous myocardial infarction and angina, fourteen subjects with typical angina pectoris and twenty subjects with left anterior chest pain and abnormal exercise electrocardiograms was 109, 92, 38 and 66 patients years respectively. One subject died during the time interval of this study. The last recorded evaluation placed him in the IFG, no change exercise ECG group.

DISCUSSION OF THIS STUDY

With the advent of quantitative exercise electrocardiography (3), a new dimension, time, has been added to the testing of cardiac function. Previously, follow-up studies of presumed normal or abnormal populations were dependent on either incidence rates of new coronary events or mortality data (2-5). Both types of evaluation require relatively long time intervals to obtain significant numbers. In addition presumed normal populations contain many subjects with subclinical heart disease which can only be uncovered by exercise testing (4, 5, 9), or coronary arteriography.

The development of standard methods of multilevel exercise tests of physical fitness and standardized method of recording and quantitative analysis of the exercise electrocardiogram has made it possible to compare an individual with himself over a time interval. This is now feasible not only in regard to the ECG and to the heart rate response traditionally used by effort physiologists as a measure of aerobic capacity, but also in regard to exercise blood pressure whose product with heart rate is an indirect measure of myocardial oxygen consumption.

The present study demonstrates that participation in a regular supervised program of physical exercise influenced favorably both physical fitness and the exercise ECG of selected subjects with arteriosclerotic heart disease. Improvement of these parameters was found to be a direct function of adherence to the prescribed exercise program.

Occasionally there was discordance between adherence to the exercise program, and change in physical fitness. The basic reason for lack of improvement in the heart rate and blood pressure responses is the inadequate adaptation of the subject to muscular exercise. Two important factors may account for this failure: (a) inadequate design of the training program with less than optimal stressing of the cardiovascular-skeletal muscular system during the exercise periods, or (b) an inability of the organ systems (cardiovascular, neurogenic or endocrine) to adapt because of disease or dysfunction. For example, in one of the subjects the inability of an organ system to adapt was due to severe atherosclerosis of all three major coronary arteries which precluded the development of intercoronary collaterals.

The biologic significance of the relationship between changes in the quantitative exercise electrocardiogram and physical fitness has not yet been established. The present study indicates a positive correlation since the exercise ECG improved in the Improved Fitness Group and deteriorated in the No Change or Worse Fitness Groups. The concordance suggests that changes in these parameters reflect either the structural or functional status of the underlying disease process—progression, stability, or reversal.

At the present time information is not yet available about the extent of collateral arterialization or regression of the atherosclerotic process in the coronary arterial circulation in ASHD subjects studied before and after physical conditioning. However, the physiological effects of physical conditioning of ASHD subjects has been demonstrated in the present and other studies (24). Enhanced fitness is associated with a lower heart rate and blood pressure and larger stroke volume during exercise (24).

It seems reasonable to assume that the improvement of the exercise ECG is related to the enhancement of physiologic function. Since inadequacy of the oxygen supply to the myocardium produces displacement of the ST segment and changes its slope, improvement of the exercise ECG of the conditioned subject suggests that the myocardial oxygen needs have been satisfied. This may occur either by augmenting the oxygen supply or by reducing the needs. The lack of data for the former possibility has already been cited. The reduction of myocardial oxygen needs for the same external work load is suggested by the reduction of exercise heart rate and blood pressure—whose product has been shown to be proportional to the oxygen uptake by the myocardium (18, 19). The similarity of the effects of beta-adrenergic blocking agents (25) and of physical conditioning suggests that the latter influences the storage and/or the release of catecholamines of the heart during exercise and rest.

Since myocardial oxygen need is a function of both heart rate and blood pressure, it was expected that the change in physical fitness as measured by HR X SBP would have a higher correlation than the heart rate alone, with the changes in the ECG parameters. This was not found. The change in fitness as measured by heart rate alone had a significant correlation with the change in the ST J displacement, whereas the change in fitness as measured by the HR X SBP did not.

Perhaps the product of heart rate and brachial artery systolic cuff pressure is not as good an indicator of myocardial oxygen needs or uptake because the blood pressure at the proximal aorta is not necessarily assessed accurately by the cuff pressure at the brachial artery (26). Another possible reason for the lack of correlation is that the systolic blood pressure of subjects with arteriosclerotic heart disease may be extremely labile and more unpredictable than the heart rate.

The product of the heart rate and brachial systolic blood pressure likewise may not be as good a measure of physical fitness as heart rate. This may account for the apparent paradox in which the Worsened Fitness Group (WFG) appeared to deteriorate although initially more fit than the Improved Fitness Group (IFG) when characterized by the blood pressure or BP X HR response to exercise. However, the fitness as measured by derivatives of heart rate alone, i.e., Work Load 150 or Predicted Maximum Oxygen Uptake was similar (Table 23-I). Deterioration of the physical fitness of the WFG was due primarily to deterioration in blood pressure response to exercise whereas improvement in physical fitness of the IFG was caused by improvement in both blood pressure and heart rate responses to exercise.

Comparison of our data with that of Lester *et al.* (10) reveals that, as expected, the exercise ECG responses of more of our subjects with arteriosclerotic heart disease fall into the borderline and abnormal categories (48 per cent). The differences between our subjects and his screened normal population is even more striking when one considers that his subjects were exercised to their maximum, whereas our subjects were exercised at submaximal levels. The average heart rate response of our subjects was only 127. If our subjects with normal responses (52 per cent) had been exercised to higher work intensities surely many would have shifted to the abnormal category. Many subjects failed to attain higher work levels because of subjective tiredness or leg fatigue (20). In a recent study of middle-aged Finnish businessmen a significant per cent also were unable to achieve a heart rate of 150 on the bicycle ergometer, usually because of the onset of chest pain (21). This is a practical consideration which must be taken into account in the design of exercise tests for the middle-aged, sedentary, population with arteriosclerotic heart disease.

Our study population consists mostly of middle and upper class businessmen and professionals. Their physical fitness (23.8 ml O_2/kg B.W./min) is low when compared to a similar economic group in Finland (21), as well as when compared to the more fit Swedish population (8). This undoubtedly reflects the extreme sendentary habits of the study population.

The results of the present study are in agreement with other investigators regarding the relatively greater sensitivity of the ECG taken during exercise compared with the ECG taken during recovery (20, 27, 28). Although the ECG recorded during recovery is as effective in identifying abnormal responses, as the ECG recorded during exercise, the latter is clearly superior in identifying borderline responses. Neither alone however is as good as the combination of both.

The changes which occur in the ECG taken during exercise are more easily related to the physiologic demands of exercise than those occurring during recovery at which time the effects of recovery are added to the residue of exercise. The physiological changes which occur during the recovery period are more unpredictable than the changes during exercise especially if the subject remains in the upright position. The sudden expansion of venous capacity from relaxation of the skeletal muscles in the legs and abdomen causes transient peripheral pooling of venous blood and a sudden reduction of venous return to the right heart (12). How these changes affect the balance between myocardial blood supply and oxygen demand are difficult to quantitate in the individual subject.

The present study has shown that exercise electrocardiography can be quantitated by using techniques which are currently available and do not involve the use of computers. It requires standard type and intensity of work and standard recording and analysis of the ECG. Physical conditioning has a predictive effect on the exercise electrocardiogram of subjects with arteriosclerotic heart disease, tending to normalize it, i.e., decrease ST J displacement, and increase the slope of the ST segment. The improvement may have been accomplished by decreasing the metabolic demands placed on the heart for any amount of total body work, or by changing some intrinsic property of the myocardium or its blood supply. To determine whether this effect of physical conditioning on the exercise electrocardiogram has biological significance in arresting the progression of the disease, more data especially from follow-up mortality studies are needed.

Conclusions regarding the mortality data of the present study will be deferred until completion of a future report dealing with over 240 ASHD subjects.

SUMMARY

Exercise electrocardiograms of one-hundred men with arteriosclerotic heart disease, mean age forty-eight years were analyzed prior to, and after an average of thirty-three months participation in a program designed to enhance physical fitness.

Principles of quantitative exercise electrocardiography were applied using standard intensities of exercise on a bicycle ergometer, and standard recording and standard quantitative analysis of the electrocardiogram. The ST J displacement and slope of the 0.08 second ST segment were measured according to the method of Lester *et al.* (10).

Physical fitness (as measured by change in heart rate $\times$ systolic blood pressure product) improved in 64 per cent. Improvements in heart rate, systolic blood pressure, work load 150 and predicted maximal oxygen uptake also occurred. Physical fitness improved in a similar percentage of subjects with initial normal, borderline or abnormal exercise ECG.

Changes in the exercise ECG were related to changes in physical fitness especially in subjects with initial borderline or abnormal exercise ECG. Improvement in the exercise ECG occurred in 79 per cent of subjects with initial borderline or abnormal exercise ECG whose physical fitness improved. Similarly deterioration of the exercise ECG occurred in 70 per cent of subjects with initial normal exercise ECG whose physical fitness worsened.

In the subjects with improved exercise ECG the mean ST J displacement decreased from 1.74 ± 0.34 mm to 0.78 ± 0.16 mm ($p <$ 0.001). The mean slope increased from 0.16 ± 0.18 mv/sec to 0.91 ± 0.13 mv/sec ($p <$ 0.001).

In the subjects with deteriorated exercise ECG the mean ST J displacement increased from 0.90 ± 0.15 mm to 1.22 ± 0.16 mm ($p <$ 0.025). The mean slope decreased from 1.06 ± 0.15 mv/sec to 0.25 ± 0.16 mv/sec ($p <$ 0.001).

The present study demonstrated that a supervised program of physical conditioning improved both physical fitness and the exercise ECG of subjects with arteriosclerotic heart disease. Improvement of the latter parameter was reflected by a decrease in ST J displacement and an increase in the slope of the 0.08 second ST segment. Improvement in both physical fitness and the exercise ECG are a direct function of adherence to the exercise program.

REFERENCES

1. HELLERSTEIN, H.K.; PROZAN, G.B.; LIEBOW, I.M.; DOAN, A.E., and HENDERSON, J.A.: Two step exercise test as a test of cardiac function in chronic rheumatic heart disease and in arteriosclerotic heart disease with old myocardial infarction. *Amer J Cardiol, 7*:234, 1961.

2. MATTINGLY, T.W.: The postexercise electrocardiogram. *Amer J Cardiol, 9*:395, 1962.

3. ROBB, G.P., and MARKS, H.H.: Postexercise electrocardiogram in arteriosclerotic heart disease. *JAMA, 200*:918, 1967.

4. RUMBALL, A., and ACHESON, E.D.: Latent coronary heart disease detected by electrocardiogram before and after exercise. *Brit Med J, 1*:423, 1963.

5. BRODY, A.J.: Master two step test in clinically unselected patients. *JAMA, 171*:1195, 1959.

6. SCHEUER, J., and BRACHFELD, N.: Coronary insufficiency: relations between hemodynamic, electrical, and biochemical parameters. *Circ Res, 18*: 178, 1966.

7. BLACKBURN, H.: The electrocardiogram in cardiovascular epidemiology:

problems in standardized application. *Ann NY Acad Sci, 126*:882, 1965.

8. ÅSTRAND, I.: Aerobic work capacity in men and women with special reference to age. *Acta Physiol Scand, 49* (suppl.) :169, 1960.

9. DOAN, A.E.; PETERSON, D.R.; BLACKMON, J.R., and BRUCE, R.A.: Myocardial ischemia after maximal exercise in healthy men. *Amer Heart J, 69*:11, 1965.

10. LESTER, F.M.; SHEFFIELD, L.T., and REEVES, J.T.: Electrocardiographic changes in clinically normal older men following near maximal and maximal exercise. *Circulation, 36*:5, 1967.

11. SHEFFIELD, L.T.; HOLT, J.H., and REEVES, J.T.: Exercise graded by heart rate in electrocardiographic testing for angina pectoris. *Circulation, 32*: 622, 1965.

12. LI, Y.B.; TING, N.; CHIANG, B.; ALEXANDER, E.R.; BRUCE, R.A., and GRAYSTON, T.J.: Electrocardiographic response to maximal exercise. *Amer J Cardiol, 20*:541, 1967.

13. HELLERSTEIN, H.K.; HORNSTEN, T.R.; GOLDBERG, A.N.; BURLANDO, A.G.; FRIEDMAN, E.H.; HIRSCH, E.Z., and MARIK, S.: The influence of active conditioning upon coronary atherosclerosis. *Atherosclerotic Vascular Disease*. New York, Appleton, 1967, chapt. 10, p. 115.

14. HELLERSTEIN, H.K., and HORNSTEN, T.R.: Assessing and preparing the patient for return to a meaningful and productive life. *J Rehab, 32*:48, 1966.

15. ELISBERG, E.I.: Heart Rate Response to the valsalva maneuver as a test of circulatory integrity. *JAMA, 186*:200, 1963.

16. VON DOBELN, W.A.: A simple bicycle ergometer. *J Appl Physiol, 7*:222, 1954.

17. ARBAQUEZ, R.F.; FREIMAN, A.H.; REICHEL, F., and LaDUE, J.S.: The precordial electrocardiogram during exercise. *Circulation, 22*:1060, 1960.

18. KATZ, L.N., and FEINBERG, H.: The relation of cardiac effort to myocardial oxygen consumption and coronary flow. *Circ Res, 6*:656, 1958.

19. SARNOFF, S.T.; BRAUNWALD, E.; WELCH, G.H.; CASE, R.B.; STAINSBY, W.N., and MACRUZ, R.: Hemodynamic determinants of oxygen consumption of the heart with special reference to the tension-time index. *Amer J Physiol, 192*:148, 1958.

20. SALZMAN, S.H.; HELLERSTEIN, H.K.; FEIL, G.H., and MARIK, S.: Serum cholesterol and capacity for physical work of middle aged sedentary males. *Lancet*, 1967, p. 1348.

21. HERNBERG, S.: Serum cholesterol and capacity for physical work. *Lancet*, 1964, p. 441.

22. ROBB, G.P.; MARKS, H.H., and MATTINGLY, T.W.: The value of the double standard two step exercise test in the detection of coronary disease. *Trans Assoc Life Insur Med Dir Amer, 40*:52, 1957.

23. HILL, A.B.: *Principles of Medical Statistics,* New York, Oxford U.P., 1966, p. 137.

24. ASMUSSEN,E.: Muscular exercise. In *Handbook of Physiology.* Amer. Physiol. Soc., Washington, D.C., 1965, Vol. II, chapt. 36, sect. 3 (Respiration), p. 966.

25. BRAUNWALD, E.; SONNENBLICK, E.H.; ROSS, J. JR.; GLICK, G., and EPSTEIN, S.E.: An analysis of the cardiac response to exercise. *Circ Res, XX* (suppl. I) and *XXI* (suppl. I): 44, 1967.

26. MARX, H.J.; ROWELL, L.B.; CONN, R.D.; BRUCE, R.A., and KUSUMI, F.: Maintenance of aortic pressure and total peripheral resistance during exercise in heat. *J Appl Physiol, 22*:519, 1967.

27. ROSENFELD, I.; MASTER, A.M., and ROSENFELD, C.: Recording the electrocardiogram during the performance of the master two-step test. *Circulation, 29*:204, 1964.

28. BELLET, S., and MULLER, O.F.: The electrocardiogram during exercise. *Circulation, 32*:477, 1965.

PART SIX

THE POPULATION FREQUENCY, RELATIONS, DIAGNOSTIC POWER AND VALIDITY FOR CORONARY DIAGNOSIS OF THE ISCHEMIC EXERCISE ELECTROCARDIOGRAPHIC RESPONSE

24

Electrocardiographic Responses to Maximal Exercise in American and Chinese Population Samples

Robert A. Bruce, E. Russell Alexander, Y. B. Li, B. N. Chiang, Nong Ting and T. R. Hornsten *with assistance of* R. Taylor *and* V. Hofer

It is a distinct privilege to be invited to participate in this conference on "Measurement in Exercise Electrocardiography" in honor of an outstanding investigator in the field, Dr. Ernst Simonson. After an extensive survey of exercise electrocardiography, he noted that the "overall diagnostic value of the ECG response to exercise for the detection of heart disease exceeds that of any other electrocardiographic procedures used in addition to the routine 12 lead ECG" (1). As is already evident from this program, his studies have stimulated many research developments in biophysics, pathophysiology, clinical testing and cardiovascular epidemiology.

MULTISTAGE TEST OF MAXIMAL EXERCISE

Before presenting observations on ECG responses to maximal exercise in healthy men from various population samples, it is pertinent to describe the background observations which prompted these studies. A single-stage treadmill test of quite moderate severity had been used for years to appraise functional capacity of ambulatory cardiac patients (2). Whereas a low work load was deliberately chosen to avoid any hazard to these patients, experience demonstrated that it was indeed maximal for the most impaired patients who could not complete

Note: These studies have been supported by Grant-in-Aid CD-00066 from the National Center for Chronic Disease Control, USPHS, and Grants-in-Aid HE 09302 and 09303, National Heart Institute, USPHS.

the prescribed ten minutes effort. Since the stress was so mild for others with little or no impairment, it often failed to differentiate their performance from that of normal subjects. Accordingly, a multistage test was introduced in 1963 (3). It was subsequently modified to provide intermediate increments in speed and grade of walking and running, every three minutes, until a self-determined end-point of exhausting fatigue, dyspnea, aching or weakness of the legs, dizziness or chest pain was attained by each person tested. Oxygen costs, expressed as milliliters per kilogram of body weight per minute, for the first four submaximal workloads for healthy men are displayed in Figure 24-1. Since the energy expended is work against gravity, rather than resistance as it is with bicycle ergometers, it is proportional to body weight. When oxygen intake is divided by body weight, smaller standard deviations are obtained, regardless of appreciable inter-individual differences in both variables.

It should be noted that before any subject or patient is tested, he is examined clinically and electrocardiographically to exclude those who have an acute myocardial or pulmonary illness in the active phase. Secondly, the patient and the exercise electrocardiogram are monitored professionally throughout the test; if untoward signs, such as ataxic

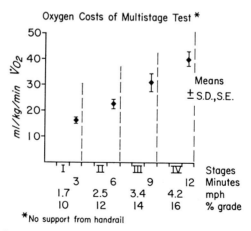

FIGURE 24-1. Oxygen costs in milliliters per kilogram of body weight per minute for the first four stages of the multistage treadmill test of maximal exercise. As maximal exertion is approached, for either a normal subject or a cardiac patient, oxygen uptake does not continue to increase linearly with further increments in the work load but attains a plateau.

TABLE 24-I
PREVALENCE OF LIMITING SYMPTOMS
WITH THE MULTISTAGE MAXIMAL EXERCISE TEST

	Normals	*Cardiacs*
Number of Tests	892	2586
Dyspnea	57%	53%
Weakness and/or Pain in Legs	45%	34%
Fatigue	31%	41%
Chest Pain	1%	24%

gait, change in sensorium or ventricular tachycardia (three or more consecutive beats) occur, the test is stopped. With these precautions in the selection and supervision of individuals tested, safety with respect to significant complications has been assured in over 5000 tests.

The prevalences of the three major limiting symptoms were nearly the same for either normal subjects or ambulatory cardiac patients who have been tested (Table 24-I). The frequency of chest pain, however was 24 per cent in the cardiac patients, versus only 1 per cent of the normal subjects. Multiple limiting symptoms were more frequently observed in cardiac patients.

ANALYSIS OF THE BI-POLAR EXERCISE ELECTROCARDIOGRAM

A single bi-polar precordial lead from the V_5 position to the inferior tip of the right scapula has been used to record the exercise ECG. This "distorted" lead represents an obliquely oriented "lead I," with left precordial preponderance. A separate electrode grounds the patient. The recordings are standardized so that 1 millivolt equals 10 mm deflection, with a Sanborn direct-writing electrocardiograph.

Examples from the records of the Cardiac Work Evaluation Clinic demonstrate several important points about the ECG changes observed with this lead system in patients with clinically established ischemic or coronary heart disease. First, JM was a forty-eight-year-old male who had recovered from two myocardial infarcts. He was able to complete the second stage of exercise when he stopped because of chest pain (Fig. 24-2). The precordial ECG showed ST segment depression during maximal exertion and initial recovery which persisted for over three minutes after exertion. The maximal heart rate was only 138 per minute. In the second example of KFS (Fig. 24-3), a fifty-nine-year-old white male with healed myocardial infarction, exer-

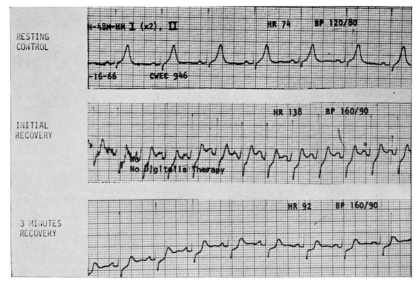

FIGURE 24-2. Bipolar precordial lead electrocardiograms recorded at rest, during submaximal and maximal exercise, initial recovery and three minutes later in a patient (JM, 48 M) with two previously healed myocardial infarcts. Note the ST segment depression, which is not quite horizontal in this lead system, along with the occurrence of chest pain with this exertion.

tion was stopped at eighty seconds of the second stage because of dyspnea and fatigue. Although no pain occurred, there was definite ST segment depression which progressed to T wave inversion three minutes after exertion. In the third example, (Fig. 24-4), a sixty-four-year-old male, RC, with healed myocardial infarction completed one minute of the third stage when he stopped because of angina, dyspnea and fatigue, yet there was no significant ST depression after this more strenuous exertion. The maximal heart rate was only 126 per minute, however. In the fourth example (Fig. 24-5), a thirty-seven-year-old male with healed myocardial infarction had been treated with digitalis. Because of dyspnea, fatigue and leg weakness, he was able to walk for only two minutes in the second stage of the test. Although he denied chest pain, the bi-polar precordial ECG recorded marked ST-T changes during and after exertion. Finally, a fifty-three-year-old healthy male (Fig. 24-6), with no clinical evidence of heart disease, completed seventy-five seconds of the fourth stage when he

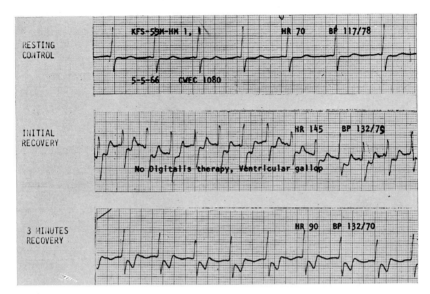

FIGURE 24-3. Similar electrocardiograms recorded before, immediately after and three minutes after maximal exercise in a patient (KFS, 59 M) with healed myocardial infarction. Exertion was limited by dyspnea and fatigue. Despite marked ST segment depression, progressing from horizontal to downsloping with inverted T waves in the same lead system, he was not aware of any chest discomfort or pain. He was not under treatment with digitalis.

stopped because of dyspnea and fatigue with no chest pain. His maximal heart rate was 187 per minute. Again, in the initial recovery period, ST segment depression of more than 2 mm was recorded. These five examples illustrate the variations in ST forces of ventricular repolarization which are observed with angina pectoris, healed myocardial infarction and even occasionally, in healthy asymptomatic middle-aged men. Not all patients with angina or healed infarction show this response. Conversely, ST depression is usually accentuated in those ischemic patients who are under treatment with one of the digitalis glycosides. In contrast to methods employed by others, it has been the practice in this laboratory to utilize a single precordial lead and to note the changes recorded. It is possible that more typical or marked changes in ST forces might be recorded in other leads in some instances. Occasionally such changes might be missed in this single bi-polar lead.

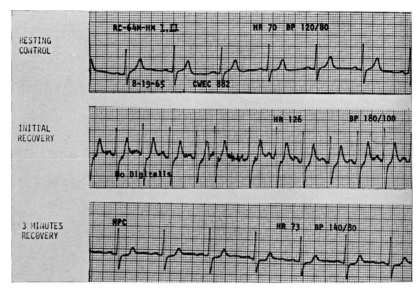

Figure 24-4. Precordial electrocardiograms recorded before, during and after maximal exertion in a patient (RC, 64 M) with angina pectoris and healed myocardial infarction. Despite the reproduction of chest pain or angina, as well as dyspnea and fatigue, there was no significant ST change observed in this lead system. A single nodal premature beat was recorded however.

Preliminary studies of healthy men in Seattle revealed no significant ST segment depession of 1 mm or more in normal young men. Occasional middle-aged men over forty years of age did exhibit this response (Fig. 24-6). Actually the age-specific prevalence increased with advancing age, and this followed, rather than preceded, a significant reduction in maximal oxygen intake (Fig. 24-7) (4). On direct comparison with the double Master two-step test, only two out of 201 normal men showed this response, but eighteen revealed it with the multistage test of maximal exercise (5). Another comparison in Chinese men showed a threefold difference which was attributed to the much lower exertional heart rates attained with the double Master two-step test (6).

Observer variability in intrepretation of this ST response to maximal exercise was excessive when Blackburn submitted thirty-eight tracings from this laboratory to fourteen cardiology experts in seven medical centers (7). Indeed, the reported prevalence of "positive"

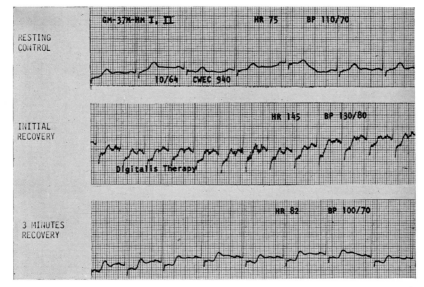

FIGURE 24-5. Precordial lead electrocardiograms in another patient (GM, 37 M) with healed myocardial infarction who became dyspneic, fatigued and weak after two minutes of exertion at the second stage. There was no chest discomfort. In this instance, the marked ST-T changes were attributed to the effects of digitalis therapy.

responses with undefined criteria ranged from as low as 5, to as high as 55 per cent! Unanimous agreement by all fourteen observers was obtained on only seven normal, and one abnormal, tracings. The mean estimate was 10.8 per cent. Thus, needs for rigid criteria and objective analysis were clearly documented.

In order to meet these needs, in addition to improving the ECG signal to background noise ratio during vigorous exercise, a computer averaging technique was introduced (8). In each instance, 100-beat samples for each period of observation before, during and after exercise were averaged, digitized and calibrated. Statistical analysis of the serial standard deviations of averaged voltages for each 10 msec interval defined the minimal variance, and hence maximal reproducibility, for the PR reference voltage and the ST voltage deviations. With this improved objective analysis, it has been possible to examine three different loci of the ST segment by both the empirical clinical criterion (1 or more millimeters deflection) and another criterion de-

TABLE 24-II
COMPARISON OF POSTEXERCISE (MAXIMAL) RESPONSES
Classifications by Computer Measurements

Loci: mv Criteria: Classification:	ST₂ (40-59 msec)				ST₃ (70-79 msec)				ST₄ (40-79 msec)				Prevalences
	≤ —.063*		≤ —.100		≤ .004*		≤ —.100		≤ —.041*		≤ —.100		
	—	+	—	+	—	+	—	+	—	+	—	+	
Classification of Visual Interpretations (≤ —.100mv) { —	71	23	86	8	70	24	87	7	73	21	90	4	82.5%
{ +	1	19	3	17	0	20	13	7	1	19	7	13	17.5%
Computer: Prevalences %	36.9		21.9		38.5		10.0		35.0		14.9		
Specificity (True Negatives) %	75.6		91.5		74.4		92.5		77.5		95.6		
False Positives %	24.4		8.5		25.5		7.5		22.4		4.3		
Sensitivity (True Positives) %	95.0		85		100		35		95		65		
False Negatives %	5.0		15		0		65		5		35		
Misclassified %	21.1		9.6		21		17.6		19.3		9.6		
Chi-square	35.2		53.0		38.5		11.6		38.2		47.9		
Discrimination of abnormal response:	Maximal				Moderate				Intermediate				

Prevalences in relation to visual interpretations by clinical method

Material: 4th annual examination of middle-aged American men (YMCA cohort), Hornsten *et al*, 1967

Methods: Computer averaging (ref. 8), 100 beat samples, differential triggering R downslope for minimal variance (ref. 2), at 3 loci, as specified, after nadir of S in bipolar precordial ECG lead.

Voltage Criteria: *Statistical: 99% confidence limits for entire sample; Visual (clinical) ≤ —0.100 millivolts

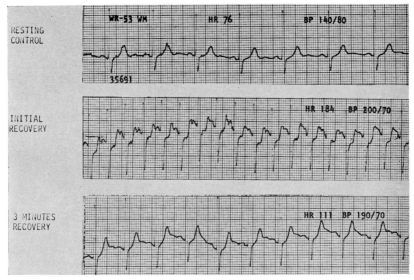

FIGURE 24-6. Precordial lead electrocardiograms recorded in a healthy middle-aged male (WR) who was able to continue effort into the fourth stage of the test for seventy-five seconds. He was limited by dyspnea and fatigue, with a maximal heart rate of 187 per minute. Note the ST segment depression which appeared transiently in the tracing immediately after this exertion. There was no chest discomfort or pain.

fined by the 99 per cent confidence limit (Table 24-II). The optimal classification in relation to visual interpretation of electrocardiographic responses was achieved by use of the clinical criterion at either 50 to 59 msec (ST_2) or 40 to 79 msec (ST_A) after the nadir of the S wave. With the former, only 10 per cent were misclassified; whereas the specificity for true negatives was 91 per cent, the sensitivity for true positives was 85 per cent. The 2 x 2 relationship of computer classifications to visual interpretations had a chi-square of 53 (P < .001). When interpretations by American and Chinese colleagues in the cooperative international study (*to be cited below*) were compared, only 6 per cent were misclassified (chi-square 109, P < .001). Actually, classification of the ST responses in these prevalence studies has been by visual interpretation of the strip chart recording of the ECG. Objective computer analysis has been utilized to study the quantitative magnitudes and time courses of the responses. From the direct comparisons cited above, reasonably reliable classifications of

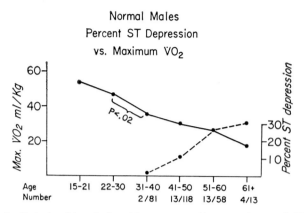

FIGURE 24-7. Relationship of the rising age-specific prevalence of ST segment depression to the maximal oxygen intake of healthy men. Note the significant decrement in mean oxygen intake in the years prior to the appearance of ST segment depression (4).

the ECG responses have been made by visual interpretation when a fixed criterion of at least 1 mm depression of the ST segment has been utilized. Such depression, on a standardized tracing, may exhibit an upslope, horizontal line, or downslope from ST to T wave in this particular bi-polar lead.

Because of the depression of the ST junction and initial ST forces of ventricular repolarization, which is proportional to heart rate, and varies with posture, as noted by Sjöstrand in 1950 (9), any excessive depression during exertion must be defined quantitatively in relation to the normal limits for the observed heart rate. With objective computer measurements of the ST_2 voltage, it has been possible to define the means as well as the standard deviations of these responses for submaximal and maximal exercise (Fig. 24-8). Four important points should be noted from this analysis. First, there is a progressive depression with increasing workloads and tachycardia which is nearly linear for submaximal loads. As maximal exertion is approached, the slope of this relationship is altered, reflecting some myocardial adjustment. Whether this represents metabolic responses to changes in intracardiac pressure and/or coronary circulation is unknown. Second, in this lead system, the mean ST_2 voltage in normal men at maximal exertion is below -0.1 mv which is often cited as the clinical criterion for the

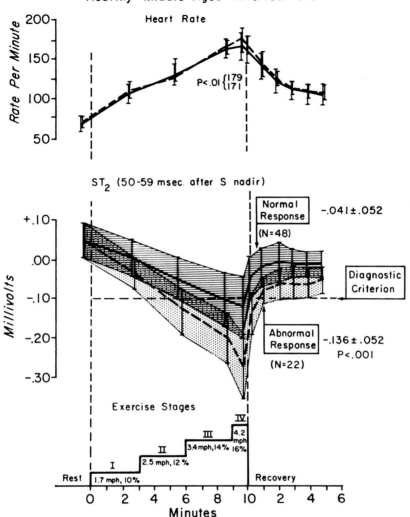

Differentiation of Myocardial Responses in
Healthy Middle-Aged American Men

FIGURE 24-8. Means ± standard deviations of heart rates and quantitated ST_2 voltage responses in two groups of healthy middle-aged men. Although of similar age (53.9 ± 5.9 and 53.6 ± 7.5 years, respectively), they differ in respect to postexertional ST segment response to graded exercise up to maximum. Progressive depression of ST_2 with increasing heart rate (Sjöstrand effect) in those with the normal responses (upper zone) is exaggerated by even greater depression for similar heart rate in the twenty-two men with abnormal postexertional ST segment deprssion which is attributed to transient myocardial ischemia. Note that in immediate recovery, ST_2 voltage changes markedly out of proportion to a minor decrease in heart rate but restoration of normal values is delayed in the men with abnormal response which exceeds the diagnostic criterion of ⩽ −0.10 mv.

diagnosis of an ischemic response. Therefore, even greater depression must be found before an abnormal response during exertion can be identified. Patients or healthy subjects who show ST depression after exertion usually exhibit more marked depression during the exercise. Third, ST_2 and ST_3 voltages return toward the resting baseline level immediately (within the time necessary to sample 100 consecutive heartbeats) after maximal exertion. Since this occurs before there is a significant reduction in heart rate, it may reflect striking changes in myocardial performance due to the sudden reduction of venous return and diminished diastolic filling of the ventricles. Conversely, exertional ST segment depression is not just a function of tachycardia *per se,* but reflects altered myocardial performance as well. Fourth, with respect to discrimination of abnormal from normal responses, there is less overlap of standard deviations for the ST_2 responses than with the ST_3 responses. The optimal location for voltage differentiation thus is confined to 0.05 to 0.06 seconds after the S nadir in this lead system. This may be slightly earlier than the midpoint of the QT interval as reported by Blomqvist for the X, Y, Z coordinates of the Frank lead vectorcardiogram (10).*

With further refinements in computer triggering which reduce variance (12), statistical analysis now suggests that ST responses during 75 per cent of maximal exertion may become as reliable as those observed after maximal effort. For purposes of classification of subjects in epidemiological surveys, measurements by computer methods will be necessary to define the subtle quantitative changes in the presence of marked respiratory variation of the baseline. Just as submaximal stress tests do not provide as high a proportion of positive ST responses after exertion, visual interpretation of the changes during exercise will not provide as many positive responses.

FREQUENCY OF ELECTROCARDIOGRAPHIC RESPONSES TO MAXIMAL EXERCISE IN POPULATION SAMPLES OF MIDDLE-AGED MEN

Ultimately the predictive value of ST segment depression after maximal exertion in healthy middle-aged men may be assessed by the

---

* A quantitative comparison of the changes in the bipolar and X, Y and Z leads is now in progress to clarify this relationship (11).

frequency of clinical manifestations of coronary heart disease in longitudinal follow-up studies. So far, with only four years of follow-up, too few events have occurred to make any definitive statement. In the meantime, comparison of the age-specific prevalence from grossly different population samples might be informative. For this purpose, parallel studies utilizing similar criteria for selection and methods of testing have been conducted on American men in Seattle and Chinese men in Taipei, Taiwan. The former group was drawn from a previously defined roster of men who were members of the Seattle YMCA or members of selected departments of the University of Washington (5, 20). After excluding a few with clinical manifestations of cardiac disease, there were 163 men of forty to fifty-nine years of age who were found to be healthy on two separate examinations ranging from two to four years apart. Of these, eighteen had resting blood pressures in excess of 159 mm Hg systolic and/or 94 mm Hg diastolic, but none had evidence of heart disease.

With the collaboration of the cardiology staff of the National Defense Medical Center in Taipei, Chinese men of forty to fifty-nine years of age from both upper and lower socioeconomic classes were invited to participate in a parallel study. After exclusion of a few with heart disease on a single examination, there were 1527 healthy volunteers. In the lower socioeconomic group, there were eighty-one enlisted military personnel (13) and 100 pedicab-men (14) reported in detail elsewhere. In the upper socioeconomic group, there were 1346 men who were drawn from rosters of civilian bank and power company managers and executives, as well as senior military officers of the rank of colonel or higher (15). These Chinese groups were of particular interest because the frequency of coronary heart disease has been reported to range from 2 to 5 per cent of all types of cardiovascular disease admitted to military and civilian hospitals in Taipei (13).*

All subjects were interviewed and examined physically, by chest x-ray, by 12-lead electrocardiogram, and by a series of laboratory

---

*Another group of 210 American men, both civilian and military personnel who were temporarily in residence in Taipei have been studied by Gutman, Ting, Watten and Alexander (16). A report of the pertinent details of this group is in preparation.

TABLE 24-III

FREQUENCY DISTRIBUTIONS OF ST SEGMENT DEPRESSION

≤ −0.1 millivolt after multistage treadmill test of maximal exercise in healthy men from diverse population samples, utilizing Sanborn electrocardiographic recording of bi-polar precordial lead in all instances

Age Groups, Years	40-44	45-49	50-54	55-59	40-59
American Men					
In Seattle (A)	(4/48) 8.3%	(6/54) 11.2%	(8/39) 20.5%	(6/22) 27.3%	(24/163) 14.7%
Chinese Men in Taipei (according to socioeconomic status)					
Upper (B)	(15/462)	(28/456)	(38/354)	(13/74)	(94/1346) 7.0%
Lower (C, D)	(3/61)	(1/54)	(3/35)	(2/30)	(9/181) 5.0%
Both Groups	(18/523) 3.4%	(29/510) 5.7%	(41/389) 10.5%	(15/104) 14.4%	(103/1527) 6.7%

(A) Fourth annual examination YMCA cohort, second examination campus personnel, Hornsten *et al*, 1967.
(B) Senior officers, managers and executives, Ting and Alexander, 1967.
(C) Enlisted men, Alexander *et al*, 1965.
(D) Pedicab-men, Chiang *et al*, 1967.

tests, including determination of serum cholesterol by standardized methods. Then each was tested by the multistage test to maximal exertion, as described earlier. Because of the unexpected occurrence of postexertional dizziness and syncope in some of the first Chinese subjects to be tested, the initial recovery period after maximal exertion was modified to permit walking at 1 mph on the level for two minutes to avoid orthostatic symptoms (from pooling in dilated dependent venous capacitance vessels [6]).

The percentage frequencies of ST segment depression of at least 1 mm are shown in Table 24-III for each of the population samples which have been examined. They are arranged according to national origin, place of residence and/or socioeconomic classification, and age distributions. The highest prevalence of 14.7 per cent for men of forty to fifty-nine years of age was observed in the American men residing in Seattle. This group is not likely to represent the population at large, however. Within the twenty-year range of forty to fifty-nine years of age, there is a rising age-specific prevalence for those who resided in Seattle.

Chinese men residing in Taipei have been subdivided into socioeconomic classes because of the more frequent clinical manifestations of coronary heart disease in those of the upper socioeconomic class. Dietary restrictions imposed by meager earnings of those in the lower socioeconomic classes, especially when combined with habitual physical conditioning by occupational necessity, as in the pedicab drivers, may be expected to reveal the potentiality for ischemic heart disease less frequently. Both of these groups, within the ages of forty to fifty-nine years, have lower frequencies of postexertional ST segment depression than American men (Table 24-III). The tendency for a progressive rise in age specific prevalence is apparent in the larger number of men in the upper socioeconomic class. This is not clearly apparent in the lower class of Chinese men; it is likely that self-exclusion, especially from arduous work in older men who may have become symptomatic from cardiovascular or other disease, is an important selective factor.

Another provocative observation is the greater frequency of delayed ST segment depression in the Chinese. This was an unexpected clinical observation (6) which has been confirmed by averages of computer measurements of the ST_2 voltage time course after maximal

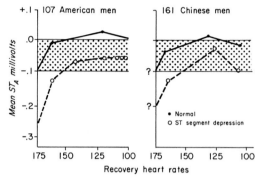

TIME COURSES OF AVERAGED POSTEXERTIONAL
(MAXIMAL) ECG RESPONSES

FIGURE 24-9. Comparison of the average quantitative ST$_A$ voltages during cardiac deceleration after maximal exertion in 107 American men and 161 Chinese men. Note that the upper solid lines for men with normal ECG responses are well within the normal range (*shaded zones*) for all periods of observation in recovery. The broken lower lines represent the voltage-time course for those men who exhibited an abnormal ST segment depression. In the case of the American men, this abnormality was present only during *initial* recovery. In the Chinese men who were abnormal, this voltage showed a secondary fall at the end of five minutes of observation. See text for comments.

exertion (Fig. 24-9). In the Chinese, the mean ST$_2$ voltage shows a delayed fall which exceeds the minor tendency observed in American men in Seattle.* Nevertheless, it should be noted that the predominant vascular problem in the American population is coronary atherosclerosis, which affects the proximal epicardial portion of these vessels. In the Chinese, as in the Japanese, the predominant problem is hypertensive disease, which primarily affects the small, distal arteries in the myocardium if the vasculature of the heart is involved. Although the time course of the ST depression, which seems to be delayed in the Chinese men, may reflect a minor modification in the testing procedure after maximal effort, it is of great interest that Japanese investigators utilizing the double Master two-step test also emphasize the importance of ST depression a few minutes after cessation of exercise (17).

---

*Preliminary analysis of data on American men tested in Taipei suggests that this delayed response represents a difference related to the modified method of testing, which permits the men to walk at 1 mph and 0 per cent grade for two minutes after maximal exertion.

RELATIONSHIPS OF ST RESPONSES TO RISK FACTORS

In this brief summary of data on several groups of men, only a few variables may be selected to indicate the possible relationships of ST segment depression after maximal exercise to other associated risk factors. In Table 24-IV, mean ages of Chinese and American men selected are comparable. Yet the American men are constitutionally taller and heavier. They also tend to have, on the average, slightly higher systolic and diastolic blood pressures at rest than the Chinese. Of particular interest is the significantly higher concentration of serum cholesterol. Chinese men of the lower socioeconomic classifications weigh less, tend to be slightly shorter, and have a lower mean cholesterol concentration than Chinese men selected from the upper socioeconomic classes. These data strengthen the earlier preliminary impression (18) that the apparent prevalence of ST segment depression after maximal exertion in these population samples varies with the cholesterol concentration and the apparent frequency of clinical manifestations of ischemic heart disease.

The possible relationship of ST response to maximal exercise to risk

TABLE 24-IV

PHYSICAL CHARACTERISTICS AND RISK FACTORS

Healthy men from diverse population samples selected for
maximal exercise testing of ST response

	American Men in Seattle	Chinese Men in Taipei	
		Upper SES*	Lower SES*
Number of Men	163	1346	181
Age, years	48.2±5.1**	47.1±4.5	47.5±6.8
Height, cm	178.0±6.8***	168.2±5.3	166.2±5.9***
Weight, kg	79.4±100***	62.5±9.0	58.9±8.3***
Systolic blood pressure, mm Hg.	126±18	127±18	122±21***
Diastolic blood pressure, mm Hg.	83±10**	80±11	76±11***
Cholesterol, mg%	238±39***	198±35	176±33***
Duration of maximal exercise, sec	591±85***	481±90	606±112#***
Maximal heart rate	177±11***	172±16	172±16
ST depression	14.7%	7.0%	5.0%

* SES represents socioeconomic status

\# 100 pedicab-men only, since duration of others was longer due to holding handrail for support.

** P < .01 } in relation to upper socioeconomic class of Chinese men
*** P < .001 }

factors has also been examined longitudinally in the American YMCA men (19). Initially the reproducibility of this response on the follow-up examination one year later was 95 per cent (20). With subsequent longitudinal observations, there have been changes in both directions (19), yet 89 per cent of the men continue to exhibit either negative or positive ST responses to maximal exercise. Of the few who have shown changes, there have been interesting differences in the mean values of associated variables (Table 24-V). Thus, of eight who reverted from positive to negative, the cholesterol concentration averaged 211 mg%. Conversely, in thirteen who changed from negative to positive, the resting blood pressures were higher, and the mean cholesterol concentration was the highest of all four subgroups. Whereas it may be distressing that the mean cholesterol concentrations were virtually identical—and in an intermediate range—for the 155 men who were consistently negative and for ten men who were consistently positive, the latter were also significantly older. Possibly these findings are consistent with the observation of others that with older age groups, the relative importance of cholesterol as a risk factor dinimishes (21).

EFFECTS OF PHYSICAL TRAINING ON ECG RESPONSES TO EXERCISE

One of the contemporary questions about the prevention of ischemic heart disease due to coronary atherosclerosis is whether habitual physical activity, either by occupational necessity or recreational desire, exerts a protective role, or functions as a negative risk factor. Now that the preclinical phase of a prolonged and progressive vascular disease can be assessed, it is quite pertinent to investigate this possibility. Two feasibility studies have been conducted in this laboratory (22). In the first, six normal men and one male patient with angina pectoris of forty-one to sixty-nine years of age were studied before and after several weeks of "steady state" training. The latter consisted of twenty-minute periods of walking upgrade on the treadmill at an average work load of 73 per cent of the measured maximal oxygen intake. This was performed three times weekly for ten weeks. The second experiment involved eight asymptomatic healthy men of forty-one to sixty-six years of age. They performed "interval training" of walking

TABLE 24-V

RELATIONSHIPS OF ASSOCIATED VARIABLES TO
ELECTROCARDIOGRAPHIC RESPONSES IMMEDIATELY AFTER MAXIMAL EXERCISE
IN THIRD ANNUAL EXAMINATION OF AMERICAN MEN (YMCA COHORT) (19)

Classification of ECG Responses	Consistently Negative	Reversion from Positive to Negative	Conversion from Negative to Positive	Consistently Positive
Number of Men	155	13	8	10
Age, years	46.5 ± 6.9**	50.0 ± 8.6	50.9 ± 7.2	54.4 ± 10.2 **
Height, cm	178.9 ± 6.4*	175.7 ± 5.5	176.3 ± 5.8	173.5 ± 7.0*
Weight, kg	80.3 ± 10.1	78.9 ± 13.8	79.3 ± 10.2	78.8 ± 11. 7
Systolic Blood Pressure, mm Hg	127 ± 14**	130 ± 18	147 ± 33**	133 ± 22
Diastolic Blood Pressure, mm Hg	84 ± 8*	87 ± 9	91 ± 9*	87 ± 9
Cholesterol, mg%	226 ± 40*	211 ± 44*	257 ± 39*	224 ± 23
Triglyceride, mg%	88 ± 57	53 ± 17*	81 ± 30*	99 ± 45**
Duration of exercise (secs.)	651 ± 102**	630 ± 194	620 ± 93	541 ± 131**
Change in ST_2†				
Change in Heart Rate	—.5 ± .5**	—.4 ± .6	—1.4 ± .8	—1.3 ± .5**

* P < .05 } by t test for comparison of the paired values for the variable specified.
** P < .01 }
† microvolts per heart beat

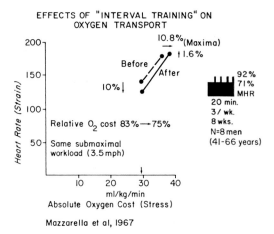

EFFECTS OF "INTERVAL TRAINING" ON
OXYGEN TRANSPORT

Mazzarella et al, 1967

FIGURE 24-10. Changes in average heart rates and minute oxygen intake per kilogram of body weight in eight asymptomatic men who were tested at a submaximal and a maximal work load before and after "interval type" of training for eight weeks. (See text for details.) Note the same absolute oxygen intake for the same submaximal work load, but the fall in relative oxygen cost due to the 10.8 per cent increase in maximal oxygen intake. Heart rate for submaximal exertion diminished whereas that for maximal effort hardly changed.

for four minutes on a gradual incline, and one minute on a steep incline, repeated three times for a total twenty minutes at average work loads of 71 and 92 per cent of maximal heart rate. Again, there were three periods per week for eight weeks. Slightly greater changes in most, but not all, men were obtained with the second program. Average changes in the stress (absolute oxygen intake per kilogram of body weight) to the strain on the circulation (heart rate) at the same submaximal and altered maximal work loads before and after training are shown in Figure 24-10. Because the maximal oxygen intake (denominator) increased about 10 per cent, the relative cost or percentage ratio of submaximal exercise for the same load and absolute oxygen intake (numerator) decreased from 83 to 75 per cent. Concomitantly, submaximal heart rate declined 10 per cent. A similar stress-strain analysis of the myocardial performance under the same conditions is shown in Figure 24-11. In this context, the heart rate is the measure of the stress imposed on the heart muscle. The computer measured ST_2 voltages represent the strain observed in the early phase of repolarization during systolic contraction of the

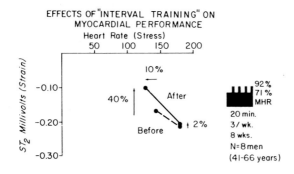

Mazzarella et al, 1967

FIGURE 24-11. Changes in average heart rate and ST_2 voltage before and after physical training in the same eight men. Note the 10 per cent decrease in submaximal heart rate and 40 per cent change in ST_2 voltage. At maximal exertion, however, the average rate and voltage for these men were not altered significantly.

ventricles. Although submaximal heart rate (stress) is 10 per cent less after this interval training program, the ECG strain observed is 40 per cent less than before. Stated differently, at exactly the same submaximal work load, there was less ST segment depression; indeed, it was hardly beyond the normal range of response described by the Sjöstrand effect of tachycardia (9). The slope of the relationship of ST_2 to heart rate was altered. Despite this improvement for submaximal effort, there was some improvement in three men but no significant difference, on the average for all men at maximal exertion. Thus, some subtle palliation of the alleged ischemic response at submaximal effort was achieved, but the absolute strain with maximal stress was not altered. If these findings were extrapolated to clinically symptomatic coronary heart disease, a parallel change would be beneficial since all but peak loads in ordinary daily activities are conducted at submaximal stresses. It should be noted, furthermore, that in neither of these feasibility studies did all men improve; in each instance, the ST changes were slightly accentuated, rather than diminished in one subject. Thus, physical training of ischemic persons will necessitate some medical supervision.

In addition to these short-term intervention experiments with physical training are the observations on habitual physical activities. In healthy Americans in Seattle subdivided according to physical activity status, there has been no significant difference in the prevalence of ST segment depression after maximal exertion (20). Nevertheless, the lowest prevalence of this response was found in the Chinese pedicab-men who are chronically conditioned by occupational activity and who have much lower serum cholesteral concentrations (14).

DISCUSSION

In these studies, the principle recognized by Simonson that the exercise electrocardiogram exceeds the value of the resting ECG (1) has been extended to encompass maximal exertion in population samples usually considered to be at either high or low risks for coronary heart disease. Although the ECG observations have been limited to a single bi-polar lead system to explore the potentialities of continuous monitoring by this technique, refinements in objective quantitative measurements have been introduced to assess the accuracy of visual interpretations, the time course of responses, and even preliminary experimental studies of the stress-strain analysis of responses to physical training in healthy middle-aged men with preclinical, if any, coronary heart disease.

The wisdom of maximal exercise testing evolved from years of moderate stress testing of ambulatory clinical patients with ischemic heart disease (2). Continuing the same principles of preliminary physical and electrocardiographic examination (3) to exclude any who should not be tested, especially if in an active phase of myocardial infarction, and providing professional monitoring during the test (42), safety has been achieved while the feasibility and practicality have been demonstrated.* The particular type of exercise (steps, bicycle or treadmill ergometer) is less important than the principles of a multistage test with progressive increments in work load with

---

*Quite recently, after the presentation of this material at the symposium, the first exception to these principles was demonstrated when a normal male of 42 years of age, with normal exercise performance and ECG responses to maximal exertion, suddenly developed an hyperacute myocardial infarction while taking a shower 10-15 minutes after the exertion. Cardiac arrest from ventricular fibrillation occurred within 20 minutes, but he was successfully resuscitated. He was monitored carefully in the coronary care unit for one week and thereafter he had an uneventful convalescence (43).

sufficient time for step-wise physiological adaptation. The advantages of the treadmill procedure are twofold: work against gravity is directly proportional to body weight (if support from holding or leaning on the handrails is not allowed); involuntary regulation of the rate of energy expenditure is provided. Thus, the treadmill, as emphasized by Dr. Henry L. Taylor, is really a laboratory and a clinical tool of remarkable precision. Indeed, it has been possible to repeat measurements of maximal oxygen intake within 2 per cent—which is equal to that observed for maximal heart rate. On direct comparison, higher ventilation and slightly greater oxygen intakes have been observed in the same subjects with the treadmill than with the bicycle (23). Possibly the latter imposes a partial splinting of the shoulder girdle muscles which may restrict ventilation. A more important factor may be the vigorous displacements of the diaphragm by the abdominal viscera with running. In view of pressor responses to sustained contractions, vigorous grasping of the handle-bar of a bicycle ergometer may alter the blood pressure response (24).

Thus, each technique for exercise testing has its advantages and disadvantages, but the ability to achieve reproducible work loads should be a dominant consideration in the interests of scientific data. From other studies, the oxygen intake with the multistage treadmill test increases nearly linearly with time during submaximal loads (11), and a normal time of two to three minutes to reach a plateau can be demonstrated even in cardiac patients (25). Furthermore, measurements of maximal oxygen intake with the multistage test are virtually identical to those of the classical Taylor method of running at 7 mph for two and three-quarter minutes (26). The additional advantage of the multistage test is that maximal effort can be achieved in a single test, even the first trial, with any motivated and ambulatory patient or normal subject. The most effective means of differentiating cardiacs from normals, however, is the total oxygen intake (3).

The ST segment depression observed with the single bipolar precordial lead electrocardiogram is found in most, but not all, patients with ischemic heart disease. The selected clinical examples demonstrate the variations encountered in magnitude, time-course and pressure or absence of chest pain or angina. Failure to observe this response may suggest that a different lead axis would be more informative. Nevertheless, gradual disappearance over months and years after clinically established myocardial infarction suggests the possible role of collateral circulation. Studies reported by others indicate a frequent correlation with significant coronary occlusive disease documented by coronary arteriography (27). Indeed, the sensitivity of the ST segment response (1 mm or more for 0.08 sec during or after exercise) was 84 per cent, with a specificity of 100 per cent (chi-square 16.4). (Failure to observe this response in the presence of occluded left anterior descending artery in a recent challenging case of a young woman with only slight impairment of exercise capacity was associated with considerable collateral flow from the right coronary artery [11].) The presence of ST segment depression after exercise is often attributed to myocardial ischemia, as noted by Simonson (1). Yet it is important to emphasize that this response is nonspecific in relation to etiology of heart disease, for it is observed in one quarter of the patients with valvular heart disease, and some of the patients with hypertensive disease (3). It is accentuated by treatment with digitalis (3) which increases the rate of systolic contraction (dp/dt), but treatment to moderate toxicity in normal young men has been without effect, even at maximal exertion (28).

In healthy men, where symptoms and signs of heart disease are excluded by examination, and there is no treatment with digitalis, the presence of this ECG response may represent a potentiality for subsequent clinical manifestations of disease in the future (5). Until sufficient data are accumulated with years of follow-up observations, which are in progress, the pathologic specificity and differentiation from the effects of aging remain in doubt. Again, as noted earlier by Simonson, "perhaps the best overall criterion is the number of abnormal exercise responses in addition to the number of abnormal ECGs in rest found in unselected, large population samples" (1). It is in this context that preliminary sampling of markedly different populations has been initiated to gain further insight.

Comparison of population data is hazardous when limited to small samples with incomplete epidemiological and clinical studies. Nevertheless, pathophysiologic differences apparent in these pilot studies warrant further comment. Serum cholesterol levels for the American men in this study may be slightly lower than other studies (29), while those for the Chinese men are typical of healthy men in Taiwan (30). They are also consistent with the unusually low prevalence of myocardial infarction in that country. For example, Tsai *et al.* at the National Taiwan University Hospital collected seventy-three cases of myocardial infarction in six years between January 1, 1954, and December 31, 1959 (31). Ratio of males to females was 5.6 to 1.0, and the average age was fifty-seven years. Infarction occurred more commonly in "leading citizens" with "less physical activity," and the annual prevalence increased each year. This unusually low prevalence for a major civilian hospital in a city of one million inhabitants suggests that many patients may not be obtaining medical care in a hospital. Yet comparative prevalences of acute coronary artery disease in the 801 Army General and Veterans General Hospitals in Taipei were 1.8 and 3.0 per cent of all cardiovascular disease between 1958 and 1963, while the frequency for private patients admitted to the Center Clinic was 11 per cent (32). Recent studies by Lee and associates, who collected autopsy specimens of hearts from several parts of the world and utilized standard methods of examination, clearly indicate that myocardial infarction is rare in some parts of Africa and the Orient (33). At autopsy the prevalence of cardiovascular disease was 7 per cent at the National Taiwan University Hospital versus 10 per cent for Chiba University Hospital in Japan and 44 per cent for Columbia University Hospital in New York City (34). Furthermore, the vast majority of the autopsies in Taipei showed only mild arteriosclerosis, yet age distributions were not significantly different from those in other localities.

It is now apparent that even maximal exercise testing of middle-aged men is feasible, with the precautions already cited, and that rather provocative differences can be elicited. It is impossible to state at this point whether such differences reflect, even very roughly, any differences in coronary arterial perfusion of the myocardium. Whereas previously widespread use of coronary arteriography in the absence of clinical disease formerly could not be justified, perhaps it can be now. In the interim, there has been gratifying technological improvement resulting in clearer demonstrations of the vascular anatomy with risks fading almost to the vanishing point. Yet the procedure is not quite as simple and repeatable as serial maximal exercise tests. The latter, however, may identify the individuals, rather than population samples, who should be studied in this manner.

Until further correlated anatomical information in healthy persons becomes available, it is also noteworthy that there appears to be some relationship between risk factors for coronary heart disease and this transient postexertional ST segment response. The relationship is more apparent in American men, who usually have a greater risk for this disease, than it is in Chinese men. When spontaneous changes in ST response occur longitudinally in a few years, it is impressive to note significant differences in mean values of risk factors in the very small number of men who have changed (19).

The age-specific prevalence of ST segment depression in healthy middle-aged Caucasians varies directly with selective factors in sampling, work loads, methods and criteria, as well as aging. It varies inversely with maximal oxygen intake. Roughly similar or higher frequencies have been found by computerized vectorcardiographic studies of Swedish men (10), and scalar ECG studies on Americans in Chicago (35) and in Philadelphia (36). Conversely, lower frequencies were found in Birmingham (37) with a near maximal test, and possibly a higher yield is apparent with the maximal. All of these utilized more than one lead system, and some (37) delayed recording in recovery for a few seconds until the subject had assumed the supine posture. The very low prevalence reported for 1449 middle-aged working men who were studied during moderate work loads (38) illustrates the need for more strenuous exercise testing. From the very diversity of approaches now available, suitable criteria for more effective standardization will certainly emerge in the future. Some of the principles important to standardization have already been published elsewhere (39-41).

Not only the testing procedures need standardization, but so do the criteria for, and exclusions from, selection for study. In the absence of clinical manifestations of disease, description of the physical characteristics, risk factors and even physical conditioning become important attributes in the analysis of relationships.

The role of physical activity and physical training may be assessed more critically by the combined use of maximal exercise testing and quantitative computer analysis of the ST response in this single bipolar ECG lead. Indeed, with only two types of observation to exercise on a treadmill—the ECG and oxygen intake—it is possible to appraise the changes in the stress-strain relationships of both the body as a whole and the heart muscle. Since submaximal energy expenditure is virtually predictable, the main determinant is the ECG which provides both the heart rate and the ST responses. Hopefully, with development of a suitable special purpose computer, the myocardial stress-strain analysis may become available in the future as a direct reading on-line instrument. This remains as an appropriate challenge to our biophysical collaborators, just as the demonstration of the feasibility becomes a challenge to cardiologists and, along with epidemiologists, radiologists and pathologists, to initiate similar studies to assist in the ultimate definition of the role of exercise electrocardiography in heart disease control and prevention. The enthusiastic interest of Ernst Simonson should hasten our efforts.

SUMMARY AND CONCLUSIONS

A multistage technique to elicit maximal exercise performance of either ambulatory cardiac patients or healthy subjects has been described in terms of its oxygen costs per kilogram of body weight. The relative frequencies of symptoms, physical signs and ECG responses indicated that chest pain and ST segment depression were commonly observed in cardiac patients. Examples of variations in ST responses in a single bi-polar precordial lead to such effort in selected patients with clinical manifestations of coronary heart disease were contrasted with atypical responses observed in some healthy middle-aged men. The latter clearly reveals an age dependency which follows a significant reduction in maximal oxygen intake with age. The magnitude of observer errors, a method of computer analysis and the apparent accuracy of visual interpretation of responses for classification of men have been cited. Details of the relationship of quantitative ST voltages to heart rate and work load have been described. Pending eventual definition of the relationship of ST depression of at least 1 mm after maximal exertion to any future clinical manifestations of coronary heart disease, a series of observations have been made on healthy middle-aged American and Chinese men who represent populations with unusually high and low clinical incidence of coronary disease. The overall prevalence and the age-specific prevalences of this response were lower in the Chinese, particularly those in the lower socioeconomic class, than in Americans residing in Seattle. Parallel differences have been found in risk factors associated with coronary heart disease. Longitudinal studies on Americans reveal satisfactory reproducibility, yet in a few who showed changes in this response, there have been parallel differences in cholesterol and blood pressure.

It is concluded that this ECG evidence of transient myocardial ischemia may provide an opportunity for earlier detection of coronary heart disease in healthy middle-aged men. Certainly, maximal exercise testing and ECG analysis is feasible for both experimental clinical and epidemiological studies. The preliminary observations on two different population samples are sufficiently provocative to warrant further studies to define the predictive value of maximal stress testing in earlier detection of ischemia heart disease.

The effects on whole body performance and myocardial performance before and after physical training of middle-aged adults have been described in terms of separate stress-strain relationships. Whereas maximal oxygen intake can be increased, both submaximal heart rate and quantitative ST_2 changes were diminished by such training, which involved twenty minutes of submaximal exertion three times a week for two months or more.

REFERENCES

1. SIMONSON, E.: Use of the electrocardiogram in exercise tests. *Amer Heart J, 66*:552, 1963.

2. BRUCE, R.A.: Evaluation of functional capacity and exercise tolerance of cardiac patients. *Mod Conc Cardiovasc Dis, 25*:321, 1956.

3. BRUCE, R.A.; BLACKMON, J.R.; JONES, J.W., and STRAIT, G.: Exercise testing in adult normal subjects and cardiac patients. *Pediatrics, 32*(II): 742, 1963.

4. BLACKMON, J.R., and BRUCE, R.A.: Unpublished observations, 1965.

5. DOAN, A.E.; PETERSON, D.R.; BLACKMON, J.R., and BRUCE, R.A.: Myocardial ischemia after maximal exercise in healthy men. *Amer Heart J, 69*:11, 1965.

6. LI, Y.B.; TING, N.; CHIANG, B.N.; ALEXANDER, E.R.; BRUCE, R.A., and GRAYSTON, J.T.: Electrocardiographic response to maximal exercise. Treadmill and double Master exercise tests in middle-aged Chinese men. *Amer J Cardiol, 20*:541, 1967.

7. BLACKBURN, H., and a Committee: The exercise electrocardiogram. Differences in interpretation. *Amer J Cardiol, 21*:871, 1968.

8. BRUCE, R.A.; MAZZARELLA, J.A.; JORDAN, J.W., JR., and GREEN, E.: Quantitation of QRS and ST segment responses to exercise. *Amer Heart J, 71*:455, 1966.

9. SJÖSTRAND, T.: The relationship between the heart frequency and the ST level of the electrocardiogram. *Acta Med Scand, 138*:111, 1950.

10. BLOMQVIST, G.: The Frank lead exercise electrocardiogram. *Acta Med Scand, 440* (suppl.):178, 1965.

11. HORNSTEN, T.R., and BRUCE, R.A.: Unpublished observations, 1967.

12. TAYLOR, R.R.; BRUCE, R.A.; HOFER, V., and HORNSTEN, T.R.: Variance reduction of computer averaged ECG responses to maximal exercise. Unpublished observations, 1967.

13. ALEXANDER, E.R.; TING, N.; GRAYSON, J.T.; LU, C.; LI, Y.B., and BRUCE, R.A.: Pilot study of ischemic heart disease on Taiwan. *Arch Environ Health, 10*:689, 1965.

14. CHIANG, B.N.; ALEXANDER, E.R.; BRUCE, R.A., and TING, N.: Physical characteristics and exercise performance of pedicab and upper socio-economic classes of middle-aged Chinese men. *Amer Heart J, 76*:760, 1968.

15. TING, N., and ALEXANDER, E.R., Personal communication, 1967.

16. GUTMAN, ROBERT A.; ALEXANDER, E.R.; LI, Y.B.; CHIANG, B.N.; WATTEN, RAYMOND, H.; TING, NONG, AND BRUCE, ROBERT A.: Determinant factors in delayed ST response to maximal exercise among selected American men in Taiwan. In preparation, 1969.

17. TAKAHASHI, H.; IWATSUKA, T.; OHASHI, I., and HOTTI, S.: Some observations of the ST depression in the exercise electrocardiogram. *Jap Heart J, 4*:105, 1963.

18. BRUCE, R.A.: Comparative prevalence of segmental ST depression after maximal exercise in healthy men in Seattle and Taipei. *Physical Activity and the Heart.* Karvonen, M.J., and Barry, A.J. (Eds.), Springfield, Thomas, 1967.

19. MOST, A.S.; HORNSTEN, T.R.; HOFER, V., and BRUCE, R.A.: Exercise ST changes in healthy men. *Arch Int Med, 121*:225, 1968.

20. DOAN, A.E.; PETERSON, D.R.; BLACKMON, J.R., and BRUCE, R.A.: Myocardial ischemia after maximal exercise in healthy men: One year follow-up of physically active and inactive men. *Amer J Cardiol, 17*:9, 1966.

21. KEYS, A.: The age trend of serum concentrations of cholesterol and of S_f 10-20 ("G") substance in adults. *J Geront, 7*:201, 1962.

22. MAZZARELLA, J.A.; SKINNER, J.S.; EVANS, T.R., and BRUCE, R.A.: Effects of physical training on electrocardiographic responses to exercise. In preparation, 1967.

23. BRUCE, R.A.; JONES, J.W., and STRAIT, G.: Anaerobic metabolic responses

to acute maximal exercise in male athletes. *Amer Heart J, 67*:643, 1964.

24. DONALD, K.W.; LIND, A.R.; McNICHOL, G.W.; HUMPHREYS, P.W.; TAYLOR, S.H., and STAUNTON, H.P.: Cardiovascular responses to sustained (static) contractions. *Circ Res, 20-21* (suppl. I):15, 1967.

25. BLACKMON, J.R.; ROWELL, L.B.; KENNEDY, J.W.; TWISS, R.D., and CONN, R.D.: Physiological significance of maximal oxygen intake in "pure" mitral stenosis. *Circulation, 36*:497, 1967.

26. ROWELL, L.B., Personal communication, 1967.

27. MASON, R.E.; LIKAR, I.; BIERN, R.O., and ROSS, R.S.: Multiple-lead exercise electrocardiography. Experience in 107 normal subjects and 67 patients with angina pectoris, and comparison with coronary arteriography in 84 patients. *Circulation, 36*:517, 1967.

28. BRUCE, R.A.: Unpublished observations, 1966.

29. KEYS, A., and FIDANZA, F.: Serum cholesterol and relative body weights of coronary patients in different populations. *Circulation, 22*:1091, 1960.

30. TSAI, H.S.; WU, C.C., and CHEN, J.S.: Cholesterol level in patients with coronary atherosclerotic heart disease. *J Formosa Med Assoc, 61*:1031, 1962.

31. TSAI, H.S.; YEN, T.S.; CHEN, C.M., and WU, T.L.: Clinical observations on myocardial infarction in 1954-1959 hospital material. *J Formosa Med Assoc, 59*:608, 1960.

32. TING, N., Personal communication, 1964.

33. LEE, K.T.; NAIL, R.; SHERMAN, L.A.; MILANO, M.; DEDEN, C.; IMAI, H.; GOODALE, F.; NAM, C.S.; SCOTT, R.F.; SNELL, E.S.; DAOUD, A.S.; JARMOLYCH, I.; JAKOVIC, L., and FLORENTIN, R.: Geographic pathology of myocardial infarction. *Amer J Cardiol, 13*:30, 1964.

34. LIU, J.H.: Reports of Institute of Pathology, National Taiwan University, 1967, No. 8, p. 1.

35. BERKSON, D.M.; STAMLER, J., and JACKSON, W.: The precordial electrocardiogram during and after strenuous exercise. *Amer J Cardiol, 18*:43, 1966.

36. BILLET, S.; ROMAN, L., and NICHOLS, G.J.: Correlation of the electrocardiographic exercise test and blood cholesterol. *Amer J Cardiol, 17*: 43, 1966.

37. LESTER, F.M.; SHEFFIELD, L.T., and REEVES, T.S.: Electrocardiographic changes in clinically normal older men following near maximal and maximal exercise. *Circulation, 36*:5, 1967.

38. BLACKBURN, H.; TAYLOR, H.L.; VASQUEZ, C.L., and PUCHNER, T.C.: The electrocardiogram during exercise. Findings in bipolar chest leads in 1449 middle-aged men, at moderate work levels. *Circulation, 34*:1034, 1966.

39. BLACKBURN, H.: The electrocardiogram in cardiovascular epidemiology: Problems in standardized application. *Ann NY Acad Sci, 126*:882, 1965.

40. BLACKBURN, H.; TAYLOR, H.L.; OKOMOTO, N.; RAUTAHARJU, P.; MITCHELL, P.M., and KERKHOF, A.C.: Standardization of the exercise electro-cardiogram, a systematic comparison of chest lead configurations employed for monitoring during exercise. In *Physical Activity and the Heart*. Karvonen, M.J., and Barry, A.J. (Eds.), Springfield, Thomas, 1967, chapt. 9, p. 101.

41. Report of a Committee on Electrocardiography, American Heart Association: Recommendations for standardization of leads and of specifications for instruments in electrocardiography and vectorcardiography. Charles E. Kossmann, M.D., Chairman. *Circulation, 35*:583, 1967.

42. Addendum to Fox, S.M., and SKINNER, J.S.: Some planning in the United States for further studies to define the relationship between physical activity and coronary heart disease. In *Physical Activity and the Heart*. Karvonen, M.J., and Barry, A.J. (Eds.), Springfield, Thomas, 1967, chapt. 20, pp. 245-248.

43. BRUCE, R. A.; HORNSTEN, T. R., AND BLACKMON, J. R.: Myocardial infarction after normal responses to exercise. *Circulation, 38*:552, 1968.

DISCUSSION

Dr. Taylor: Ordinarily the physiologist classifies "maximal oxygen intake" as that rate of work which will produce a plateauing of the oxygen intake; that rate of work beyond which another increment will produce no increase in the oxygen intake. On the continuous step-up tests I sometimes have difficulty being sure that a plateau has existed, and I'm also having difficulty in knowing whether people have gone to maximal oxygen intake or to an end-point which isn't quite as reproducible. I wonder if you would have any impressions as to which kinds of work stresses you are dealing with here?

Dr. Bruce: With certain patients, I do not think it is wise to push to supramaximal work, because of the possibility of fibrillation—we have never seen this, and hope we never will.

It is possible to demonstrate a plateau; we are cautious in trying to document the plateau.

Dr. Taylor: I am not questioning your procedure. I think that it is useful, though, to make this distinction between talking about going to maximal oxygen intake or to maximum work capacity. I think that the two can be, in some people, at least, a little different. Do we have any questions from the floor, Dr. Lepeschkin?

Dr. Lepeschkin: One important point. When an arrhythmia develops during exercise testing, should the subject lie down or remain standing and continue work? It seems to me that in the person lying down, this would increase the flow to the heart and stretching of the heart muscle, and the chances of the arrhythmia persisting are even greater; while in the upright position, of course the stroke output is less and the heart rate is faster, and we know that, as Dr. Brooks told us, a fast heart rate suppresses the ectopic beat. I would like to know what your experience is.

Dr. Bruce: You have touched on an interesting point, Dr. Lepeschkin. It has been our practice in patients we see in the cardiology clinic and test in this manner, that we have them sit down on a chair placed on the treadmill after their maximal exertion, rather than lying down. Once in a while we have to have them lie down when they may become light-headed or faint and do not have enough cardiac output and cerebral blood flow. I presume this because they recover as soon as they lie down; and this suggests the possibility of venous pooling in the veins in the lower limbs.

It is interesting from a different point of view that premature beats, arrhythmias, are far more prevalent in Americans than they are in the Chinese. I was very much struck by this when I went to Taiwan and was amazed how hard it was to find a premature beat. Dr. Chiang, when he first looked at our American tracings, made the opposite observation; he was surprised to see so many of them, not that they were frequent, but so many people had isolated ventricular beats here and there. In terms of the postural aspects, again, in the Chaing, when he first looked at our American tracings, made the opposite observation; he was surprised to see so many of them, not venous pooling, and would have to lie down. But on lying down, they still did not show evidence of arrythmia. So there are other aspects of this in addition to the apparent irritability of the myocardium.

Dr. Taylor: Dr. Bruce mentioned that in all these work procedures they were careful not to have the subject touch the treadmill handrail. I want to underline this, because if you take the trouble to test this, on normals, at least, just putting a hand on the rail will cut the oxygen consumption by around 10 per cent in a great many situations. This is a practical point which I think needs to be emphasized.

25

Correlation of Graded Exercise Electrocardiographic Response with Clinical and Coronary Cinearteriographic Findings

ROBERT E. MASON, I. LIKAR, R.O. BIERN *and* R.S. ROSS

The exercise electrocardiogram (ECG) has certain advantages over other tests for coronary insufficiency. It is simple in that it is non-invasive of the internal environment and mechanical structures of the heart, and, as described below, does not necessitate sophisticated equipment. It is reasonably safe in that it can be adjusted to the tolerance of each individual patient, and can be monitored during the test. The information it provides is current, and in many ways more valuable than that derived from long-range follow-up and autopsy studies. Through our opportunity to perform this test on a group of patients being studied concurrently by coronary cinearteriography, we have been able to compare each of these parameters with the clinical diagnosis, and thus to gain some information as to the accuracy of each of these three parameters.

The method we have used in our graded exercise stress test has been published in some detail (1). We wished to obtain information from multiple scalar leads both during and after exercise to determine whether information might be available from such records which had

Note: This investigation was supported in part by U.S. Public Health Service Research Grant HE-05584-CV from the National Heart Institute, and by Clinical Center Grant FR-35 from the Division of General Medical Sciences.

Work was done while Dr. Likar was a Fellow in Medicine, supported by Graduate Training Grant 2 TI HE-5159 from the National Heart Institute; Dr. Biern was a U.S. Public Health Service Research Fellow, supported by Grant 5-F2-HE-22,894 from the National Heart Institute and Dr. Ross was the recipient of a Career Development Award 5 K3 HE-3795 from the National Heart Institute.

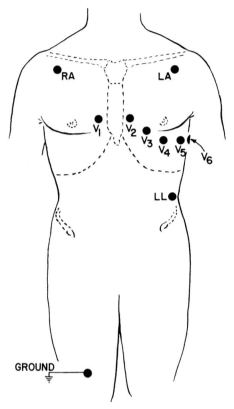

FIGURE 25-1. Placement of electrodes for recording multiple-lead electrocardiograms at rest and during exercise.

been absent or only partially represented in the simple precordial monitoring leads used in many laboratories. Satisfactory limb leads cannot be recorded during exercise with electrodes placed in the usual position at the periphery of the limbs due to the interference caused by muscle potential. Therefore we explored the surface of the body to determine what electrode placement would give limb leads closely resembling those obtained from standard electrode placement and yet be as free as possible from muscle potential interference. We found the placement indicated in Figure 25-1 was the closest to this ideal, giving scalar leads virtually identical in form to standard leads and varying minimally in amplitude from them. The arm electrodes are placed in the infraclavicular fossae 2 cm below the clavicle and medial

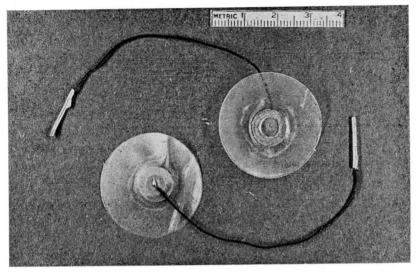

FIGURE 25-2. Top and bottom views of disposable electrode.

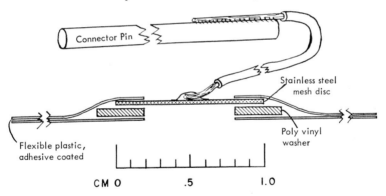

FIGURE 25-3. Cross-section diagram of electrode.

to the respective deltoid muscle. The left leg electrode is placed roughly midway between the costal margin and the iliac crest in the anterior axillary line. The precordial electrodes are then placed in the usual V positions, permitting one to record a 12-lead electrocardiogram with appropriate multiple channel equipment. It should be noted that if augmented unipolar leads are to be recorded simultaneously, loss of amplitude may occur unless buffer amplifiers are built into the circuit.

Considerable experimentation has been conducted on electrodes for use in exercise stress electrocardiograms. The electrode we have developed obviates the great majority of problems we have encountered with other types of electrodes. It is depicted in Figures 25-2 and 25-3. It is very small, flat and of low mass, each weighing less than 0.5 gm. It consists of a stainless steel mesh disc sandwiched between two thin layers of flexible plastic, and separated from the skin by a washer of flexible plastic 0.5 mm thick. This washer prevents electrode-skin contact which would produce abrupt shifts of the baseline. Due to its construction there is minimal tendency for the electrode to vary in its relationship to the surface of the skin during the motions of exercise. Hence the baseline shifts secondary to such motions are less than with any electrode we have tested. It is inexpensive to manufacture and disposable after a single use and therefore very convenient.

We have administered stress in the form of external work. We fully agree with other colleagues reporting in this symposium that the form of the external work is of little importance and have interested ourselves primarily in administering work which is readily measurable and which is adaptable to the particular problems of the patient at hand. We have used the Lanoöy bicycle ergometer (2) but find that a fair percentage of American patients are unable to operate a bicycle ergometer. Others in the cardiac division (3) have developed an escalator ergometer which has proven very useful and helpful in our work. The work has been begun at the general level of the double two-step test for the individual (4), but in order to permit the circulation to reach a steady state has been continued for a five-minute period instead of three minutes as in the double two-step test. If the subject at that time is tolerating the work well the load has been increased at intervals of three minutes until one of the following four end-points is reached:

1. Pain of the degree of the usual daily anginal attack.
2. Fatigue.
3. Heart rate 90 per cent of the expected maximum for his age group (5).
4. Positive ischemic response in the monitored ECG.

The criterion we have used for a positive test is 1.0 mm of ischemic ST segment depression, lasting 0.08 seconds or longer. By "ischemic" we mean that the ST segment must be absolutely horizontal or downsloping for this period of time (6). This is an arbitrary criterion but

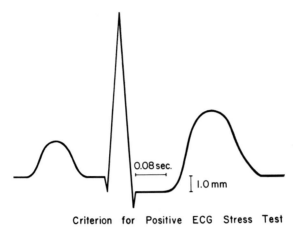

Criterion for Positive ECG Stress Test

FIGURE 25-4. Criterion for positive ECG stress test. The ST segment during or after exercise must be depressed 1.0 mm or more for 0.08 seconds or more and have a flat or downsloping configuration.

one reasonably recognizable by the observer and, in our opinion, a very significant and abnormal change (Fig. 25-4). Records have been read by two observers with the identifying information obscured at a point in time remote from the recording for the purpose of the present report.

The coronary cinearteriograms have been carried out by Dr. R. S. Ross and his colleagues using the Sones technique in which each coronary artery in turn is catheterized and individually injected with radiopaque material. A movie is taken of the fluoroscopic screen, showing the progress of the radiopaque material through the coronaries in two different planes. The cine lesions are classified as follows:

Class 0. No visible abnormality.
Class 1. Minimal narrowing.
Class 2. 50 per cent narrowing of one artery.
Class 3. Multiple severe narrowings.
Class 4. Complete occlusion of one or more arteries.

Two hundred subjects have been studied by the graded exercise electrocardiographic stress test described above and concurrently by cinearteriography. From these 200 patients we have eliminated for the present study those with any condition which might be expected to interfere with the ST segment response to exercise, namely subjects taking digitalis, those with ventricular conduction defects such as bundle branch block and Wolff-Parkinson-White syndrome, those with blood pressure exceeding 160/100, those with endocardial, myocardial or pericardial disease, those with congestive failure, anemia, or electrolyte disturbances, and finally all those whom we would consider clearly on clinical grounds and response to exercise to be vasoregulatory hyperreactors (7). These subjects show an exaggerated response of the ST segment to changes in position and to exercise, this response being normalized by propranolol.

We are left then with 164 subjects, the results of whose tests are now to be described. Seventy-one patients on careful clinical evaluation have been found to have typical Heberden's angina pectoris. Twenty-two patients have been diagnosed as having atypical angina. The clinical picture in these patients is very strongly indicative of angina pectoris but is atypical in some particular feature such as character or distribution of the pain or failure to respond promptly to nitro-

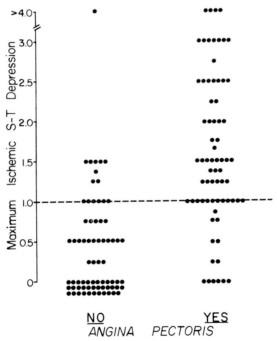

FIGURE 25-5. Comparison of response to exercise in 142 patients having typical angina pectoris with those not having angina.

glycerin. Finally there are seventy-one subjects classified as "other." These subjects are not considered to be normal in that each was considered to have sufficient chest discomfort or abnormality in his response to the two-step test to justify coronary cinearteriography. Arteriography carries a slight but very definite risk, and has not been done in our hands to any subject considered absolutely normal.

As a result of this study we have three parameters for comparison: the response to graded exercise electrocardiographic stress test, the results of the cinearteriogram, and the classification by careful clinical diagnosis. It is of interest to take each pair of these parameters in turn for analysis. In Figure 25-5 is graphed the electrocardiographic response to exercise on the vertical axis. The group of patients who have typical angina are on the right and those who are considered not to have clinical coronary insufficiency on the left. The atypical angina subjects are eliminated from this graph. It is seen that the majority of patients with angina have an exercise test which is positive (on or above the broken horizontal line indicating 1.0 mm of ischemic segment depression). Conversely those without angina show a majority of negative responses. The following table indicates the figures observed:

Ischemic ST	*Sensitivity* (for classical angina)		*Specificity* (for noncardiac chest complaint)	
⩾ 0.5 mm	.89	63/71	.55	39/71
⩾ 1.0 mm	.82	58/71	.79	56/71
⩾ 1.5 mm	.52	37/71	.92	65/71

Figure 25-6 uses the same clinical classification shown in the previous figure with the response distributed according to the arteriographic class. Here it can be seen that patients with typical angina pectoris (shown on the upper level) in the great majority of instances will be found to have severe coronary artery disease by arteriography. To be specific, forty-six of the seventy-one in this group have a complete occlusion of at least one coronary artery, and sixty-eight of the seventy-one fall into cine classes 2, 3 and 4, whereas only three are in classes 0 and 1. The group without angina (*shown on the lower level*) conversely contains only twelve instances of significant arteriographic lesions.

The whole population of 164 subjects is included in Figure 25-7.

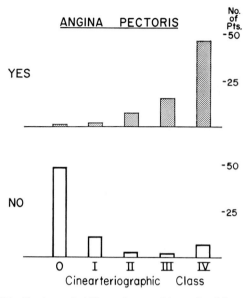

FIGURE 25-6. Distribution of 142 patients with and without typical angina pectoris according to the results of cinearteriogram.

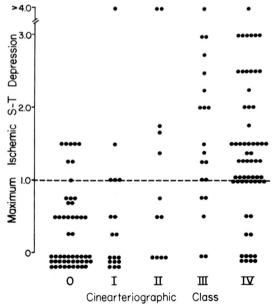

Figure 25-7. Comparison of results of cinearteriography in 164 patients with ECG response to exercise.

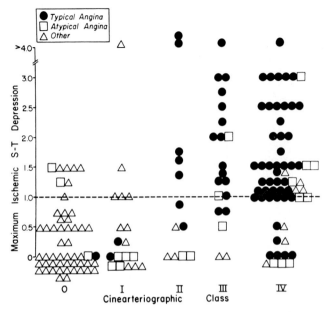

FIGURE 25-8. Same distribution as in Figure 25-7, further identified by indication of clinical diagnosis.

The ECG response to exercise is indicated on the vertical axis and the subjects distributed according to arteriographic class on the horizontal axis. The patients with a positive ECG response to exercise in the majority of instances have severe arteriographic disease and those with a negative response to exercise mostly fall into arteriographic classes indicating minimal involvement of the coronaries. The categories are divided as follows:

Ischemic ST	*Sensitivity for Cine II-IV*		*Specificity for Cine 0-1*	
$\geqslant$ 0.5 mm	.83	78/94	.60	42/70
$\geqslant$ 1.0 mm	.74	70/94	.81	57/70
$\geqslant$ 1.5 mm	.44	41/94	.90	63/70

For a criterion of $\geqslant$ 1.0 mm ischemic ST this corresponds to 26 per cent "missed cases" of distinct coronary artery disease and 19 per cent "false positives."

All three parameters are combined in Figure 25-8. This represents the same scatter of patients as in the previous figure, but each is now identified according to his clinical diagnosis (typical, atypical and other). In summary, this graph indicates that the majority of the subjects with angina have a positive ECG test and severe coronary lesions demonstrated by the arteriogram, but not all of them. The majority of patients with positive ECG tests have clinical angina pectoris and severe disease by the arteriogram, but not all of them. The majority of patients with severe arteriographic lesions have a positive ECG response to exercise and clinical angina pectoris, but not all of them.

The correlation between these parameters then is not perfect. Each parameter has certain complicating features which would tend to keep it from correlating perfectly with either of the others. The electrocardiographic stress test, in addition to the multiple problems of recording and interpretation mentioned by other collaborators in this symposium, may under certain circumstances be more sensitive or less sensitive than the other parameters in a given subject. For example, it is perfectly possible and even quite probable that one can feel pain from a mass of ischemic muscle too small to show a change in the peripheral electrocardiogram. Furthermore, it has been demonstrated in dogs (8) that the flow through a coronary artery must be reduced at least 30 per cent below the normal level before there is any abnormality demonstrable in the ECG at the periphery. The flow must be reduced 75 per cent before severe ECG changes are demonstrated routinely, a finding quite compatible with the results of the present study in humans.

The clinical diagnosis of angina pectoris is a notoriously difficult one even in the hands of experienced clinicians. It is in a sense the diametric opposite of the diagnosis reached by double blind process in that it is a double subjective process. The subject must recognize and describe his discomfort and then the clinician must ask appropriate questions and interpret the description of the patient to establish the diagnosis in the face of his own inherent bias.

The cinearteriogram has certain unavoidable limitations. It can only show lesions down to a certain size. Statistically, the majority of significant coronary artery disease occurs in arteries of the size that it delineates adequately. Cinearteriographers however, recognize that this technique demonstrates lesions much better than it demonstrates flow. Flow can be determined in this technique only by the rate of filling and the rate of emptying of the vessels involved, and is exceedingly difficult to quantitate in comparison with subsequent autopsy studies. In all likelihood cinearteriography underestimates the amount of vascular disease in most subjects. During this technique the radio-paque material injected is a very unphysiological hypertonic material and there is quite possibly a difference in the flow through the coronary arteries of this material as compared to the flow of normal blood.

Each of these three parameters then looks at a different facet of the central disorder, myocardial ischemia. One cannot anticipate a perfect correlation among the three parameters. The correlation demonstrated is very instructive. Much work is being done in each of these three fields to improve the techniques, but it may not be possible for any of these techniques to give the full story in an individual. The combination of all three techniques may be much more valuable. It is clear that the work being reported in this symposium will improve the accuracy and precision of instrumentation in the electrocardiographic stress test. Our work, I believe, points out that as cardiologists we must not lose sight of our desire to improve the overall diagnostic accuracy of tests for myocardial ischemia. We may continue to require considerable information from other techniques and other sources, and cannot rely on the electrocardiographic stress test alone.

REFERENCES

1. Mason, R.E., and Likar, I.: A new system of multiple-lead exercise electrocardiography. *Amer Heart J, 71*:196, 1966.
2. Lanooy, C., and Bonjer, F.H.: A hyperbolic ergometer for cycling and cranking. *J Appl Physiol, 9*:499, 1956.
3. Talbot, S.A.; Likar, I., and Harrison, W.K., Jr.: Exercise escalator for electrocardiographic studies in patients with coronary heart disease. *Amer Heart J, 72*:35, 1966.
4. Master, A.M., and Rosenfeld, I.: Criteria for the clinical application of the "two-step" exercise test: Obviation of false negative and false positive responses. *JAMA, 178*:283, 1961.
5. Robinson, S.: Experimental studies of physical fitness in relation to age. *Arbeitphysiologie, 10*:251, 1938.
6. Myers, G.B., and Talmers, F.N.: Electrocardiographic diagnosis of acute myocardial ischemia. *Ann Intern Med, 43*:361, 1955.
7. Mason, R.E.; Likar, I.; Biern, R.O., and Ross, R.S.: Multiple-lead exercise electrocardiography: Experience in 107 normal subjects and 67 patients with angina pectoris, and comparison with coronary cinearteriography in 84 patients. *Circulation, 36*:517, 1967.
8. Wegria, R.; Segers, M., and Krating, R.P.: Relationship between reduction in coronary flow and appearance of electrocardiographic changes. *Amer Heart J, 38*:90, 1949.

Concluding Remarks

CHANDLER McC. BROOKS

As SOMEWHAT OF AN outsider I probably have the expected obtuseness and acuteness which characterizes the amateur. As I have listened to presentations and discussions, I have reached some conclusions and formulated some questions.

1. Last night Dr. Simonson said that when Hitler and the Nazis came into power it was thought they would last only six months or so. They remained. It is obvious now that the computers are here to stay. Please do not extend the analogy.

Since every institution must have its computer center, they will be used in medicine and physiology. Therefore, the question is no longer *whether;* it is *how.* We must overtake instrumentation and put it to *proper use* in electrocardiography.

2. It is rather axiomatic in medicine that even if one does not know what he is doing, if he does it well, consistently and repetitively, he will be accepted and some patients at least will be convinced they have been saved. Higher success is attained, we think, if procedures are reasonable.

All one has to do in exercise electrocardiography is to accept standardized procedures, conventions and then collect data. Out of these largely arbitrary procedures something worthwhile is sure to result. Whether it will be the best possible depends upon wise selection of these conventions.

Certainly, a methodology of diagnosing cardiac abnormalities will succeed, especially if that methodology creates, aggravates, awakens, these abnormalities. I say this because it is obvious that some procedures discussed could, if in inexperienced hands or too computer-dependent in decision to terminate, do harm. I am sure all of us are aware of this but this has been assumed and not discussed in detail.

3. If one reaches conclusions on a pragmatic basis and obtains quantitative data by methodology, this is fine, but transfer back to

[456]

physiology may be extremely difficult unless physiology is initially considered. Ultimately, one is driven to judging what is going on in the heart. It is here that I have felt some dissatisfaction with what I have heard.

a. I think the exclusion of variation by seeking only the "characteristic configuration" of any state is hazardous. The ultimate "characteristic change" is only half the story. It is my opinion that surveillance of variation and its changes would give an earlier and more sensitive clue to developing or present abnormality. For example, fluctuations in P-R values precede block and averaging them out would not help an early diagnosis of conduction failure.

b. One should be very careful with the screening out of noise or interference with the biological signal. Certainly, some elements of cardiac muscle reactions are so similar to skeletal muscle "noise" that they would be eliminated by any filter used to block skeletal muscle electrical signals. It is apparent that all persons here are aware of this problem.

c. I suggest that the attempt to identify "fiduciary points" should involve consideration of the lability of the process creating the marking signal, that giving the fiduciary point. Some processes, the rise of the R wave or the entry process, are less labile than others. In heart action regenerative depolarization is little modified except by extremely abnormal and unusual circumstance. The terminal phases of repolarization also are relatively rigid, but conduction speeds, duration of the plateau are extremely changeable. I think it would be impossible to identify regularly and reliably the beginning, midportion or any component of the T wave.

The QRS or the whole ECG complex, as seen, is just an average of many potential balances between paired reference electrodes and the average is of varied process at diverse places. The sophistication of instrumentation may exceed the reliability of basic methodology—indirect recording from fluctuating processes in a fluctuating conductor situation.

d. Since one deals with a cyclical event and desires it to assay the normality of events in the cycle, two fiduciary points are needed. The beginning and end must be identified so that analysis by segments of time can be made proportionate to fluctuating total time. I believe the group is seeking to trigger from events, but they cannot be reliably identified by time from any one fiduciary point because in changing they change durations disproportionately. I know of no easy solution to suggest.

4. Although I am certain that all present recognize that not only events in the heart affect the monitors during exercise, but also the heart position and its contacts with good and bad conductors. These changes do not produce noise, but somehow they must be calculated in any attempt to judge myocardial changes. A change in conductor contact could, in my opinion, reverse a T wave in some leads at least. All present are more competent to deal with this problem than am I —my point is merely that as a problem for this methodological development, it was not discussed.

5. Finally, I might make some remarks about biological processes being in continual flux with no absolutely steady states or absolute repetition. All measurements are only relatively correct for any other instant in time. I could suggest definitions for your questions relative to the meaning of precision and accuracy. There is a danger of language-meaning difference in these cooperative enterprises in which engineers, physiologists and physicians invade one another's fields. I will say, that despite all the differences one can see and imagine, this present group of Biomedical - Cardiographic - Physiological - Physicist - Engineers inspires one's confidence. Their ultimate goals will be attained, I am sure.

This has been a most interesting meeting indeed, and I am certain it has been a very productive one. I wish to thank Dr. Simonson for having such nice friends and for having attained the age and distinction to catalyze such a conference. I wish to express my gratitude to Dr. Blackburn and the Minnesota Heart Association for their generosity and the excellence of their plan. I am certain I speak for all others in expressing our high appreciation of your efforts and your goals.

On Missing and Catching Boats

ERNST SIMONSON
*On the Occasion of Ernst Simonson Day, September 28, 1967,
The Minneapolis Club*

MY SCIENTIFIC CAREER started with missing the boat. As an undergraduate student with pharmacologist Otto Riesser at Greifswald in Germany, it was suggested that I continue his investigations of acetylcholine-induced muscle contraction. Acetylcholine was even then a remarkable substance. Immersion of a frog gastrocnemius or sartorius muscle into an extremely weak solution of 1:100,000, and as I found out, of 1:1 million, and occasionally 1:10 million, would produce a contraction equal in magnitude to the maximum contraction of a twitch elicited by maximum electrical stimulation. On slow immersion of the muscle the contraction started as soon as the Ringer-acetylcholine solution reached the level of the nerve entrance, and would last for hours. Obviously, the effect was located in the myoneural junction rather than in the muscle fiber, and there were no detectable action currents during the contraction. We thought, of course, that acetylcholine might be the contraction substance. However, I dismissed this idea because electrical stimulation applied at the height of the acetylcholine contraction produced a sizeable twitch; the combined amplitude of twitch and acetylcholine contraction greatly exceeded the size of the maximum contraction to either (*Arch. f. exper. Pathol. &
Pharmakol., 96, 1923*). We rather believed that acetylcholine acted on a hypothetical substrate for muscle tone, and assumed as did other physiologists at that time, that there is a dual function of the skeletal muscle: contraction and tone, each with its own substrate. Twelve years later, Brown, Dale and Feldberg demonstrated in cats and dogs by arterial injection of acetylcholine that acetylcholine is, indeed, the contraction substance and thus established the basis for the theory of cholinergic transmission which is now generally accepted. If our interest had not been diverted to other problems this discovery might have been in our grasp. It comes as little and late consolation that the

[459]

theory of cholinergic transmission for muscle contraction has been doubted recently by Rieker, 1966.

At that time instead I became intrigued with the problems of muscle tone. After injection of scopolamine stimulation of the frog gastrocnemius *in situ* with a single shock produces a "tonic" after contraction, i.e., after the fast twitch the contraction is maintained near or somewhat below the maximum amplitude for many seconds. This phenomenon is abolished by spinal cord section. It is reproduced by mechanical stimulation of the midbrain (*Pflug. Arch. Physiol. 203*: 1924; *205*:1925). The after-contraction was not associated with action currents, in this respect similar to the acetylcholine contraction. The pathways were explored as well as effect of electrolytes and drugs on this phenomenon. From here I was tempted to go into neurophysiology or neurosurgery, extending the results to more detailed studies on mammals. However, in connection with my work on muscle tone, I became increasingly interested in the physiology of muscle contraction and muscular work and so went into exercise physiology.

At that time, in the early twenties, the physiology of muscle contraction was in an exciting phase of development subsequent to the fundamental discoveries of Hill and Meyerhof. Under the impact of their theory, and Hill, Long and Lupton's investigations in man, I started to study in greater detail the dynamics of oxygen intake during work and recovery (O_2 debt) and was aided by the award of a Rockefeller Fellowship. Since application of the Hill-Meyerhof theory was new, it was a good time to start work in this field; nearly every result was bound to be a discovery.

The University of Greifswald had through several centuries a distinguished medical faculty. In my time there Morawitz was Professor of Medicine and the founder of the modern theory of blood coagulation. He was followed by H. Straub. Hugo Schulz was Professor of Pharmacology, succeeded by Otto Riesser in 1923. Hugo Schulz was an excellent historian and unorthodox thinker and impressed deeply nearly everybody with whom he came in personal contact. He published very little and yet had a strong influence on the direction, thinking, philosophical attitude and approach of outstanding clinicians such as August Bier and Sauerbruch, who were Professors of Surgery, in succession in Greifswald. Having, during his long lifetime, seen so many biomedical theories come and go, he had acquired an understandable attitude of wait and see. One of his bon mots was: *Der Theologe ist, im Vergleich zum Mediziner, ein WaisenKnabe was das Dogma anbelangt* (The theologian compared to the physician is an orphan as far as dogma is concerned). There was also Paul Grawitz, the last surviving associate of Virchow. He must have been in his eighties; at that time there was no mandatory retirement age at German universities. His name is preserved in the description of the Grawitz tumor, but to his last day he doubted the migration of leukocytes discovered by Cohnheim, the most brilliant of Virchow's associates. Grawitz would tell us of his student days in the pre-antiseptic era. If needles or silk for surgery did not appear to be quite clean, one would wipe them off on one's coat. He claimed surprisingly little happened.

Friedberger, succeeding Loeffler the discoverer of the diphtheria bacillus, first described anaphylactic shock. There also was Bleibtreu, Professor of Physiology, the last surviving associate of Pflüger. Edgar Atzler as assistant and Gunther Lehmann working in his department as graduate student were the core of the Institut für Arbeitsphysiologie founded in 1925 by Rubner at the University of Berlin, later, in 1928, transferred to Dortmund. I also worked as an undergraduate student in this department, and my very first paper, observations on cardiac motion, originated from there (*Pflüg. Arch. Physiol. 165*, 1922). Although I never was a member of the Institut für Arbeitsphysiologie, common interests and personal friendship connected me with Edgar Atzler (to his early death) Gunther Lehmann, and E. A. Müller. In these formative years Riesser's enthusiasm for biological problems was infectious.

Like the University (which celebrated its 500th anniversary a few years ago) Greifswald was an old city. Most of the houses dated from 1800 and earlier. The cobblestone pavement was designed to prevent traffic which it did effectively. There was a saying that in case of a world catastrophe one should go to Greifswald because everything would happen there one hundred years later.

In 1928, I was invited by Physiologist Albert Bethe at the University of Frankfurt/Main to develop *Arbeitsphysiologie* (Industrial Physiology) at his department. This was the first division of Industrial

Physiology at any German University. Bethe, one of the great physiologists of the first half of the twentieth century perhaps is best known in the United States as editor of the *Handbuch der Normalen and Pathologischen Physiologie*. I worked also with Ludwig Ascher and organized a Department of Industrial Physiology at the Institute of Social Hygiene. Ascher was one of the leading German statisticians in social medicine, specializing in Industrial Health. I investigated energy expenditure in foundry workers, the first investigations of this type under conditions of industrial work. For this purpose I developed a new respiration apparatus, designed for minimum interference with job performance and employing the "Teilstrom" principle (partial air currents). Francis G. Benedict's letter on the occasion of this was a wonderful appreciation. This principle was later applied to the respiration apparatus of the Max Planck Institute.

Working in Bethe's department of "Animalische Physiologie" were Dr. Ernst Fischer and Professor Wilhelm Steinhausen. Professor Gustav Embden was Professor of "Vegetative Physiologie," working on biochemical changes of muscle contraction, and was an early opponent of Hill-Meyerhof. Thus, there was in Frankfurt a most stimulating atmosphere for work on muscle and exercise physiology. In one of many talks with Professor Wilhelm Steinhaussen on physiology and physiologists he advised me, "If you wish to make a good career, you must have a polemic with a famous author, but, never never win!"

Without intentionally heeding this advice, I soon after became involved in a polemic with A. V. Hill, who had a few years earlier, received with Meyerhof, the Nobel prize for their work and theory of muscle contraction.

One of the impressive features of the Hill-Meyerhof theory was that every thing fitted together so perfectly: the heat production in muscle contraction and the biochemical changes as were known at that time, and the dynamics of gaseous exchange during muscular work. It was assumed that metabolic processes continue unchanged during work, so that the oxygen deficit at the beginning of work corresponds exactly to the oxygen debt after work. As mentioned, my work in Greifswald was largely stimulated by the work of Hill and Meyerhof. In Greifswald, I had concentrated mainly on the rate of recovery from oxygen debt. In Frankfurt, I started to investigate the processes of

the beginning of exercise. It seemed that the pieces did not fit together as well as it appeared in the work of Hill, Long and Lupton
due to the fact that the biochemical processes in the first few minutes
of work are different from those after the steady state has been reached.
The oxygen debt cannot be predicted from the oxygen deficit in the
beginning of work. H. Hebestreit and Emanuel Hansen (later Director
of the Institute of Gymnastic-Theory in Copenhagen) joined me in
this work, assisted also by Sophie Schemel, who later became my wife
(*Pflüg. Arch., 225*:498, 1930). A. V. Hill objected to these results:
"They preceeded to make experiments on the efficiency of muscular
work which, were the results correct, would indeed have brought the
edifice tumbling in ruins" (*Physiol. Rev., 12*:1932). The results are
actually the basis for the so-called "warm-up period." I continued
this work later in Kharkov, USSR, expanding the results to different
types of work and exploring details of the mechanism, with applications to industrial work, to athletics and to disease. The basic results
have been repeatedly confirmed, particularly by Scandinavian workers,
and E. A. Müller, Institut für Arbeitsphysiologie in Dortmund, has
proposed this be called the Simonson effect. Despite A. V. Hill's pre-
dictions, his edifice still stands, although some repairs were needed.
There is no question but that Hill's investigations with Long and
Lupton were the most stimulating event in the physiology of exercise
in the past fifty years.

A second polemic in which I became involved was concerned with
the fusion frequency of flicker (FFF). The famous author who
started this polemic was Selig Hecht, who had laid the groundwork
for the present theory of vision. The fusion frequency of flicker
(FFF) is that rate of successive light flashes, on increasing frequency,
where the sensation of flicker disappears and becomes plain light. It
was used since the mid-nineteenth century as one of the fundamental
methods for investigation of basic visual parameters such as brightness, contrast, size of illuminated area, etc. From personal discussions
with the great Russian physiologists I. P. Pavlov and particularly A. A.
Ukhtomskii, I thought that FFF may be related to the Wedenskii-
Ukhtomskii theory of excitability, based on the importance of the
time parameter. (The effective time parameter, the refractory period
of trains of repeated stimuli, has some relationship to Lapicque's

chronaxie, and was extensively studied in muscle tetanus and reflexes by the Russian authors). Later, using the FFF in patients with central nervous, metabolic and circulatory disorders, with Norbert Enzer and Samuel Blankstein participating in this work at Mount Sinai Hospital, Milwaukee, Wisconsin, we found significantly lower FFF in these patients than in normal subjects. Thus, the FFF showed depression of excitability of visual pathways, and possibly, in general, of the central nervous system in these conditions. I presented the results at the meeting of the American Physiological Society in Chicago in 1943 where Selig Hecht objected violently. His criticism was, indeed, devastating. He could not conceive that this method could be sensitive to other than strictly visual parameters, in other words, that visual pathways are functionally integrated with the state of the CNS. I received a few letters with some expressions of condolence, together with the assertion that Selig Hecht had exceeded the limits of reasonable argumentation. Since our investigations the FFF has been used in numerous studies of physiological and pathological stresses, and the sensitivity of this method to a variety of stresses has been confirmed.

Another polemic, and I really never intended to be a controversial person, involved the whole Illuminating Society. Joseph Brozek and I, in the Laboratory of Physiological Hygiene, studied the effect of illumination level on strenuous visual performance. For about five decades illuminating societies of all countries have maintained that there is no limit to the beneficial effect of increase of the illumination level. We found that there is a definite brightness optimum beyond which performance decreases. This optimum was somewhat below the recommended levels for this type of work, but was, at 100 foot-candles, still quite high. I should mention that the Illuminating Society invited me to present my results at their annual meeting 1950.

Thus, I did get involved in polemics with famous authors, as my friend Wilhelm Steinhausen asked me to do, but I followed only the first half of the advice, since my results happen to have been confirmed elsewhere. Whether this helped or damaged my career I do not know.

Coming back to my work at the University of Frankfurt there was much interest in the development of Arbeitsphysiologie not only in

Germany but also in Russia. The Russian government sent several young physiologists to work with me. One of them, Peter I. Dolgin, had, unknown to me, an influential government position. I soon got an invitation to come to Russia first for a visit. I remember some details of this visit, in February, 1930, quite distinctly. When Peter Dolgin showed me the sights of Kharkov I carried my Leica on a shoulder strap. He said, "You cannot do this here, somebody may cut the strap with a scissors." We went to the Meeting of the Soviet Physiological Society in Rostov. There Dolgin took me out in a sleigh-ride to see the new tractor plant, about twelve miles from Rostov. We were huddled in blankets and furs, but the bitter cold penetrated everything; since then I know the meaning of the phrase "frozen stiff." When we arrived, the plant was closed. At an evening banquet, a dancer (artists are frequently invited to Russian banquets) performed "The Dying Swan." When she collapsed, as is proper for a dying swan, Rossovki, Professor of Physiology at the University of Rostov, rushed to the stage and offered first aid.

As a result of this visit I was offered a position as Scientific Director of the Institute of Industrial Physiology, of the Ukrainian Commissariate of Labor in Kharkov. At that time there was an active exchange of visiting scientists between Germany and the USSR, similar to the present exchange program between the National Academy of Sciences in Washington and the Academy of Sciences, USSR. My contract was for two years, renewable for another two years. I consulted the German Auswärtige Amt, who were in favor of my going, as was Professor Bethe and other members of the Medical Faculty of the University of Frankfurt. So I left, in the summer of 1930, with the blessings of the Dean.

At that time life in Russia was not too different from life in Germany or other Western Countries except for the scarcity of things. The "foreign specialists," however, had a special store available, a somewhat awkward situation. While the government was, of course, Communist, there was at that time not much influence noticeable in private life or in research. The Russian people are extremely hospitable, generous, and like to have a good time, and we found many good personal friends. Before we went to Russia, we were frightened by some articles of well-known reporters who did not see a smiling face in Russia. Of course, this was nonsense. After coming to the United States, we found that the Russian people in their general mentality and attitude to life are very close to the American people, and any separation of peoples on the basis of different forms of government is artificial and regrettable. One way to help to bridge this is by communication between scientists, and I have continually tried to contribute to this end by reviews of Russian cardiovascular research, and by participation in the Translation Supplement of the Federation of American Societies of Experimental Biology.

We found in Russia that the language was not quite as formidable as it had looked printed. The progress of my wife was facilitated by our housekeeper. My wife often had reason to be upset with her. By the winter semester, 1933, I was able to give lectures in Russian and was appointed as Professor of Normal Physiology at the First Medical Institute of Kharkov, one of the oldest Universities in Russia.

My friend G. V. Volbort, Chairman of the Department of Physiology, was in a poor state of health from chronic nephritis, so we shared the course in normal physiology. Volbort gave me frequent good advice. When I started my lectures on metabolism, he warned me not to mention that the metabolic rate of the Chinese is lower, because this would conflict with the rigid Marxist theory that all races are equal; in any case, many students might feel that way. Although ultimately I would probably prove my point, it would be wise to avoid endless discussions. Volbort spoke from experience.

In Kharkov, I continued my work in Exercise and Industrial Physiology, and became interested in intermediary carbohydrate metabolism.

Professor Volbort, one of Pavlov's early associates, gave me much background information about Pavlov and his work, and introduced me personally to the great scientist. In Leningrad I met also Professor Ukhtomsky, whom I regard as one of the great physiologists of this century, although very little is known outside Russia of his work. Thus, I became increasingly interested in CNS problems.

Up until this time, 1934, the choice of topics for a Russian researcher was liberal. There was some emphasis on practically applicable results, but it was later recognized that in a planned economy biological research could not be left out. So a planning system was set up and all research plans had to be submitted to the center (Gosplan) in Moscow. With this, scientific planning came into closer scrutiny, not only in regard to the technical scientific aspects, but also in regard to consistency with the basic political philosophy of dialectic materialism. Unfortunately the interpretations of this philosophy were variable. Before approval, which took three to four months, no budget was available for any research project. This has some similarity with the NIH granting procedure, but the staffing of the planning center in Moscow was far inferior to the NIH set-up. There was also much less elasticity in planning as well as in the execution of research. As I learned from colleagues, most intentionally underestimated the number of experiments in their submitted budgets so that their associates would get an award if their output exceeded the estimated number. I was told that most of the planning staff in Moscow would not be able to estimate how many experiments were actually needed for a certain project and therefore their only evaluation criterion was whether the number of experiments performed was above or below the approved estimate. A remarkable red tape system was developed which I believe was not quite equalled elsewhere. Occasionally, this is a consolation when I am overwhelmed here with progress reports or grant applications.

These were all growing pains in the rapid expansion of biomedical research which I expect have been overcome by now or considerably reduced in any case. Excellent work is now being done in Russia as it has been in the past. J. Brozek and I recently reviewed the trends of Soviet biomedical research (*Science*, 1965).

Unfortunately, the situation in Russia deteriorated with the seizure of power in Germany by Hitler. Since I could not return to Germany, I stayed longer than originally intended. The Russians recognized the true character of the Nazi regime from the very beginning. Hitler said on many occasions that he needed *Lebensraum* in the East and the Russians took his word for it. Suspicion has always been a typical feature of Russia, going back several centuries. The Soviet leaders expected that Hitler would use subversion. Therefore, they suspected that everybody was a potential Nazi spy. Stalin's purges which started about 1933 and continued to the outbreak of war were to a large part due to the menace from Nazi Germany. I kept politically aloof, never going to any political meetings and we felt, as "foreign specialists," reasonably safe, at least for some time.

In early 1937, I was offered a top position at the Ukrainian Academy of Science in Kiev, under condition of acceptance of Russian citizenship. This we were not prepared to do, so we decided to leave. It was not an easy time during the depression and influx of German scientists into all free countries. However, our decision was facilitated by the situation as it developed in the summer of 1937. Nobody, but nobody, could feel safe. All foreigners were suspected as spies, together with Red Army officers and high party officials. I know of one professor of medicine who submerged into obscurity by accepting a job as a technician. When we left, about 25 per cent of the medical faculty of the University of Kharkov had been arrested. None of our personal or professional friends would acknowledge us in the street, for fear they would be implicated in case of our arrest. As a matter of fact, nothing happened to us, but one could not possibly know what would happen and we lived through several anxious weeks.

My wife, our son Walter (then one and one-half years old) and I arrived in Prague in August, 1937. Prague is a beautiful city, and at that time, Czechoslovakia was a true liberal democracy. I was promised a good position as head of the Department of Industrial Physiology of the Central Psychotechnical Institute of Czechoslovakia. I met Josef Brozek at the branch of the Institute in Znin. Seven years later we came together again at the Laboratory of Physiological Hygiene in Minneapolis; a small world indeed. We would have enjoyed staying in Czechoslovakia. The new department of Industrial Physiology was planned to be on the fifth floor of a building of the Institute for which construction had already started. However, one year later, Hitler started the trouble in the Sudetenland which terminated in Munich, and interrupted everything. It was clear that we could not stay in Prague, so I applied for an American visa. While we were waiting for it, I received an offer of a good position at the Sorbonne in Paris from Professor Henry Laugier, Director of the Department of Industrial Physiology (*Travail Humain*). I was very inclined to accept it, since I had no position in the United States or elsewhere in prospect. My wife then made the most crucial and best decision of my life. She said, "This fellow Hitler comes ever after you, first Germany, then Russia, now Czechoslovakia. Paris is much too close for comfort. We go to America."

In 1959, I met Henri Laugier at the International Physiology Congress in Buenos Aires. He said that they never could understand why I did not accept the excellent position at the Sorbonne. History should have given him the answer.

We arrived in New York in April, 1939. I went to work at Mount Sinai Hospital, Milwaukee with Norbert Enzer, who was Director of Pathology and very much interested in Industrial Health. The position and funds for research were modest; it was, of course, still the time of depression.

From theoretical and practical considerations, I started to work with flicker fusion, applied to the measurement of CNS fatigue. The practical considerations were very simple, it was cheap to build the equipment around a Cenco rotator costing about $35.00. The whole apparatus came to about $60 to $70. We found a quite consistent drop of the FFF at the end of the working day, more or less parallel with the subjective sensation of fatigue. Amphetamine and Pervitin reversed the drop of FFF and abolished the subjective fatigue. So we were bold enough to propose the FFF as test for CNS fatigue. (*J. Ind. Hygiene and Toxicol.*, 23:83, 1941). With this, we started a large controversial literature which still continues. Three years later, on the basis of a series on the effect of alcohol, we retracted our conclusion of parallelism between subjective fatigue and drop of FFF since the effects of alcohol on the FFF were correlated to the blood concentration but not to subjective sensations (*Amer. J. Clin. Pathol.*, 14: 333, 1944). It is remarkable that in the large literature reference is made only to our first publication but not to the reversal in the following paper. In any case we can say that rarely in the history of medical research has such a large literature started with so little investment. Working with flicker fusion, I naturally became interested in vision, particularly retinal functions, and extended my work to light and dark adaptation. However, we were not able to get any sizeable research funds. On a limited scope, I continued some work on exercise, but found surprisingly little interest in industrial physiology in the United States and only in a small number of laboratories was systematic work on exercise in progress.

So early in 1942, Norbert Enzer said "Ernst, you will go into electrocardiography. Research grants or not, there will always be clinical application, and the literature is tremendous and growing. Besides, we need in the very near future an electrocardiographer at the Hospital, since Dr. Frisch will go into the Army."

Actually, at that time electrocardiography was in a state of relative stagnation. A few years earlier, Sir Thomas Lewis, who laid, with Einthoven, the groundwork for clinical electrocardiography, decided that the cream was taken off, and not much left to do. So he changed his field and started to work on pain. It was fortunate that Norbert Enzer had more confidence in electrocardiography than Sir Thomas, though admittedly on much less information.

As an introduction, I attended Louis Katz's excellent course in electrocardiography at Michael Reese Hospital, Chicago. Electrocardiography fascinated me from the beginning, and has been my major field for the past twenty-six years.

In the summer of 1944, Ancel Keys and Maurice Visscher invited me to the University of Minnesota, on the basis of a grant from the Foundation for Infantile Paralysis, which was shared by the Laboratory of Physiological Hygiene and the Department of Physiology. In the Department of Physiology, I worked on nerve and muscle fatigue in rats after an interval of nearly twenty years since my work in Greifswald. At the Laboratory of Physiological Hygiene I developed an instrument for determination of the elasticity coefficient in man, for clinical application to poliomyelitis patients. In 1947, Ernest Frank, the biophysical engineer, approached me at the Federation meeting and said that he had confirmed my values of the elasticity coefficient with an entirely different method. We did not know at that time that we both would go into vectorcardiography a few years later. Another satisfaction from this work was the letter (in English) from a German clinician who asked: "How is it possible to become an elastometer" (*Bekommen*, in German, is of course "to get"). I have reason to believe that the Foundation for Infantile Paralysis was less satisfied. A member of the central office of the Foundation, visiting the Laboratory, said somewhat reproachfully that the development of the elastometer over the past two years had cost the Foundation $25,000 (which included salaries). This was, of course, long before grant inflation, and although it was not said, there was a definite implication that this was gross overpayment. From their point of view this was probably the case.

This grant terminated shortly after, and I came full time to the Laboratory of Physiological Hygiene. It was an exciting place at an exciting time. After the end of the wartime semi-starvation experiment in conscientious objectors, we had numerous discussions about which direction to go but we always had, as before, teamwork in mind. We considered exercise and athletics, industrial physiology and several other potential projects, but decided to start the longitudinal cardiovascular degeneration (CVD) project, which is still going on now twenty-one years later. At that time, Josef Brozek and I started also the work on visual fatigue which I mentioned earlier.

The scientific and personal contact among the senior staff with Ancel Keys as director, and Henry Blackburn and Henry Taylor closest to my work in electrocardiography and exercise, was always close. Without their encouragement and constructive criticism my accomplishments would not have been possible.

After I had been working in electrocardiography for about fifteen years, I passed through a similar crisis as had Sir Thomas Lewis. I have always been intrigued with visual perception because of its complexity, and I accepted a part-time appointment in the Department of Ophthalmology. The time with Erling Hansen, John Wendland and other members of the department was pleasant, enjoyable, and I believe reasonably productive. However, I came back to electrocardiography within a short time and wrote my book *Differentiation Between Normal and Abnormal in Electrocardiography*. Charles Kossman wrote the preface and Ancel Keys, to whom the monograph was dedicated, wrote the introduction. What I have tried to accomplish in my experimental work and in the book was to develop a basis for quantitative electrocardiography and therefore I ventured into vectorcardiography quite early, in 1951. My association with Otto H. Schmitt in vectorcardiographic research was and is most enjoyable and rewarding.

One of the most satisfactory aspects of electrocardiography is its clinical application. My appointment as consultant at the Veterans Administration Hospital and the Mount Sinai Hospital gave me this outlet. Frequent discussions with my friend Reuben Berman contributed much to a perspective of clinical application.

Other topics of major research activity over the past two decades were peripheral circulation, aging and response to physiological stresses. My activity in aging was penalized by making me the chairman of the 17th Annual Meeting of the Gerontological Society in Minneapolis, October, 1964.

Taken all in all, I could not have dreamed of better facilities for my work, and I will always be thankful to Dr. Gaylord Anderson, Director of the School of Public Health, and Ancel Keys, Director of the Laboratory of Physiological Hygiene, for the support of my work. I have had most generous grant support from the NIH.

After mandatory retirement from the University, I continue my work in electro and vectorcardiography at Mount Sinai Hospital, jointly with Otto H. Schmitt in the Department of Biophysics and with a slant to clinical application which has been too long delayed. The perspectives for development of this work, at Mount Sinai Hospital seem to be excellent.

Probably, I have been involved in too many problems, but I have found, whatever I started, important problems still open, in spite of the tremendous literature. My major fields have been exercise physiology and electrocardiography. I am working now, supported by a NIH grant, on what I hope will be a comprehensive monograph on Performance and Fatigue.

This conference on quantitative exercise electrocardiography blends perfectly with my major interests and experience, and I wish to thank most sincerely my good friend Henry Blackburn with his committee Arnold Adicoff, Reuben Berman, James Dahl, Otto Schmitt and Naip Tuna for its organization. Somehow I feel that this honor is the high point of my career.

Author Index

[473]

Subject Index

[480]